# Anatomy
## *of*
# Love

A Natural History of Mating,
Marriage, and Why We Stray

COMPLETELY REVISED AND UPDATED

## Helen Fisher, PhD

W. W. Norton & Company
*Independent Publishers Since 1923*
New York • London

For information about permission to reproduce selections from this book, write to Permissions, W. W. Norton & Company, Inc., 500 Fifth Avenue, New York, NY 10110

For information about special discounts for bulk purchases, please contact W. W. Norton Special Sales at specialsales@wwnorton.com or 800-233-4830

Manufacturing by Quad Graphics
Book design by Dana Sloan
Production manager: Louise Mattarelliano

ISBN: 978-0-393-28522-2

W. W. Norton & Company, Inc.
500 Fifth Avenue, New York, N.Y. 10110
www.wwnorton.com

W. W. Norton & Company Ltd.
Castle House, 75/76 Wells Street, London W1T 3QT

1 2 3 4 5 6 7 8 9 0

FOR LOVERS EVERYWHERE

*And in memory of Ray Carroll*

# CONTENTS

# Here's to Love!

*Journalist:* Why do you only write about relationships?
*Nora Ephron:* Is there something else?

I was recently traveling in the highlands of New Guinea in the back of a pickup truck, talking with a man who had three wives. I asked him how many wives he would like to have. There was a pause as he rubbed his chin. I wondered: Would he say five? Ten? Twenty-five wives? He leaned toward me and whispered: None.

We are a pair-bonding species. Some 85% of cultures permit a man to have several wives, but few men actually build a harem. A man has to have a lot of goats, cows, land, money, or other impressive resources to get several women to share his wedding bed. Even then, having more than one wife can be a toothache. Co-wives fight; sometimes they even poison one another's children. We are built to rear our babies as a team of two—with a lot of helpers near the nest.

This book is the story of that monumental human passion: to love. As well as all of the spinoffs of our basic human reproductive strategy: how we court; who we choose; how we bond; why some are adulterous and some divorce; how the drive to love evolved; why we have teenagers and vast networks of kin to rear our young; why a man can't be more like a woman and vice versa; how sex and romance drastically altered with the invention of the plow; and, in the last chapter, a new look at future sex.

When W. W. Norton invited me to do a second edition of this book, I gaily said yes, thinking this was a privilege and an easy job. The first version had taken me ten years to write; I thought this revision might take ten days. Then I read the book—and swiftly realized that I had to update almost all of it.

So I have now added a great deal of data and ideas, including data on all of our brain-scanning experiments on romantic love, rejection in love, and long-term love; my new data on the biology of personality and why you fall in love with one person rather than another; new information on adultery, love addiction, sexual selection, and mate choice; the newest statistics on worldwide patterns of divorce; my theory on the development of morality across the life course; my hypothesis about our modern dating habits—what I call "slow love,"; and a wealth of new data on future sex, collected in collaboration with Match.com.[1] I also added references for my additions (and retained most of the original references) and two of my questionnaires as additional appendices.

Journalist David Gergen once called me "America's last optimist." There is much to cry about, but there is also much to celebrate—including our inexhaustible human drive to love. Technology is changing how we court. But it can't change love. Romantic love and attachment emanate from the most primitive regions of the brain, near those that orchestrate thirst and hunger. And as Plato aptly wrote in *The Symposium*: "The God of love lives in a state of need." Love is a need, a craving, a drive to seek life's greatest prize: a mating partner. We are born to love. Indeed, if we survive as a species, we will still fall in love and form pair-bonds a million years from now.

This book traces the trajectory of this indestructible human passion. And it ends on a high note. I firmly believe that if there ever was a time in human evolution when we have the opportunity to make happy partnerships, that time is now.

Here's to love,
*Helen Fisher*

# ANATOMY OF LOVE

# 1

## Games People Play

### Courting

Moved by the force of love,
fragments of the world seek out one another
so that a world may be.

—PIERRE TEILHARD DE CHARDIN

In an apocryphal story, a colleague once turned to the great British geneticist J. B. S. Haldane and said, "Tell me, Mr. Haldane, knowing what you do about nature, what can you tell me about God?" Haldane replied, "He has an inordinate fondness for beetles." Indeed, the world contains over 300,000 species of beetles.

I would add that "God" loves the human mating game, for no other aspect of our behavior is so complex, so subtle, or so pervasive. And although these sexual strategies differ from one individual to the next, the essential choreography of human courtship, romance, love, and marriage has myriad designs that seem etched into the human psyche, the product of time, selection, and evolution.

They begin the moment men and women get within courting range—with the way we flirt.

### Body Talk

Irenäus Eibl-Eibesfeldt, a German ethologist,[1] noticed a curious pattern to women's flirting behavior. Eibl-Eibesfeldt had used a camera with a secret lens so that when he directed the camera straight ahead, he was actually taking pictures to the side. This way he could focus on local sights and catch on film the unstaged facial expressions of people near him. In his travels to Samoa, Papua, France, Japan, Africa, and Amazonia, he recorded numerous flirting sequences. Then, back in his laboratory at the Max Planck Institute for Behavioral Physiology, near Munich, Germany, he carefully examined each courting episode, frame by frame.

A universal pattern of female flirting emerged. Women from places as different as the jungles of Amazonia, the salons of Paris, and the highlands of New Guinea apparently flirt with the same sequence of expressions.

First, the woman smiles at her admirer and lifts her eyebrows in a swift, jerky motion as she opens her eyes wide to gaze at him. Then she drops her eyelids, tilts her head down and to the side, and looks away. Frequently she also covers her face with her hands, giggling nervously as she retreats behind her palms. This sequential flirting gesture is so distinctive that Eibl-Eibesfeldt is convinced it is innate, a human female courtship ploy that evolved eons ago to signal sexual and/or romantic interest.

Other gambits people use may also come from our primeval past. The coy look is a gesture in which a woman cocks her head and looks up shyly at her suitor. A female possum does this too, turning toward her suitor, cocking her snouty jaw, and looking straight into his eyes. Animals frequently toss their heads in order to solicit attention. Courting women do it regularly; they raise their shoulders, arch their backs, and toss their locks in a single sweeping motion. Albatrosses toss their heads and snap their bills between bouts of nodding, bowing, and rubbing bills together. Mud turtles extend and retract their heads, almost touching noses. Women are not the only creatures who use their heads to flirt.[2]

Men also employ courting tactics similar to those seen in other species. Have you ever walked into the boss's office and seen him leaning back in his chair, hands clasped behind his head, elbows high, and chest thrust out? Perhaps he has come from behind his desk, walked up to you, smiled, arched his back, and thrust his upper body in your direction? If so, watch out. He may be subconsciously announcing his dominance over you. If you are a woman, he may be courting you instead.

The "chest thrust" is part of a basic postural message used across the animal kingdom—"standing tall." Dominant creatures puff up. Codfish bulge their heads and thrust out their pelvic fins. Snakes, frogs, and toads inflate their bodies. Antelope and chameleons turn broadside to empha-size their bulk. Mule deer look askance to show their antlers. Cats bristle. Pigeons swell. Lobsters raise themselves onto the tips of their walking legs and extend their open claws. Gorillas pound their chests. Men just thrust out their chests.

When confronted by a more dominant animal, many creatures shrink. People turn in their toes, curl their shoulders, and hang their heads. Wolves tuck their tails between their legs and slink. Subordinate lobsters crouch. And many species bow. A bullied codfish curls its body downward. Liz-ards move their whole bodies up and down. Deferential chimpanzees nod their heads so rapidly and repeatedly that primatologists call it bobbing.

These "crouch" and "loom" positions seen in a host of creatures are often manifest in courtship too. I recall a cartoon in a European magazine. In the first box a man in swimming trunks stands alone on an empty beach—his head sags, his stomach protrudes, his chest is concave. In the next box, an attractive woman is shown walking along the beach past the man; now his head is erect, his stomach sucked in, his chest inflated. In the last box, the woman is gone and he has resumed his normal, sad-sack pose. It is not uncommon to see men and women swell and shrink in order to signal importance, defenselessness, and approachability.

## The "Copulatory" Gaze

The gaze is probably the most striking human courting ploy. Eye lan-guage. In Western cultures, where eye contact between the sexes is per-mitted, men and women often stare intently at a potential mate for about two to three seconds during which their pupils may dilate—a sign of extreme interest. Then the starer drops his or her eyelids and looks away.[3]

Eye contact seems to have an immediate effect. The gaze trig-gers primitive parts of the human brain, calling forth one of two basic emotions—approach or retreat. You cannot ignore the eyes of another fixed on you; you must respond. You may smile and start conversa-tion. You may look away and edge toward the door. But first you will probably tug at an earlobe, adjust your sweater, yawn, fidget with your eyeglasses, or perform some other meaningless movement—a "displacement gesture"—to alleviate anxiety while you make up your mind how to acknowledge this invitation, whether to flee the premises or stay and play the courting game.

This look, known to ethologists as the copulatory gaze, may well be embedded in our evolutionary psyche. Chimpanzees and other primates gaze at enemies to threaten them; they look deeply into one another's eyes in order to reconcile after a battle too. The gaze is also employed before coitus, as seen among bonobos, or "pygmy" chimpanzees—apes closely related to the common chimp but smaller and perhaps smarter. Several of these almost human creatures live in the San Diego Zoo, where males and females copulate regularly. But just before intercourse the couple spends several moments staring deeply into each other's eyes.[4]

Baboons gaze at each other during courtship too. These animals may have branched off of our human evolutionary tree more than twenty-five million years ago, yet this similarity in wooing persists. Anthropologist Barbara Smuts said of a budding baboon courtship on the Eburru cliffs of Kenya, "It looked like watching two novices in a singles bar."[5]

The affair began one evening when a female baboon, Thalia, turned and caught a young male, Alex, staring at her. They were about fifteen feet apart. He glanced away immediately. So she stared at him—until he turned to look at her. Then she intently fiddled with her toes. On it went. Each time she stared at him, he looked away; each time he stared at her, she groomed her feet. Finally Alex caught Thalia gazing at him—the "return gaze."

Immediately he flattened his ears against his head, narrowed his eyelids, and began to smack his lips, the height of friendliness in baboon society. Thalia froze. Then, for a long moment, she looked him in the eye. Only after this extended eye contact had occurred did Alex approach her, at which point Thalia began to groom him—the beginning of a friendship and sexual liaison that was still going strong six years later, when Smuts returned to Kenya to study baboon friendships.

Perhaps it is the eye—not the heart, the genitals, or the brain—that is the initial organ of romance, for the gaze (or stare) often triggers the human smile.

⌒

"There is a smile of love / And there is a smile of deceit," wrote poet William Blake. Actually human beings have at least eighteen distinctive types of smiles,[6] only some of which we use while courting. Both men and women use the "simple smile," a closed-mouth gesture, when they greet a familiar passerby. In this expression, the lips are closed but stretched, and no teeth are showing; the gesture is often combined with a nod to express acknowledgment. People who smile at you like this will probably not pause to get acquainted.

The human "upper smile" signals stronger interest. In this expression, you expose your upper teeth to show your positive intentions. The upper smile is often combined with a one-sixth-of-a-second eyebrow flash, in which the eyebrows are raised, then quickly dropped. Eibl-Eibesfeldt has seen this upper smile among Europeans, Balinese, Amazonian Indians, and Bushmen of southern Africa, and he reports that it is used in all sorts of friendly contacts—including flirting. Chimps and gorillas use this half smile when they play. But they show their bottom teeth rather than their top ones. In this way they conceal their dagger-like upper fangs, canine teeth with which they threaten one another.

The "open smile," in which the lips are completely drawn back and both upper and lower teeth are fully exposed, is what we often use to "pick up" one another. Former president Jimmy Carter's smile is a remarkable example. Carter was courting our minds, our votes, our opinions; had he coupled this "super smile" with the sequential flirt, the coy look, the head toss, the chest thrust, or the gaze, his intentions would have been unmistakably sexual instead.

The "nervous social smile," another type of human grin, plays a distinctly negative role in courtship. It stems from an ancient mammalian practice to bare one's teeth when cornered. I once saw a marvelous example of it during a television appearance. My host was being verbally assailed by her other guest. She could not be impolite or leave the set. So she pulled her lips back and exposed both rows of firmly clenched teeth. Then she froze, holding this nervous grin.

Chimpanzees employ the nervous social smile, the "bared teeth" display, when confronted by a superior. They use it to express a combination of fear, friendliness, and appeasement. We make the nervous social smile in difficult social situations too, but never when courting. So if a potential lover grins at you with clenched teeth, you can be fairly sure that he or she is thinking less of wooing than of surviving the introduction.

## Universal Courting Cues

Despite the obvious correlations between the courting gestures of humans and those of other animals, it has taken over a century of investigation to prove that human beings around the world actually do share many of the same nonverbal cues. Darwin was the first to wonder about the heritability of human facial expressions and body postures. To confirm his suspicion that all men and women use the same gestures and poses to express basic human emotions, he sent a query to colleagues in remote areas of the Americas, Africa, Asia, and Australia in 1867.

Among his many questions about the aboriginals were these: "When a man is indignant or defiant does he frown, hold his body and head erect, square his shoulders and clench his fists?" "Is disgust shown by the lower lip being turned down, the upper lip slightly raised, with a sudden expiration?" "When in good spirits do the eyes sparkle, with the skin a little wrinkled round and under them, and with the mouth a little drawn back at the corners?"[7]

Scientists, journalists, missionaries, and friends from around the world replied yes to Darwin's queries, and he became convinced that joy, sorrow, happiness, surprise, fear, and several other human feelings were expressed in panhuman gestural patterns inherited from a common evolutionary past. These nonverbal cues included the human smile. As he later wrote in his book *The Expression of the Emotions in Man and Animals* (1872), "With all the races of man the expression of good spirit appears to be the same, and is easily recognized."

More than a hundred years later psychologist Paul Ekman and his colleagues confirmed Darwin's conviction that the same basic facial postures are used by various peoples around the world. When he showed pictures of American faces to Fore tribesmen of New Guinea, Sadong villagers of Sarawak, Brazilians, and Japanese and asked them to identify the expressions, these diverse men and women easily recognized the expressions of sorrow, surprise, disgust, fear, and anger—as well as the smiling grin.[8]

Smiling, it seems, we were born to do. Some infants begin to imitate their mother's smile within thirty-six hours after birth, and all babies begin social smiling at about three months of age.[9] Even children born blind and deaf burst into radiant grins, although they have never seen this facial gesture in those around them.

Like the smile, the sequential flirt, the coy look, the head toss, the chest thrust, and the gaze are probably all part of a standard human repertoire of gestures that, used in certain contexts, evolved to attract a mate.

Could these courting cues be part of a larger human mating dance?

David Givens, an anthropologist, and biologist Timothy Perper have proposed this. Both scientists spent several hundred hours in American cocktail lounges watching men and women pick each other up. Givens did his work in the pubs around the University of Washington campus in Seattle. Perper sipped his beer, stared at young singles, and took notes in the Main Brace Lounge, the Homestead, and other bars in New Jersey, New York, and eastern Canada. Both scientific voyeurs found the same general pattern to the courting process.[10]

According to these investigators, American singles-bar courtship has several stages, each with distinctive escalation points. I shall divide them into five. The first is the "attention-getting" phase. As soon as they enter the bar, both men and women typically establish a territory—a seat, a place to lean, a position near the bar, door, or dance floor. Once settled, they begin to attract attention to themselves.

Tactics vary. Men tend to pitch and roll their shoulders, stretch, stand tall, and shift from foot to foot in a swaying motion. They also exaggerate their body movements. Instead of simply using the wrist to stir a drink, men often employ the entire arm, as if stirring mud. And the whole body is employed in hearty laughter—made loud enough to attract those around them. Thus simple gestures are embellished, overdone.

Then there is the swagger with which men often move to and fro. Male baboons on the grasslands of East Africa also swagger when they foresee a potential sexual encounter. A male gorilla walks back and forth stiffly as he watches a female out of the corner of his eye. This parading gait is known to primatologists as "bird-dogging." Males of many species also preen. Human males pat their hair, adjust their clothes, tug their chins, or perform other self-clasping or grooming movements that diffuse nervous energy and keep the body moving.

Older men often use different props, advertising their availability with expensive jewelry, clothing, and other accoutrements that spell success. But all of these signals can be reduced to one basic, three-part message: "I'm here; I'm important; I'm harmless." What a difficult mixture of signals to give out simultaneously—importance *and* approachability. Yet men succeed; women regularly court men.

"It is better to be looked over than overlooked," Mae West once said. Women know it. Women begin the attention-getting phase with many of the same maneuvers that men use: smiling, gazing, shifting, swaying, preening, stretching, moving in their territory to draw attention to themselves. Often they incorporate a battery of feminine moves as well. They twist their curls, tilt their heads, look up coyly, giggle, raise their brows, flick their tongues, lick their upper lips, blush, and hide their faces in order to signal, "I am here."

Some women also have a characteristic walk when courting; they arch their backs, thrust out their breasts, sway their hips and strut. No wonder many women wear high-heeled shoes. This bizarre custom, invented by Catherine de' Medici in the 1500s, unnaturally arches the back, tilts the buttocks, and thrusts the chest out into a female come-hither pose. The clomping noise of their spiky heels helps draw attention too.

With this high-heeled gait, puckered lips, batting eyes, dancing brows, upturned palms, pigeoned toes, rocking bodies, swaying skirts, and gleaming teeth, women signal approachability to men.

# Grooming Talk

Stage two, the "recognition" stage, starts when eyes meet eyes. Then one or the other potential lover acknowledges the demarche with a smile or slight body shift, and the couple move into talking range.[11] This can be the beginning of the romance.

But it is nowhere near as risky as the next major escalation point: stage three, talk. This idle, often meaningless conversation known as "grooming talk" is distinctive because voices often become higher, softer, and more sing-songy—tones one also uses to express affection to children and concern for those in need of care.

Grooming talk starts with such benign statements as "How do you like your iPhone?" or "How's the food?" The icebreakers are as varied as the human imagination, but the best leads are either compliments or questions, since both require a response. Moreover, *what* you say often matters less than *how* you say it. This is critical. The moment you open your mouth and speak, you give away your intentions with your inflection and intonation. A high-pitched, gentle, mellifluous "hello" is often a sign of sexual or romantic interest, whereas a clipped, low, matter-of-fact, or perfunctory "hi" rarely leads to love. If a prospective mate laughs somewhat more than the situation calls for, she or he is probably flirting too.

Talking is dangerous for an important reason. The human voice is like a second signature that reveals not only your intentions but also your background, education, and intangible idiosyncrasies of character that can attract or repel a potential mate in moments. Actors, public speakers, diplomats, and habitual liars know the power of vocal tones, so they regularly modulate their voices. Movie actors raise their voices almost an octave to adopt sweet, flowing tones when "flirting" on the set. And smart liars avoid fibbing on the telephone, a purely auditory medium where subtle inconsistencies in emphasis and intonation are easily discerned. We are taught from childhood to control our facial expressions, as when our parents tell us to "smile for Grandma." But most of us are unconscious of the power of the voice.

In fact, when Match.com and I surveyed 5,000-plus single Americans in 2013, among our questions was, "Do you judge a potential date by any of the following?" Singles do: foremost is their date's grammar (83%); then their self-confidence (78%); then their teeth (76%). With your grammar, you reveal much about your upbringing; with your self-confidence, you parade your mental stability; with your teeth, you show your age and health. No wonder the voice is so important in the pickup. And there are payoffs to an attractive voice: men and women with an appealing voice have more sex partners;[12] some have more children too.[13]

Both Givens and Perper saw many potential love affairs go astray soon after conversation started.[14] But if a couple weathers this perceptual onslaught—and each person begins to listen *actively* to the other—they often move to stage four: touch.[15]

~

Touching begins with "intention cues"—leaning forward, resting one's arm toward the other's on the table, moving one's foot closer if both people are standing, or stroking one's own arm as if to stroke the other's. Then the climax: one person touches the other on the shoulder, the forearm, the wrist, or some other socially available body part. Normally the woman touches first, grazing her hand along her suitor's body in the most casual but calculated manner.

How insignificant this touching looks; how important this touching is. Human skin is like a field of grass, each blade a nerve ending so sensitive that the slightest graze can etch into the human brain a memory of the moment. The receiver notices this message instantly. If he flinches, the pickup is over. If he withdraws, even barely, the sender may never try to touch again. If he ignores the overture, she may touch once more. But if he leans toward her, smiles, or returns the gesture with his own deliberate touch, they have surmounted a major barrier well known in the animal community.

Most mammals caress when courting. Blue whales rub each other with their flippers. Male butterflies stroke and rub their mate's abdomen as they couple. Dolphins nibble. Moles rub noses. Dogs lick. Chimpanzees kiss, hug, pat, and hold hands. Mammals generally stroke, groom, or nuzzle prior to copulation.

Touch has been called the mother of the senses. No doubt this is true, for every human culture has codes that indicate who may touch whom and when, where, and how. Imaginative and resourceful in their variety, these touching games are basic to human courting. So if our pair continue to talk and touch—bobbing, tilting, gazing, smiling, swaying, flirting— they usually achieve the last stage of the courtship ritual: body synchrony.

## Keeping Time

Body synchrony is the most intriguing component of the pickup. As potential lovers become comfortable, they pivot or swivel until their shoulders become aligned, their bodies face to face. This rotation toward each other may start before they begin to talk or hours into conversation, but after a while the man and woman begin to move in tandem. Briefly at first. When he lifts his drink, she lifts hers. Then they desynchronize. In time, however, they mirror each other more and more. When he crosses his legs, she crosses hers; as he leans left, she leans left; when he smooths his hair, she smooths hers. They move in perfect rhythm as they gaze deeply into each other's eyes.

This beat of love, of sex, of eternal human reproduction, may be interrupted at any moment. But if the two are to pass on the thread of human life, they will resume their tempo and continue their mating dance. Couples that reach total body synchrony often leave the bar together.

Is the five-part pickup universal to men and women? We do not know. Certainly not everybody in the world exhibits all of the behavior patterns that Givens and Perper found in American singles joints. People in most societies do not meet in bars or clubs. Some do not even court one another openly; instead, their marriages are arranged. And few anthropologists have studied the postures, gestures, and expressions that men and women in other cultures use when they interact.

But there is a great deal of ancillary evidence to suggest that some of these patterns are universal to humankind.

In Borneo, for example, a Dusun woman often cocks her head and gazes at a potential lover. When she passes him the rice wine at a party, she casually touches him on the hands as well.[16] In fact, most travelers know that you do not have to speak the local language to flirt success-fully. The gaze, the smile, the gentle touch seem to be integral to wooing everywhere on earth.

There is more evidence that body synchrony is universal to human courtship. In almost every society where men and women are allowed to choose their lovers, singles meet at parties or festivals and dance. And what is dancing but rhythmic gestures, tandem body movement.

The traditional Medlpa of New Guinea even ritualized this mimicry. Among these people unmarried girls met potential spouses in a *tanem het*, a common room in their parents' house. Several potential spouses, dressed from head to toe in finery, assembled and sat in pairs. The "head rolling" festivities began as couples sang. Then potential partners swayed their heads, rubbed foreheads and noses, and bowed to each other repeat-edly, all to a throbbing beat. To the Medlpa, synchrony was harmony. They believed that the better one partner kept the other's time, the more likely the couple was suited to each other.[17]

Actually, body synchrony is basic to many social interactions— courtship being only one. A student of anthropologist Edward Hall took a camera to a playground in the American Midwest and, crouching behind an abandoned car to watch and tape, he caught on film the children's movements as they interacted during recess. Carefully studying the filmed sequences, Hall noticed in the children's body motions a uniform, synchro-nized rhythm. Apparently all of the children played in tandem, to a beat. Moreover, one very active little girl skipped around the playground—and set the pace. Every other child unconsciously kept her time.[18]

Called interactional synchrony, this human mirroring begins in infancy. By the second day of life, a newborn has begun to synchronize its body movements with the rhythmic patterns of the human voice. And it is now well established that people in many other cultures get into rhythm when they feel comfortable together. Photographs and slow-motion films of people in cafés, railroad stations, supermarkets, cocktail parties, and other public places in diverse societies illustrate this human tendency to adopt one another's postures.

And the beat goes on. When friends are hooked up to electroenceph-alographs, which measure brain activity, the resulting tracings show that even brain waves get in sync when two people have a harmonious conversation. In fact, if you sit at the dinner table and watch carefully, you can conduct the conversation with your hand as family members talk and eat. Stressed syllables usually keep the beat. But even silences are rhythmic; as one person pats her mouth, another reaches for the salt—right on cue. Rests and syncopations, voices lowered, elbows raised, these mark the pulse of living as well as of love.[19]

Our need to keep one another's time reflects a rhythmic mimicry common to many other animals. On a number of occasions primatologist Wolfgang Kohler entered the chimp enclosure in a primate research center to find a group of males and females trotting in "a rough approximate rhythm" around and around a pole. Kohler said the animals wagged their heads as they swung along, each leading with the same foot. Chimps sometimes sway from side to side as they stare into each other's eyes just prior to copulation too.

In fact, nothing is more basic to courtship in animals than rhythmic movement. Cats circle. Red deer prance. Howler monkeys court with rhythmic tongue movements. Stickleback fish do a zigzag jig. From bears to beetles, courting couples perform rhythmic rituals to express their amorous intentions.

To dance is natural. So I think it reasonable to suggest that body synchrony is a universal stage of the human courting process: as we become attracted to each other, we begin to keep a common beat.

## Wooing Runs on Messages

Human courtship has other similarities to courtship in other creatures. Normally people woo each other slowly. Caution during courtship is also characteristic of spiders. The male wolf spider, for example, must enter the long, dark entrance of a female's compound in order to court and copulate. This he does slowly. If he is overeager, she devours him.

Men and women who are too aggressive at the beginning of the courting process also suffer unpleasant consequences. If you come too close, touch too soon, or talk too much, you will probably be repelled. Like wooing among wolf spiders, baboons, and many other creatures, the human pickup runs on messages. At every juncture in the ritual each partner must respond correctly; otherwise, the courtship fails.

In fact, Perper began to see a curious division of labor in this exchange of signals. American women generally initiated the courting sequence—starting with subtle nonverbal cues such as a slight shift in body weight, a smile, or gaze. Women began *two-thirds* of all the pickups that Perper witnessed. And the women he later interviewed were quite conscious of having coaxed a potential lover into conversation, touching him carefully here or there, enticing him ever forward with coquettish looks, questions, compliments, and jokes.

My studies of "Singles in America," done annually since 2010 with Match.com on a representative sample of the American populace (not Match.com members), clearly illustrate that today women of every age, ethnicity, sexual orientation, and region of the country still initiate pickups.[20] Indeed, they have become blatant. In 2012, 65% of 2,700-plus men reported that at least one woman had asked them out (and 92% of men were comfortable with this). Many more women most likely still use their ageless ploys to flirt—tossing their heads, stroking their hair, glancing up coyly, staring with the copulatory gaze, arching their backs, pushing out their breasts, wearing revealing clothes, strutting in high heels, and using dulcet tones.

With the rise of the Internet, women have added even more conspicuous come-hither moves. In our 2013 "Singles in America" study, 40% of women reported that they had sent a sexually explicit text or email and 36% had sent a sexy photo, while 62% of men had received a sexually vivid written message from a woman and 61% of men had received an erotic photo. Women also jam their Facebook pages and other social networking sites with evocative photos, suggestive messages, and cute emojis and emoticons—often to start the mating process.

Female forwardness is not, of course, a purely American phenomenon. In the 1950s Clellan Ford and Frank Beach, well-known tabulators of cross-cultural sex practices, confirmed that although most peoples think men are supposed to take the initiative in sexual advances, in practice women around the world actively begin sexual and romantic liaisons as well.

In fact, it is curious that Westerners still cling to the concept that men are the seducers and women the coy, submissive recipients of male overtures. This false notion is probably a relic of our long agricultural past, when women were pawns in elaborate property exchanges at marriage and their value depended on their "purity." Hence girls were strictly chaperoned, and their sex drive was denied. Today, however, Western women have regained their sexual freedom. Released from the world of arranged betrothals and sexual subservience, they are regularly pursuers too.

Eventually, however, the man must respond to the woman's overtures if the liaison is to proceed. As one woman reported to Perper, "At some point the man should get the hint and take it from there."

Men seem to sense this shift in leadership, a shift that Perper called "initiative transfer." It normally occurs just after the couple has left the bar, or club, or party. Now the male must begin his "moves"—put his arm around the woman, kiss her, and woo her into the mood for coitus.

It is interesting how well men know their role. When Perper asked thirty-one of his male informants to describe the pickup sequence, all but three skipped over the initial parts—those directed by the woman. Only one man could recall the details of who spoke first, who touched whom when, or how either partner began to express interest in the other. But all thirty-one men spoke at length about their own duties, how they started to kiss, pet, and maneuver the woman into bed.

Who, then, is the hunter, who the prey; who the seducer, who the bewitched? Clearly both partners play essential roles. If one or the other misses an important cue, the pickup ends. When all the signals are received and each responds correctly, the beat continues. But, like other animals engaged in courtship, human partners must play "on time" for the pickup to succeed.

In a peculiar way, American singles bars resemble the singles clubs of certain birds—the lek. *Lek* is a Swedish ornithological term for a piece of ground where male and female birds meet, mix, and match. Not many avian species copulate at a leking ground, but among them is the North American sage grouse. In early March male sage grouse appear at locations ranging from eastern California to Montana and Wyoming. There, on specific patches of open meadow used yearly for mating, each male establishes a tiny "display" territory where he proceeds, for several hours after dawn for about six weeks, to propagandize—strutting, preening, "booming," and puffing to advertise his importance to passing females.

Female sage grouse migrate to the leking ground after the males are settled. First a female struts through the property boundaries of these male establishments and surveys the occupants, a process that may take her two or three days. Then she rests inside the territory of an individual she finds appealing. Shortly both resident and guest begin their courting dance, adapting to each other's rhythms, parading to show their affection before they mate.

Are the antics at cocktail parties, church socials, office luncheons, bars or clubs fundamentally different from the cavorting on a leking ground? As an anthropologist, I find it difficult to ignore the fact that people and sage grouse both set up display territories, both exhibit mannerisms designed to pick the other up, and both move in synchrony before they mate. Apparently nature has a few basic rules of courtship.

## The Dinner Date

Two more universal features of wooing are less subtle: food and song. Probably no single ritual is more significant to Western would-be lovers than eating together. Rules are changing; indeed, most of us are confused about who should pay. But if the man is courting, he still generally foots the bill; if so, a woman almost instinctively knows her companion is wooing her. In fact, there is no more frequent worldwide courtship ploy than offering food in hopes of gaining sexual favors. A fish, a piece of meat, sweets, and beer are among the countless delicacies men produce as offerings.[21]

This ploy is not exclusive to men. Black-tipped hang flies often catch aphids, daddy longlegs, or houseflies on the forest floor. When a male has felled a particularly juicy prey, he exudes secretions from an abdominal scent gland that catch the breeze, announcing a successful hunting expedition. Often a passing female hang fly stops to enjoy the meal—but not without copulating while she eats. Male birds feed potential lovers too. The male common tern often brings a little fish to his beloved. The male roadrunner presents a little lizard. Male chimpanzees living along Lake Tanganyika, in eastern Africa, offer a morsel of baby gazelle, hare, or some other animal they have caught and killed. The estrous female consumes the gift, then copulates with the donor.[22]

"The way to a man's heart is through his stomach," the adage says. Perhaps. A few female mammals do feed their lovers; women are among them. But around the world courting women feed men with nowhere near the regularity that men feed women.[23] And where food is impractical or unfashionable, men give their girlfriends tobacco, jewelry, cloth, flowers, or some other small but prized gift as a token of their affection and as a mild enticement for a tryst.

"Courtship feeding," as this custom is called, probably predates the dinosaurs, because it has an important reproductive function. By providing food to females, males show their abilities as hunters, providers, and worthy procreative partners.

"If music be the food of love, play on." Shakespeare elegantly played tribute to the last primeval courting lure: melody. Singing or playing a musical instrument to attract a mate is a common practice around the world. Among the Hopi Indians of the American Southwest, men traditionally sang a complex love song to an intended. So did men among the Samoans of the western Pacific, the Chiricahua of the American Southwest, and the Sanpoil of what is today the eastern part of the state of Washington. An Apache man hoped to entice a girl by serenading her with his flute; and both men and women among the Ifugao of central Luzon, Philippines, used the lover's harp to generate ardor in a beloved.[24]

Perhaps the society most captivated by music is our own, however. From the iPods that teenagers carry through the streets to the music that blares in almost every public place, music reigns wherever men and women congregate. And when you are invited to "his" or "her" house for dinner, you can be sure you will get more than pizza or a steak; you will get music too.

As might be expected, the melodies of human courtship are echoed in the songs of the animal community. Just step outdoors on a sultry summer night to hear the din. Frogs croak. Crickets chirp. Cats howl. Insects sing. Porcupines emit a piercing whine. Alligators bellow. Throughout the animal kingdom, the rutting calls of males—from the drumming air bladder of the haddock and muted rumble of the elephant to the "chip" of a tiny gecko lizard—serve as potent courting signs.

Decades ago Otto Jespersen, the Danish philologist, even speculated that early human courting sounds stimulated the evolution of language. "Language," he said, "was born in the courting days of mankind; the first utterances of speech I fancy to myself like something between the nightly love-lyrics of puss upon the tiles and the melodious love-songs of the nightingale."[25] This sounds farfetched. There were probably several reasons why prehistoric men and women needed advanced communication. But love songs, like national anthems, can certainly "stir the blood."

I would like to think that courtship starts when "he" or "she" makes a marvelous joke about an unlikable politician, an astute comment about the world economy, or a tantalizing remark about a recent play or sports event—something humorous, intelligent. But infatuation may begin with the slight tilt of a head, a gaze, a gentle touch, a tender syllable, a slab of roast beef in a fancy restaurant, or a whispered tune during a swaying dance.

Then the body rushes forward, leaving the intellect to unravel this feeling of infatuation: "Why him?" "Why her?"

# 2

# Why Him? Why Her?

## The Drive to Love and Who We Choose

> The meeting of two personalities is like the
> contact of two chemical substances; if there is
> any reaction, both are transformed.
>
> —CARL JUNG

"For should I see thee a little moment, / Straight is my voice hushed; / Yea, my tongue is broken, and through and through me, / 'Neath the flesh, impalpable fire runs tingling." So begins a poem describing infatuation written by Sappho on the Greek island of Lesbos some twenty-five hundred years ago.

Romantic love, obsessive love, passionate love, being in love, infatuation, call it what you will—almost everybody knows the feeling. That euphoria. That torment. Those sleepless nights and restless days. Awash in ecstasy or apprehension, you daydream during class or business, forget your coat, drive past your turn, check your phone, or plan what you will say—obsessed, longing for the next encounter with "him" or "her." Then, when you meet again, his slightest gesture stops your pulse. Her laugh dizzies you. You take foolish risks, say stupid things, laugh too hard, reveal dark secrets, talk all night, walk at dawn, and often hug and kiss—oblivious to all the world as you tumble through a fever, breathless, etherized by bliss.

Despite the hundreds of thousands of poems, songs, books, operas, dramas, ballets, myths, and legends that have portrayed romantic love since before the time of Christ, despite the countless times a man or woman has deserted family and friends, committed suicide or homicide, or pined away because of love, few scientists have given this passion the study it deserves—until recently.

Sigmund Freud dismissed infatuation, as some call it, as a blocked or delayed sex urge. Havelock Ellis called romantic attraction "sex-plus-friendship," an unconvincing description of this fever. And many people have assumed that romantic passion is a mystical, intangible, inexplicable, even sacred experience that defies the laws of nature and the scrutiny of academics.

Yet, today, scientific data on this passion are collecting.

## Falling in Love

Romantic attraction is now associated with a suite of psychological, behavioral, and physiological traits.[1] Data collection largely began with the now classic dissection of this madness, found in *Love and Limerence*, by Dorothy Tennov.[2]

Tennov devised approximately two hundred statements about romantic love and asked four hundred men and women at and around the University of Bridgeport, Connecticut, to respond with "true" or "false" reactions. Hundreds of additional individuals answered subsequent versions of her questionnaire. From their responses, as well as their diaries and other personal accounts, Tennov identified a constellation of characteristics common to this condition of "being in love," a state she called "limerence."

The first dramatic aspect of romantic love is its inception, the moment when another person begins to take on "special meaning." You start to focus intently on him or her, known to scientists as "salience." It could be an old friend seen in a new perspective or a complete stranger. But as one of Tennov's informants put it, "My whole world had been transformed. It had a new center and that center was Marilyn."

Romantic love then develops in a characteristic pattern, beginning with "intrusive thinking." Thoughts of the "love object" begin to invade your mind. A certain thing he said rings in your ear; you see her smile, recall a comment, a special moment, an innuendo—and relish it. You wonder what your beloved would think of the book you are reading, the movie you just saw, or the problem you are facing at the office. And every tiny segment of the time the two of you have spent together acquires weight and becomes material for review.

At first these intrusive reveries may occur irregularly. But many said that, as the obsession grew, they spent from 85 to almost 100% of their days and nights in sustained mental attentiveness, doting on this single individual. Indeed, along with this fixation, lovers lose some ability to focus on other things, such as daily tasks, work, and school; they become easily distracted.[3]

Moreover, they begin to focus on the most trivial aspects of the adored one and aggrandize these traits in a process called crystallization. Crystallization is distinct from idealization in that the infatuated person does indeed perceive the weaknesses of his or her idol. In fact, all of Tennov's participants could list the faults of their beloved. But they simply cast these flaws aside or convinced themselves that these defects were unique and charming. As Chaucer said, "love is blynd."

Paramount in the daydreams of Tennov's infatuated informants were three overriding sensations: craving, hope, and uncertainty. If the cherished person gave the slightest positive response, the besotted partner would replay these precious fragments in reverie for days. If he or she rebuffed one's overtures, uncertainty might turn to despair and listlessness (known as anhedonia) instead. The lover would moon about, brooding until he or she had managed to explain away this setback and renew the quest.

Key incendiaries are adversity and social barriers; these heighten romantic passion and craving—a phenomenon I christened "frustration attraction."[4] The lover also suffers separation anxiety when apart from the beloved. And underlying all of this angst and ecstasy is unmitigated fear. A twenty-eight-year-old truck driver summed up what most informants felt: "I'd be jumpy out of my head," he said. "It was like what you might call stage fright, like going up in front of an audience. My hand would be shaking when I rang the doorbell. When I called her on the phone I felt like I could hear the pulse in my temple louder than the ringing of the phone."

Intense energy (hypomania) is another central trait of romantic love. Smitten lovers report trembling, pallor, flushing, a general weakness, overwhelming sensations of awkwardness and stammering, as well as one or more sympathetic nervous system reactions, including sweating, butterflies in the stomach, a pounding heart, and/or difficulty eating or sleeping.

Some even feel a loss of their most basic faculties and skills. Stendhal, the nineteenth-century French novelist, described this feeling perfectly. Recalling the afternoons he went strolling with his sweetheart, he wrote, "Whenever I gave my arm to Leanore, I always felt I was about to fall, and I had to think how to walk."[5]

Shyness, anticipation, fear of rejection, longing for reciprocity, and intense motivation to win this special person are other central sensations of romantic passion. Lovers can also become easily jealous. Some even go to extremes to protect the budding partnership, known to animal behaviorists as "mate guarding."[6]

Above all, Tennov's participants expressed the feeling of helplessness, the sense that this obsession was irrational, involuntary, unplanned, uncontrollable. As a business executive in his early fifties wrote about an office affair, "I am advancing toward the thesis that this attraction for Emily is a kind of biological, instinct-like action that is not under voluntary or logical control. . . . It directs me. I try desperately to argue with it, to limit its influence, to channel it (into sex, for example), to deny it, to enjoy it, and, yes, dammit, to make her respond! Even though I know that Emily and I have absolutely no chance of making a life together, the thought of her is an obsession."[7]

Romantic love, it seems, is a panoply of intense emotions, rollercoastering from high to low, hinged to the pendulum of a single being whose whims command you to the detriment of everything around you—including work, family, and friends.

And this involuntary mosaic of thoughts, feelings and motivations is only partially related to sex. Tennov's infatuated lovers yearned to have sex with their beloved. But their lust was overshadowed by a far deeper craving. They wanted their beloved to call, write, invite them out, and, above all, reciprocate their passion. For infatuated men and women, emotional union trumps sexual desire. In fact, 95% of Tennov's female informants and 91% of her male subjects *rejected* the statement "The best thing about love is sex."

Moreover, these feelings can erupt at any age. I discovered this when I designed my own questionnaire on romantic love and collected data on 437 Americans and 402 Japanese.[8] (See appendix A.) People over age forty-five and those under twenty-five showed no significant statistical differences on 82% of the queries.

Intense feelings of romantic love generally first occur around puberty. But even young children can experience a "crush" or puppy love.[9] The youngest love-struck person I ever met was a two-and-a-half-year-old boy. Every time a particular little girl came to his home for a play-date, he just sat beside her and stroked her hair; after she departed, he became depressed for about two hours. She was special; he was obsessed.

Why do we fall in love with Ray instead of Bill, Sue instead of Cecily? Why him? Why her? "The heart has its reasons which reason knows nothing of," contended philosopher Blaise Pascal. But scholars can provide some reasonable explanations for this hurricane of feeling.

## Odor Lures

Infatuation may be triggered, in part, by one of our most primitive traits, our sense of smell. Every person smells slightly different; we all have a personal "odor print" as distinctive as our voice, our hands, our intellect. As newborn infants we can recognize our mother by her smell, and as we grow up we come to detect over ten thousand different odors.[10] So if nature be our guide, we are probably susceptible to odor lures.

Many creatures use odors to seduce, as was made abundantly clear to the nineteenth-century French naturalist Jean Henri Fabre. Fabre had found a cocoon of the beautiful emperor moth. He brought it into his country home and left it in his study overnight. The next morning a female emerged, sparkling from metamorphosis. Fabre put her in a cage. To his astonishment forty male emperor moths flapped through his open window that evening to woo the virgin; over the next few nights more than 150 males appeared. This female moth had exuded an invisible secretion from her distended abdomen—a pheromone, the smell of which had attracted suitors from over a mile across the countryside.[11]

Since the time of Fabre's experiments, the odor lures of over 250 insect species, and of many other animals, have been found. Some of these smells—such as castoreum, from the scent glands of Russian and Canadian beavers; musk, the red jellylike pheromone of the East Asian musk deer; and civet, a honeylike secretion from the Ethiopian civet cat—have been worn by people as diverse as the ancient Greeks, Hindus, and Chinese to intoxicate a sweetheart.

But the human body may produce some powerful olfactory aphrodisiacs as well. Both men and women have apocrine glands in their armpits, around their nipples, and in the groin that become active at puberty. These scent boxes differ from eccrine glands, which cover much of the body and produce an odorless liquid, because their exudate, in combination with bacteria on the skin, produce the acrid, gamy smell of perspiration.

Baudelaire thought one's soul resided in this erotic sweat. The nineteenth-century French novelist Joris Karl Huysmans used to follow women through the fields, smelling them. He wrote that the scent of a woman's underarms "easily uncaged the animal in man." Napoleon agreed. He reportedly sent a letter to his sweetheart, Josephine, saying, "I will be arriving in Paris tomorrow evening. Don't wash."[12]

Traditionally in parts of Greece and the Balkans, some men carried their handkerchiefs in their armpits during festivals and offered these odoriferous tokens to the women they would invite to dance; they swore by the results. In fact, sweat has been used around the world as an ingredient in love potions. In Shakespeare's day, a woman held a peeled apple under her arm until the fruit became saturated with her scent; then she presented this "love apple" to her lover to inhale. And a recipe concocted by some Caribbean immigrants to the United States reads, "Prepare a hamburger patty. Steep it in your own sweat. Cook. Serve to the person desired."[13]

But can a man's smell actually trigger romantic feelings in a woman?

Perhaps. The smell of fresh male sweat elevates LH (lutenizing hormone) in women, increasing their sexual arousal. And the smell of women's vaginal fluids, known as copulins, can elevate male testosterone activity and trigger men's sexual arousal—particularly copulins emitted during ovulation. Then, following this odiferous beginning, stimulation of the genitals during sex can trigger escalation of dopamine circuits in the brain associated with romantic passion, and potentially push one over the threshold into falling in love.[14]

A woman's or a man's smell can release a host of memories too. A poignant literary evocation of this odor memory occurs in Kipling's poem "Lichtenberg," where he wrote that the smell of rain-soaked acacia trees meant home to him. No doubt you can remember the perfume of autumn leaves, a Christmas tree, the family dog, even a former lover—and all the feelings these evoke. So the right human smell at the right moment can touch off vivid pleasant memories and possibly ignite that first, stunning moment of romantic adoration.

## Odor Soup

But Americans, the Japanese, and many other peoples find body odors offensive; for most, the smell of perspiration is more likely to repel than to attract. Some scientists think the Japanese are unduly disturbed by body odors because of their long tradition of arranged marriages; men and women were forced into close contact with partners they found unappealing.[15] Why Americans are phobic about natural body smells, I don't know. Perhaps advertisers have swayed us in order to sell their deodorizing products.

But we certainly like commercially made aromas on a mate. We buy fragrant shampoos, scented soaps, aftershave lotions, and perfumes at exorbitant prices. Then smells of food, fresh air, tobacco, and smells of the office and the home all mix with our natural smells to make an odor soup. A silent label. And people respond. In a survey by the Fragrance Foundation, both men and women rated scent as an important aspect of sex appeal—giving odor an 8.4 rating on a scale of 10.[16] Like emperor moths, human beings find smells sexually exciting.

Cultural opinions about perspiration clearly vary. Climate, type of clothing, access to daily bathing, concepts of cleanliness, upbringing, and many other social variables condition one's appetite for odors. And a clear link between human bodily smells and the euphoric craving of romantic love has not been found.

But this much I propose: when you meet someone new whom you find attractive, you probably "like the smell of him," and this helps predispose you to romance. Then, once romantic passion flowers, the scent of your sweetheart becomes an aphrodisiac, a continuing stimulant to the love affair. This may be why some women like to sleep in their boyfriend's T-shirt, and nineteenth-century men often savored the handkerchief of a lover.

## Love Maps

A far more important mechanism by which human beings become capti-vated by "him" or "her" may be what is known as your "love map." Long before you fixate on Ray as opposed to Bill, Sue instead of Cecily, you have developed a mental map, an unconscious list of traits that you are looking for in your ideal partner.[17]

Children begin to develop these love maps between ages five and eight (or even earlier) in response to family, friends, experiences, and chance associations. For example, as a child you get used to the turmoil or tranquility in your house, the way your mother listens, scolds, and pats you and how your father jokes and walks and talks. Certain temperamen-tal features of your friends and relatives strike you as appealing; others you associate with disturbing incidents. And gradually these memories begin to take on a pattern in your mind, a subliminal template for what turns you off, what turns you on.

As you grow up, this unconscious love map takes shape and a compos-ite proto-image of the ideal sweetheart emerges. Then in teenage, when sexual feelings flood the brain, these love maps begin to solidify, becom-ing more specific as to details of body type, age, interests, and quirks of temperament, humor, and personality. You develop a mental picture of your perfect mate, the settings you find enticing, and the kinds of conversations and erotic activities that excite you.

So, long before your true love walks up to you in a classroom, at a shopping mall, in the office, at a coffee shop, or at a party or event, you have already constructed some basic elements of your ideal sweetheart. Then, when you actually see someone who fits within these parameters, you fall in love with him or her and project onto this beloved your unique love map. The recipient generally deviates considerably from your actual ideal. But you brush aside these inconsistencies to dote upon your own construction.

These love maps vary from one individual to the next. Some people get turned on by a business suit or a doctor's uniform, by big breasts, small feet, or a vivacious laugh. Her voice, the way he smiles, her connections, his patience, her spontaneity, his sense of humor, her interests, his aspirations, her coordination, his charisma—myriad obvious as well as tiny, subliminal elements work together to make one person more attractive than the next.

We can all list a few specific things we find appealing in a potential mate; deep in our unconscious psyche are many more.

## Looks Count

American tastes in romantic partners show some definite patterns, however. In a test of 1,031 Caucasian college students done at the University of Wyoming, men and women rated what they regarded as sexually appealing.[18] Their answers confirmed what you might expect. Men tended to prefer blondes, blue eyes, and lighter skin color, while women liked darker men. But there were some surprises. Few men liked very large breasts or the slender, boyish female figure, and almost none of the women were attracted to an extremely muscular physique. In fact, both sexes preferred the average. Too short, too tall, too slight, too "built," too pale or dark—the extremes were weeded out.

Averageness wins. In fact, psychologists recently selected thirty-two faces of American Caucasian women and, using computers, averaged all of their features. Then they showed these composite images to college peers. Of ninety-four photographs of real female faces, only four were rated more appealing than these fabrications.[19]

As you would guess, the world does not share the sexual ideals of Caucasian students from Wyoming. When Europeans first arrived in Africa, their blond hair and white skin reminded some Africans of albinos, regarded as hideous. The traditional Nama of southern Africa particularly liked dangling vulvar lips, so mothers conscientiously massaged the genitals of their infant daughters to make them hang enticingly by teenage. Women in America tend to diet to stay slim, while Siriono women of Bolivia traditionally ate continually to stay fat.

There is seemingly no end to the varieties of human body embellishments designed to trigger romantic love: stretched necks, molded heads, filed teeth, pierced noses, scarred breasts, scorched or "tanned" skin, and high-heeled shoes in which women can barely walk, the two-foot orange gourd penis sheaths of some New Guinea tribesmen, and the purple-dyed beards of distinguished Elizabethan gentlemen. Beauty truly is in the eyes of the beholder.

However, despite wildly dissimilar standards of good looks and sex appeal, there are a few widely shared opinions about what incites romantic passion. Men and women around the world are attracted to those with clear complexions. Everywhere people are drawn to partners whom they regard as clean. And men in most places tend to prefer plump, wide-hipped women to slim ones.[20]

Looks count.

So does money.

From a study of thirty-seven peoples in thirty-three countries, psychologist David Buss uncovered a distinct male/female difference in sexual preferences.[21] From rural Zulus to urban Brazilians, men are attracted to youthful, symmetrical-looking, spunky women, while women are drawn to men with goods, property, or money. Americans are no exception. Teenage girls are impressed by boys with flashy cars, and older women like men with houses, land, or other accoutrements. Hence the gentle poet will probably not attract as many women as an insensitive, rich banker.

These male/female appetites are probably innate. It is to a male's genetic advantage to fall in love with a woman who will produce viable offspring. Youth, clear skin, bright eyes, vibrant hair, white teeth, a supple body, and a vivacious personality indicate good health—vitality important to his genetic future. And it is to a woman's biological advantage to become captivated by a man who has resources and, thus, the ability to help provide for her and her forthcoming young. As Montaigne, the sixteenth-century French essayist, summed it up, "We do not marry for ourselves, whatever we say; we marry just as much or more for our posterity."

## The Chase

But let there be mystery. A degree of unfamiliarity is essential to infatuation; people almost never become captivated by someone they know extremely well—as a classic study on an Israeli kibbutz illustrates.[22]

Here infants were placed in peer groups during the day while their parents worked. Before the age of ten these children often engaged in sexual play. But as they moved into adolescence, boys and girls became inhibited and tense around one another. Then, in teenage, they developed strong brother–sister bonds. Almost none married within their peer group, however. A study of 2,769 kibbutzim marriages found that only thirteen occurred between peers; and in each of these weddings one mate had left the communal group before the age of six.

Apparently, during a critical period in childhood, most individuals lose all sexual or romantic desire for those they see regularly.

Barriers also provoke this madness. If a person is difficult to win, it piques one's interest. In fact, this element of conquest is often central to romantic love, what has become known as the Romeo and Juliet effect. If real impediments exist, these obstructions are likely to intensify one's passion.[23]

No wonder people fall for an individual who is married, a foreigner, or someone separated from them by an obstacle that appears almost insurmountable. Yet generally there must also be some slight possibility of fulfillment before one's first stirrings of romantic passion escalate into obsession.

Timing plays an important role in romantic passion too.[24] When individuals are looking for adventure, craving to leave home, lonely, displaced in a foreign country, passing into a new stage in life, or financially and psychologically ready to share themselves or start a family, they become susceptible.

Then propinquity becomes a force. As poet Ezra Pound put it, "Ah, I have picked up magic in her nearness." When the timing is right, we tend to be attracted to someone who is around.

Your childhood experiences certainly play a role as well. Some psychologists believe we gravitate to someone similar to the parent with whom we have unresolved issues; or to someone who can provide the type of attachment we had with mother; or to a mate who reflects the values and interests of our childhood friends.[25] And most of us are attracted to someone who expands our interests, ideas, experiences, and self-perception, known as "self expansion."[26]

Last, we tend to gravitate to someone of the same ethnic and socioeconomic background, an individual with the same level of intelligence, education, and good looks, and someone who shares our values and reproductive goals[27]—what anthropologists call "positive assortative mating."

But you can walk into a room where everyone is from your background; where all share your level of good looks, intelligence, and education, as well as your general social goals and values. Yet you don't fall in love with all of them. Why not?

This question led me to explore the role of biology in mate choice.

## "We Have Chemistry!"

Personality is composed of two basic types of traits: those an individual acquires through culture and experience; and those with biological underpinnings, traits of temperament. Traits of temperament are heritable, relatively stable across the life course, and linked to specific genes, hormones and/or neurotransmitter systems. Indeed, some 40–60% of your personality stems from your biology, your nature.

So, to see if your biology draws you *naturally* to particular partners, I culled from the academic literature *any* personality trait that was linked with *any* brain system.

I found only four brain systems that were each clearly associated with a specific *constellation* of personality traits: the dopamine, serotonin, testosterone, and estrogen/oxytocin systems.[28] So I designed a fifty-six-item questionnaire to measure how much you express the traits linked with *each* of these four brain systems. (See appendix B.)

Then I put this questionnaire, now called the Fisher Temperament Inventory, on the U.S. Internet dating site Chemistry.com, a subsidiary of Match.com, and on Match.com sites in thirty-nine other countries. Over fourteen million people have now taken my questionnaire. And my colleagues and I have also completed two brain-scanning experiments showing that this questionnaire is actually measuring aspects of these four temperament dimensions.[29]

Interestingly, when I examined the questionnaire scores of 100,000 men and women on Chemistry.com, I found that no two people answered these fifty-six questions the same way. I was thrilled; I have never met two people whom I thought were alike; even my identical twin and I are not totally alike. But there are patterns to nature and patterns to personality. And most important to this book, when I examined how 28,128 anonymous men and women on Chemistry.com chose their dates, I saw some of nature's scheme.

Indeed, nature plays a role in whom we choose to love.[30]

## The Biology of Mate Choice

Those men and women who were particularly expressive of the traits linked with the dopamine system tended to be drawn to people like themselves—individuals who were equally curious, creative, spontaneous, energetic, novelty-seeking and open-minded. These people are born free. Some want a partner who will leap off the couch to go adventuring with them—be it in the mountains, deserts, seas, or cities. Others want a partner who will join them at the movies, ballet, theater, or opera. Some want to explore nature; others crave new ideas or whatever captures their fancy at the moment. Plato called these men and women Artisans. I call this style of thinking and behaving "curious/energetic" and have dubbed these men and women *Explorers*.

Explorers tend to seek other Explorers—people who are (biologically) quite similar to themselves.

Those primarily expressive of the traits linked with the serotonin system are also drawn to people like themselves. These men and women tend to be traditional, calm, and cautious. They like the familiar. They follow the rules, respect authority, and enjoy plans, routines, and schedules. They tend to be modest, orderly, and conscientious. These "pillars of society" Plato called Guardians. I refer to this style of thinking and behaving as "cautious/social norm conforming" and have labeled these men and women *Builders*.

Builders seek other Builders—partners who are equally traditional.

But while Explorers are initially attracted to other Explorers, and Builders are drawn to other Builders, men and women who are foremost expressive of the traits linked with testosterone and estrogen tend to be enchanted by the other: their opposite.

Take Steve Jobs, a classic example of a man who was highly expressive of testosterone. You could see it in his face: his high forehead, heavy brow ridges, high cheekbones and chiseled jaw were all built by this largely male hormone. But testosterone also generates a constellation of personality traits, particularly spatial and math skills—from savvy with computers to engineering, music, or mechanics. These men and women also tend to be inventive, skeptical, exacting, and openly competitive, as well as direct, decisive, tough-minded, and bold. They shoot for the stars. Plato called them Rationals; I have given them the scientific term "analytical/tough-minded" and dubbed them *Directors*. Most are men, although Margaret Thatcher (and Hillary Clinton) express many of these traits.

Regardless of their gender, Directors seek their opposite: high-estrogen folk whom I have dubbed *Negotiators*.

Negotiators, foremost, express the traits linked with estrogen and the closely related neurochemical oxytocin. These people see the big picture. Known as "web thinking," another term I coined,[31] they take a more contextual, holistic, long-term view of just about everything. They are also skilled with words, savvy at dealing with people, and highly imaginative, as well as intuitive, empathetic, trusting, and emotionally expressive. Plato referred to them as Philosopher Kings, while I have placed them in the "prosocial/empathetic" temperament dimension. Most are women, although I suspect Bill Clinton is a high-estrogen man. The whole world knows he likes to talk; he is highly socially skilled; he frequently used the phrase "I feel your pain;" and in his 957-page autobiography, he wrote, "It's important to have a synthesizing mind." All are traits linked with estrogen.

Regardless of gender, however, Negotiators are particularly drawn to Directors. You've seen this combination: either the loquacious, charming woman married to the tough-minded, laconic master of the universe; or the sweet, nurturing, patient man living with the high-power, take-no-prisoners woman.

We are all expressive of all four of these temperament dimensions, of course. Nevertheless, each of us expresses some of the traits in each temperament dimension more regularly than others. And one's broad, basic style of thinking and behaving appears to play a role in that "first fine careless rapture," as Robert Browning called romantic love.[32]

## Romantic Love: A Universal Trait

Timing; barriers; mystery; similarities in background, intelligence, looks, and values; a matched love map; your broad basic biologically based style of thinking and behaving; perhaps even the right smells: this constellation of factors can make you susceptible to falling in love with him or her. Then, when that potential mate cocks his or her head, smiles, or gazes at you, you get that rush of romantic love.

This powerful attraction is not unique to Westerners either.

Andreas Capellanus, a cleric at the court of Eleanor of Aquitaine in twelfth-century France, wrote of romantic love, "Love is a certain inborn suffering derived from the sight of and excessive meditation upon the beauty of the opposite sex, which causes each one to wish above all things the embraces of the other."[33] Since then some Westerners have come to believe that romantic love is an invention of the troubadours—those knights, poets, and romantics of eleventh- to thirteenth-century France who waxed eloquent on the vicissitudes of amour.

But romantic love is far more widespread. Vatsayana, the author of the *Kama Sutra*, the classic work on love in Sanskrit literature, lived in India sometime between the first and sixth century A.D., and he clearly described romantic love between men and women. He even provided detailed instructions on how couples might court, embrace, kiss, fondle, and copulate.

Despite the Confucian emphasis on filial piety that has long saturated Chinese mores, written tales dating back to the seventh century A.D. reveal the agony of men and women torn between obedience to their elders and romantic passion for a loved one.[34] And in traditional Japan, star-crossed lovers sometimes chose double suicide, known as *shin ju*, when they found themselves betrothed to different partners.

The eastern Cherokee believed that if a young man sings to a girl at midnight, she will think about him obsessively and become irresistibly drawn to him. Yukaghir girls of northeast Siberia wrote love letters on birch bark. In Bali, men believed a woman would fall in love if her suitor fed her a certain kind of leaf incised with the image of a god who sported a very large penis.

Even peoples who deny having concepts of "love" or "being in love" act otherwise. Mangaians of Polynesia are casual in their sexual affairs; but occasionally a desperate young man who is not permitted to marry his girlfriend kills himself. The Bem-Bem of the New Guinea highlands do not admit that they feel this passion either, but a girl sometimes refuses to marry the man whom her father has chosen for her and runs away with a "true love" instead. The Tiv of Africa, who have no formal concept of romance, call this passion "madness."[35]

Love stories, myths, legends, poems, songs, love potions, love charms, lovers' quarrels, trysts, elopements, and suicides are part of life in traditional societies around the world. In fact, in a survey of 168 cultures, anthropologists William Jankowiak and Edward Fischer were able to find direct evidence for the existence of romantic love in 87% of these vastly different peoples.[36] Equally important, they found no negative evidence. In all the other societies canvassed, anthropologists had failed to inquire about this phenomenon, cases of ethnographic oversight.

## Homosexual Love

So strong is this feeling of romantic love, so basic to human nature, that it occurs in all of us—whether our love object is a member of the opposite sex or of the same gender. To be expected, gays and lesbians also fall in love.

As mentioned, I have collected data on a representative sample of Americans between 2010 and 2014. And in this sample of more than 25,000 men and women of every ethnic background, age, and part of the country, gays and lesbians reported falling in love just as often as heterosexuals. They were also equally inclined to experience love at first sight. And they were just as eager to have a committed relationship.[37]

Most revealing, in a recent brain scanning study, both heterosexual and homosexual men and women lay in the scanner while they looked at photos of their beloveds. Those of both sexual orientations showed activity in the same basic brain pathways associated with feelings of intense romantic love.[38]

This madness, this limerence, this romantic attraction, this infatuation, this rapture is a universal human trait.[39]

## Animal Magnetism

Infatuation may not be unique to people either.[40]

What first made me suspect this was an anthropological account of a home-raised American gorilla, Toto. Toto regularly came into heat for about three days in the middle of her monthly menstrual cycle. Apparently she also became infatuated with a human male. One month it was the gardener, the next the chauffeur or the butler, at whom she gazed with "unmistakable lovesick eyes."[41]

The most curious story of infatuation in another species, however, was that of a moose that seemed to fall in love with a cow in Vermont.[42] The stricken herbivore trailed his idol for seventy-six days before he gave up his amorous "come hither" gesturing. "No man can, at one time, be wise and love," wrote poet Robert Herrick. Even moose make mistakes.

In fact, the energy, focus, persistence, possessiveness, and affection of infatuation are common among our furry and feathered brethren.[43] Consorting lions show great tenderness for each other during the female's period of heat. Giraffes gently caress each other before they mate. The male fox fixates on a vixen during her two weeks of estrus, gazing at her, doggedly following her, feeding her, licking her, and protecting her before they build their den and rear their pups together. A pair of elephants often spends hours side by side during the female's period of receptivity, stroking each other with their trunks. And baboons, chimpanzees, and other higher primates show distinct preferences for specific individuals, friendships that endure even when the female is not sexually receptive.

Indeed, no free-ranging bird or mammal will copulate with anyone who comes along. They all have favorites. They are attracted to some and repelled by others—*even during the height of estrus*, their period of heat. This choosiness is well known to scientists and called by several names, including mate choice, favoritism, sexual preference, individual preference, and selective proceptivity.[44]

Moreover, most animals form this preference instantly.

## Love at First Sight

Could this ability to adore another within moments of meeting (or even before meeting, on the Internet) come out of nature? Darwin believed this attraction can be instant. Of a female duck, he wrote, "It was evidently a case of love at first sight, for she swam around the newcomer caressingly . . . with overtures of affection."[45]

Elizabeth Marshall Thomas saw the same passion, writing, "From the moment she set eyes on him, she adored him. Wanting only to be near him, to lavish her affection on him, she followed him everywhere he went. The sound of his voice made her bark."[46] Violet, her little pug, had fallen in love with her other pug, Bingo.

And primatologist Birute Galdikas writes of a male orangutan in the Tanjung Putting Reserve, Borneo, saying much the same: "From the way Throatpouch pursued her, Priscilla had sexual charm to spare. TP was instantly smitten with her. He couldn't take his eyes off her. He didn't even bother to eat so enthralled was he by her balding charms."[47]

This magnetic attraction is like a sleeping cat; it can be awakened in an instant—hence the phenomenon of love at first sight.

Love at first sight may have a critical adaptive function in nature too.

During the mating season a female squirrel, for example, needs to breed. It is not to her advantage to copulate with a porcupine. But if she sees a healthy, energetic, virile-looking male squirrel, she should grab her chance. Perhaps love at first sight is no more than an inborn tendency in many creatures that evolved to spur the mating process. Then, among our human ancestors, this instant animal attraction evolved into what we now call love at first sight.

But how has nature actually created the bodily feeling of infatuation? What is this thing called love?

## The Brain Circuitry of Love

In 1996, I embarked on a project to establish what happens in the brain when you fall deeply, madly in love.[48]

First I planned the experiment. I would collect data on brain activity (using functional magnetic resonance imaging, or fMRI) as love-smitten participants performed two separate tasks: while gazing at a photograph of their beloved, and while looking at a photograph of someone who generated no positive or negative feelings in them. Between eyeing the positive and neutral photos, they would perform a distraction task. In this case, I would cast a large number on the screen (like 6,137) and ask participants to mentally count backward from this number in increments of seven. This, I hoped, would cleanse the brain of strong emotions between exposure to the beloved and exposure to the neutral stimulus.

Then I would compare the brain activity that occurred under all three conditions.

My hypothesis? Foremost, I suspected I would find elevated activity in the brain's networks for dopamine, a natural stimulant—because this brain system generates energy, euphoria, craving, focus, and motivation, some of the core traits of romantic love.[49]

I also posited that the closely related neurochemical norepinephrine might contribute to this madness, because this neurotransmitter produces focus and motivation too, as well as some of the bodily responses of romantic love such as butterflies in the stomach, wobbly knees, and a dry mouth. And I thought low activity in the serotonin system might create the intrusive, obsessive thinking of romantic passion.

Last, I expected that many other neurochemical systems might be involved—together producing the range of emotions, motivations, cognitions, and behaviors common to romantic love.[50]

But my bets were on dopamine.

Then, with neuroscientist Lucy Brown, psychologist Art Aron, and others, I put seventeen new lovers into the brain scanner: ten women and seven men who had been madly and happily in love for an average of 7.4 months.

I will never forget the moment I first saw the results. I was standing in a darkened lab at the Albert Einstein College of Medicine. I felt like jumping in the sky. Before my eyes were scans showing blobs of activity in the ventral tegmental area, or VTA, a tiny factory near the base of the brain *that makes dopamine* and sends this natural stimulant to many brain regions.[51]

We found activity in many other brain regions, but the VTA was particularly important.[52] This factory is part of the brain's reward system, the brain network that generates wanting, seeking, craving, energy, focus, and motivation.

No wonder lovers can stay awake all night talking and caressing. No wonder they become so absent-minded, so giddy, so optimistic, so gregarious, so full of life. They are high on natural "speed."

And men feel this passion just as powerfully as women. Tennov wrote of her 800+ informants that men and women experienced this intense passion "in roughly equal proportions." My colleagues and I have now confirmed this. In our fMRI study of young happy lovers, men showed just as much activity in the VTA and other neural pathways for romantic passion as women did.

Moreover, when my colleagues redid this brain scanning experiment in China, their Chinese participants showed just as much activity in the VTA and other dopamine pathways—the neurochemical pathways for *wanting*.[53] Almost everyone on earth feels this passion.

## The Drive to Love . . . a Natural Addiction

In fact, because the VTA lies near primitive brain regions associated with thirst and hunger, I came to realize that romantic love is a basic human drive.[54] My brain scanning partner Lucy Brown has added to this perspective, saying that romantic love is a survival mechanism as crucial as the craving for water.

This drive, this survival mechanism, is also an addiction. With a reanalysis of the data, we found activity in the nucleus accumbens (unpublished data), a brain region that is part of the reward system, is fueled by dopamine, and is associated with all of the addictions—including the cravings for heroin, cocaine, nicotine, alcohol, amphetamines, gambling, sex, and food.

Moreover, we are not the only creatures that have inherited the chemistry of love. When a female prairie vole begins to express attraction to a male vole, she experiences a 50% increase of dopamine activity in parts of this reward system.[55] An increase of dopamine in the brain is also associated with mate attraction in female sheep.[56] Hence, this neural mechanism for attraction must have evolved in many species of birds and mammals—to enable individuals to prefer and focus on specific mating partners, thereby conserving valuable courtship time and energy.[57]

In most species, however, this attraction is brief, lasting only minutes, hours, days, or weeks. In humans, intense, early-stage romantic love can last much longer.[58]

## Love Blindness

There is always variation in this experience, however. Baseline activities of dopamine (as well as norepinephrine and serotonin) vary from one person to the next—potentially altering one's proclivity to fall in love and stay in love. But other brain systems can also affect romance.

For example, some of those who report they have never felt romantic love suffer from hypopituitarism, a rare disease in which the pituitary malfunctions in infancy, causing hormonal problems and "love blindness." These men and women lead normal lives; some marry for companionship; but that rapture, that heartache, is mythology to them. Moreover, schizophrenia, Parkinson's disease, and other ailments alter dopamine pathways. In fact, in the last chapter of this book, "Future Sex," I will discuss my theory that several serotonin-enhancing antidepressants, such as Prozac, Zoloft, and the newer serotonin boosters, can suppress dopamine pathways, dull the emotions, and potentially kill romantic passion.[59]

Your experiences also affect romance. You begin in childhood to like and dislike the smells in your environment. You learn to respond to certain kinds of humor. You get used to the peace or hysteria in your home. And you begin to build your love map from your experiences. Then, in teenage, you join the military, go away to college, or become otherwise displaced. These and many other *cultural* events determine *whom* you love, *when* you love, *where* you love.

But after you find that special person, it is dopamine and other natural neurochemicals in the brain that direct *how* you feel *as* you love. As usual, culture and biology go hand in hand.

Love poems; love songs; love magic; myths and legends about love; the world's great operas, plays, and ballets; our novels, articles, blogs, TV programs, and self-help books about love; the world's palaces and temples built to honor a beloved; even sweet pictorial messages of love embedded in emojis and emoticons on the Internet: all would emerge as our forebears gradually developed our big cerebral cortex, the rind of the brain with which we think.

Yet the basic brain mechanism for romantic love lies deep in the basement of the mind, in primordial brain regions linked with wanting, seeking, and motivation.

But can it last?

## The Trajectory of Love

"Love is strongest in pursuit, friendship in possession." As Emerson believed, at some point that initial ecstasy and obsession begins to wane. For teenagers a crush can last a week. Lovers who see each other irregularly, because of some barrier like an ocean or a wedding ring from another, can sometimes sustain that smitten feeling for several years.

There is some data on the general length of this intense condition, however. Tennov measured the duration of romantic love from the moment infatuation hit to when a "feeling of neutrality" for one's love object began. She concluded, "The most frequent interval, as well as the average, is between approximately 18 months and three years."

But data vary. A study that indicates serotonin activity in the blood suggests that this intoxication lasts twelve to eighteen months.[60] And in our 2012 national Match.com survey of singles, 29% of over 5,000 men and women of every age group, background, and sexual persuasion reported that this passion lasted for two to five years; 8% remained intensely in love for six to ten years, and 18% reported that they remained madly in love for over ten years.[61]

Exactly how this ecstasy and obsession decline, no one knows. I suspect that either the nerve pathways for dopamine and related neurochemicals become habituated to these natural stimulants or the production and distribution of dopamine and related neurochemicals decline. As psychiatrist Michael Liebowitz sums it up, "If you want a situation where you and your long-term partner can still get very excited about each other, you will have to work on it, because in some ways you are bucking a biological tide."[62]

This is not true in all people, of course. We all know couples who consistently maintain that they are still madly in love after many years of marriage. People find this hard to believe. But in another of our brain scanning experiments, led this time by psychologist Bianca Acevedo, we put seventeen long-married women and men into the fMRI scanner, ten women and seven men.[63] Their average length of marriage was twenty-one years; most had grown children; and all had told us that they were still in love with their spouse.

The results were astonishing: the VTA and other basic brain regions associated with early-stage intense romantic love were just as active among these long-term lovers as among our newly-in-love younger men and women.

With one exception: Our newly-in-love participants showed activity in a specific brain region associated with anxiety, whereas in our long-term lovers this angst was replaced by new activity in brain regions linked with calm and pain suppression. Acevedo and her colleagues now believe that long-term lovers can continue to feel the intensity, focus, and sexual drive of romantic love. But the obsessive, intoxicating ecstasy declines.[64]

"Love is like a fever; it comes and goes quite independently of the will." So wrote Stendhal of early-stage intense romantic passion. Why does romantic love flow and ebb? The pulse of human infatuation, like many of our courting gestures, may be part of nature's scheme—soft-wired in the brain by time, by evolution, and by ancient patterns of human bonding.

# 3

## Is Monogamy Natural?

### Of Human Bonding . . . and Cheating

Man is compos'd here of a two-fold part;
The first of Nature, and the next of Art.

—ROBERT HERRICK, "UPON MAN"

When Darwin used the term "survival of the fittest" he was not referring to your good looks or your bank account; he was counting your children. If you raise babies that have babies, you are what nature calls fit. You have passed your genes to the next generation and in terms of survival you have won. So the sexes are locked in a mating dance, endlessly adjusting their moves to complement those of the other. Only in tandem can either men or women reproduce and pass on the beat of human life.

This mating dance—our basic human reproductive strategy—began long, long ago when the world was young and our primordial ancestors evolved into two sexes.

## Why Sex?

Different species replicate differently. A few, like a variety of whiptail lizards, have done away with sex entirely. These little reptiles roam the semiarid chaparral of the American Southwest. During the breeding season, each develops eight to ten unfertilized ova, eggs that will hatch as perfect replicas of themselves. This type of asexual reproduction—parthenogenesis, or virgin birth—has its practical side. Although they do get into copulatory poses with other whiptails, triggering egg production, whiptails do not expend time or energy courting. They don't have to haul about heavy antlers like male elk to fight other courters, or outlandish tail feathers like male peacocks to woo females. They don't attract predators as do creatures who are vulnerable as they mate. Most important, they don't mix their genes with those of other whiptails, individuals that may have inferior genetic makeups. They produce offspring that carry 100% of their DNA.

Is love between the sexes necessary? Not for desert-grassland whiptails, some dandelions, blackberries, quaking aspen trees, or the asexual wild grasses. For these species, even mating has been dispensed with.[1]

Despite the enormous Darwinian advantages of asexuality, however, our ancestors and many other creatures went the way of sexual reproduction—for at least two reasons. Individuals who mate create one vital asset in their offspring: variety. A collie and a poodle may produce a puppy that looks nothing like either of its parents. This can have bad consequences; sometimes mixture produces a poor match. But recombination creates new genetic "personalities." Some will die. But some will live and overcome nature's tireless effort to weed out poor strains.

Biologists have also proposed a more subtle explanation for why our primitive forebears evolved sexual reproduction: to confuse their enemies.[2] This is known as the Red Queen hypothesis, after an incident in Lewis Carroll's book *Through the Looking Glass*.

The Red Queen takes Alice by the arm and together they run madly, hand in hand. But when they stop, they are exactly where they started. The Queen explains this bizarre situation to Alice, saying, "Now here, you see, it takes all the running you can do, to keep in the same place." Translated into evolutionary thinking, this means that creatures that change regularly remain biologically less susceptible to the bacteria, viruses, and other parasites that kill them. Thus sexual reproduction evolved to elude one's germs.[3]

But why two sexes, males and females? Why didn't our primeval progenitors choose a reproductive strategy in which any individual could exchange its genetic material with that of any other?

Bacteria do this. Organisms simply come together and exchange DNA. A can mate with B; B can mate with C; C can mate with A; everybody can mate with everybody else; bacteria have no sexual distinctions.[4] Unlike bacteria, however, the remote ancestors of human beings (and many other creatures) developed into two distinct types: females with big, sluggish eggs composed of DNA and rich, surrounding nutriments, and males with little, agile sperm stripped bare of all but genes.

No one knows how two separate sexes evolved in the primordial goo. One suggestion is that our first sexual ancestors somewhat resembled bacteria but were larger, multicellular life forms that produced sex cells (gametes) containing half their DNA. Like bacteria, each individual produced gametes that could combine with any other gamete. But some organisms disseminated big gametes surrounded by a lot of nutritious cytoplasm. Others sprayed forth smaller sex cells with less fodder. Still others propelled tiny gametes with almost no added food aboard.

All of these sexual creatures cast their sex cells into the ocean currents. When two small gametes united, however, they lacked enough nutriments to survive. When two big sex cells joined, they were too ungainly to live on. But when a lithe, little, unencumbered gamete, a proto-sperm, united with a big, nutrient-laden gamete, a proto-egg, the new organism lived through its precarious beginning. And with time two separate sexes evolved, one carrying eggs, the other transporting sperm.[5]

There are problems with this theory, as well as alternative hypotheses.[6] And, regrettably, there are no living organisms that portray the lifeways of our first sexual ancestors. But somehow, billions of years ago, individuals of two complementary strains developed. Then two separate sexes emerged. And their continually varying offspring lived and multiplied across the eons of our restless, changing past.

## Sexual Paths Our Ancestors Overlooked

It is a wonder our rude antecedents did not opt for the sex life of strawberries—creatures that, like the little whiptail lizard, can reproduce asexually; but they also engage in sexual mating. When strawberries feel secure, the patch is unexploited, and the environment is unchanging, they clone. Why bother with sex? Only when space runs out, forcing strawberries to disperse into uncharted lands, do they put forth flowers and mate. When the pioneer berries settle in, however, they start to clone again.

Earthworms have another variation of sexuality. These creatures are both male and female at the same time; they can impregnate themselves. But most hermaphroditic plants and animals go to great lengths to avoid self-fertilization, a process that has the deficits of both sexuality and asexuality.

Perhaps the most eccentric form of reproduction, by human standards, exists in species in which individuals are able to transform themselves from one sex into the other. Among these are fish that live along the Great Barrier Reef of Australia. Known as cleaner fish, or *Labroides dimidiatus*, these reef combers live in groups of one male and five or six females. If the single male dies or disappears, the most dominant female begins to metamorphose into a male. Within a few days "she" is "he."

If men and women were able to clone themselves, if we could be both sexes simultaneously, or if we could totally transform ourselves within hours from one sex into the other, we probably would not have evolved our copulatory gaze, our flirting brow, our four broad styles of thinking and behaving, or the brain physiology for romantic love. But the ancestors of human beings, like the vast majority of other living species, did not elect the sex lives of cloning strawberries, hermaphroditic earthworms or transsexual fish. Instead, we became men and women, subspecies that must mix our genes or slip into oblivion.

Copulation is not the only way that you and I ensure our genetic futures, however. A second means by which sexual organisms propagate their DNA is a process known as kin selection.[7] This is derived from a reality of nature: every individual shares his or her genetic makeup with blood relatives. From its mother the child receives half its genes; from its father, the other half. If a child has full brothers or sisters, it shares half its genes with each of them. One-eighth of its genes it shares with cousins, and so forth. So if a man or woman spends a lifetime nurturing genetic relatives, he or she is actually helping his or her own DNA. When kin survive, you survive—hence the concept of "inclusive fitness."[8]

No wonder people around the world tend to favor their genetic kin.

~

Our surest way to posterity, however, is through mating. In fact, all of our human rituals concerning courtship and mating, marriage and divorce, can be regarded as scripts by which men and women seduce each other in order to replicate themselves—what biologists call reproductive strategies.

What are these mating games?

Well, men have a few basic options, as do women; the elegance of each is that it is easily distinguished by counting heads. A man can form a pair-bond with a single wife at a time, monogyny (from the Greek *mono*, "one," and *gyny*, "female"); or he can have multiple wives at the same time, polygyny (poly means "many"). Women have two similar options: monandry (one husband) or polyandry (many husbands at the same time). Moreover, monogamy means "one *spouse*" without signifying gender; and polygamy means "several spouses" without signifying gender.[9] Last is group marriage, or polygynandry—a reproductive strategy that occurs when two or more males have a socially recognized spousal arrangement with two or more females.

As you will soon see, we are largely a monogamous species—we form pair-bonds to rear our young. But, among academics, monogamy does not necessarily imply fidelity. What is more, adultery often goes hand in hand with monogamy, as well as with other reproductive strategies.[10]

## Nature's Philanderers

Male red-winged blackbirds, for example, oversee large territories of marsh during the breeding season; several females join a single male on his patch of real estate and copulate with only him. Or so the story goes. However, scientists then vasectomized some of these males prior to the breeding season.[11] Females then joined these neutered males, copulated with them, and nested in their home ranges—nothing unusual.

But many of these females laid fertile clutches. Clearly these females had not been sexually faithful to their partner. To be positive of this, scientists took blood samples from the infant nestlings of a different sample of thirty-one female red-winged blackbirds. Almost half of all nests contained one or more chicks whose father was not the landlord. Most of these females had copulated with "floaters" or with a male that lived next door.[12]

Adultery is common in other species too. Some 90% of more than 8,000 avian species practice pair-bonding to rear their young—monogamy.[13] They must; someone must sit on the eggs continually and this individual will starve to death unless they have a mate bring them food. But ornithologists have observed extra-pair copulations, or "sneakers," in over one hundred species of monogamous birds.

Only 3% of mammals form a pair-bond to rear their young.[14] But these individuals also philander. Among them are gibbons, lesser apes that live in pairs in some of the rain forests of China, India, Indonesia, and other parts of Southeast Asia, including the islands of Sumatra, Borneo, and Java. Gibbons have long been thought to be paragons of virtue. Not so. Some females raise infants that are genetically not related to their current "spouse."[15]

Indeed, the marshes, the meadows, the forests across the earth are full of philanderers. And if you have missed the combination of monogamy and cheating in red-winged blackbirds or gibbons, surely you have noticed philandering in people.

All married men and women in the United States are, by definition, monogamous; having several spouses at the same time is against the law. According to some recent estimates, however, some 20–40% of American heterosexual married men and 20–25% of American heterosexual married women have had an extramarital affair.[16] American dating couples currently report a 70% incidence of infidelity.[17] And in a recent survey of single Americans, 60% of men and 53% of women admitted to "mate poaching," trying to woo an individual away from a committed partnership to begin a relationship with them.[18] Mate poaching is also common in thirty other cultures.[19]

It's impossible to really know how accurate any of these figures are.

But no one would deny that adultery occurs in every culture around the world.

So here's the point. Pair-bonding is only part of our basic human reproductive strategy; extramarital sex is often a secondary, complementary component of our *mixed* or *dual* mating tactics. In fact, infidelity is so widespread and persistent in monogamous avian and mammalian species, including humans, that scientists now refer to monogamous species as practicing *social monogamy*, in which partners display the array of social and reproductive behaviors associated with pair-bonding while not necessarily displaying sexual fidelity as well.

However, before I explore the amorphous tangle of human adultery, I would like to examine the human mating patterns that are quite visible—our marriage systems.[20]

Perhaps the most remarkable thing the sexes have in common is that they bother to marry at all.

Yet marriage is a near cultural universal; it predominates in almost every society in the world. In 2009, 83% of American men and 88.5% of American women had married by age 49;[21] and today 85%–90% of men and women in the United States are projected to wed.[22] From church ledgers, court records, lists, and marriage files of ninety-seven industrial and agricultural societies, the Statistical Office of the United Nations has culled data on marriage since the 1940s. Worldwide, between 2000 and 2011, an average of 90.2% of women and 88.9% of men married by age forty-nine.[23]

Marriage is also the norm where record-keepers have not arrived. Among the Cashinahua Indians of Brazil, marriage is a casual affair. When a teenage girl becomes eager to marry and gets her father's permission, she asks her husband-to-be to visit her in her hammock after the family is asleep. He must be gone by daybreak. Gradually he moves his possessions into the family home. But the marriage is not taken seriously until the girl becomes pregnant or the liaison has lasted at least a year. In contrast, Hindu parents in India sometimes suggest a husband for their daughter, and with her permission they make elaborate wedding plans.

There are several separate wedding rites. Then, long after the marriage has been consummated, the families of the bride and groom continue to exchange property according to negotiated terms.

Marriage customs vary. But from the steppes of Asia to the coral atolls of the western Pacific, the vast majority of men and women take a spouse. In fact, in all traditional societies marriage marks a critical step into adulthood; spinsters and bachelors are rare.

What are the marriage strategies of men and women? Although I will maintain that monogamy, or pair-bonding, is the hallmark of the human animal, there is no question that some men and women follow other sexual and reproductive scripts. Men are the more variable of the genders, so let's begin with them.

## Harem Building

"Hogamus, higamus, men are polygamous." So the ditty goes. Only 16% of the 853 cultures on record actually prescribe monogyny.[24] Industrial societies are among them. We are in the minority, however. A whopping 84% of all human traditional societies permit a man to take more than one wife at once—polygyny.

Although anthropologists have used a lot of ink and paper to describe cultural reasons for the widespread permissibility of this harem building, it can be explained by a simple principle of nature: polygyny can have tremendous genetic payoffs for men.[25]

The most successful harem builder on record was Moulay Ismail the Bloodthirsty, an emperor of Morocco. *The Guinness Book of World Records* reports that Ismail sired 888 children with his many wives. But even Ismail may have been surpassed. Some "hardworking" Chinese emperors copulated with over a thousand women, all carefully rotated through the royal bedroom when they were most likely to conceive. These privileged heads of state were not the only men to experience harem life, however. Polygyny was common in many West African societies, where about 25% of older men had two or three wives at once.

The most colorful example of harem building, by Western standards, is the Tiwi, who live on Melville Island, about twenty-five miles off the northern coast of Australia.

In this gerontocracy, custom traditionally dictated that all women be married—even those not yet conceived. So, after her first menstruation, a pubescent girl emerged from temporary isolation in the bush to greet her father and her future *son*-in-law. As soon as she saw these men, she lay in the grass and pretended to be asleep. Carefully her father placed a wooden spear between her legs; then he handed this ceremonial weapon to his companion, who stroked it, hugged it, and called it wife. With this simple ceremony, her father's friend—a man in his thirties—had just married all of the *unborn* daughters this teenage girl would someday bear.

Because men were betrothed to babies not yet conceived, boys had to wait until their mid-forties to make love to their pubescent wives. Young men had sex, of course; sweethearts sneaked into the bush together all the time. But young men craved the prestige and power that marriage brought. So they learned to wheel and deal, bartering promises, food, and labor for wealth and potential wives in later life. Then, as they accumulated spouses and begot children, men gained control of their daughters' unborn daughters, whom they proceeded to marry off to their friends in exchange for even more potential wives.[26] By his seventieth birthday, a rich and clever Tiwi gentleman might have collected as many as ten brides, although most had far fewer.

This traditional Tiwi marriage system worked before the coming of the Europeans. Because of the great age difference between spouses, men and women married several times. Women liked choosing new young husbands as they got older. Men and older women savored the wits and bargaining it took to manipulate marriage negotiations. And the Tiwi said that everybody enjoyed the sexual variety.

Women in most societies try to prevent their husbands from taking a junior wife, although they are less reluctant to accept a younger sister as a co-wife. Apart from the chronic jealousy and battles for attention, women married to the same man tend to war with one another over food and the other resources their mutual husband provides.

There comes a point, however, when a woman becomes willing to join a harem—a Rubicon known as the polygyny threshold.[27]

This occurred among the Blackfoot Indians of the northern plains of North America at the end of the nineteenth century. By this time warfare had become chronic and casualties were enormous, so eligible Blackfoot men were in short supply. Women needed husbands. At the same time, men needed extra wives. The horses and guns they had acquired from the Europeans enabled these Indians to kill many more buffalo than they had been able to kill on foot with bows and arrows. Successful hunters needed extra hands to tan these hides—the backbone of their trading power. This tipped the balance; unwed girls preferred being the second wife of a rich man to being the only wife of a poor one or a woman with no spouse at all.[28]

Polygyny also occurs in the United States. Although harem building is illegal here, some Mormon men take several wives for religious reasons. Their forefathers in the Church of Jesus Christ of Latter-Day Saints, founded in 1831 by Joseph Smith, originally held that men should take more than one wife. And although the Mormon Church officially turned away from polygyny in 1890, some devout fundamentalist Mormons still practice plural marriages. Not surprisingly, many of these polygynous Mormon men are also rich.[29]

If polygyny were permitted in New York, Chicago, or Los Angeles, an Episcopalian or Catholic man with $500 million could probably also attract several women willing to share his love—and his cash.[30]

So men tend to seek polygyny to spread their genes; while women join harems to acquire resources and ensure the survival of their young. *But these are not conscious motivations.* If you ask a man why he wants a second bride, he might say he is attracted to her wit, her business acumen, her vivacious spirit, or her splendid thighs. If you ask a women why she is willing to "share" a man, she might tell you that she loves the way he looks or laughs or takes her to fancy vacation spots.

But no matter what reasons people offer, polygyny enables men to have more children; under the right conditions, some women (particularly first wives) also reap reproductive benefits. So, long ago ancestral men who sought polygyny and ancestral women who acquiesced to harem life disproportionately survived, selecting for this unconscious motivation. No wonder harems crop up where they can.

## Humankind: A Monogamous Primate

Because of the genetic advantages of polygyny for men and because so many societies permit polygyny, many anthropologists think that harem building is a badge of the human animal.

I do not agree. Certainly it is a secondary *opportunistic* reproductive strategy. But in the vast majority of societies where polygyny is permitted, only about 5–10% of men actually have several wives simultaneously.[31] Although polygyny is widely discussed, it is much less practiced. Instead, the vast majority of men and women in almost every society on earth form a pair-bond, with serial monogamy the most common mating pattern.[32]

In fact, after surveying 250 cultures, anthropologist George Peter Murdock summarized the data, saying, "An impartial observer employing the criterion of numerical preponderance, consequently, would be compelled to characterize nearly every known human society as monogamous, despite the preference for and frequency of polygyny in the overwhelming majority."[33]

Around the world today the vast majority of men marry one woman at a time. And because human polygyny is regularly associated with rank and wealth, monogamy was most likely even more prevalent throughout our long hunting and gathering past, when accumulating property was impossible.[34]

❧

"Higamus, hogamus, women monogamous." Women also tend to take a single spouse—monandry. All women in so-called monogamous societies have only one husband at a time; they never have two spouses simultaneously. In so-called polygynous societies, a woman also marries only one man at a time, despite the fact that she may have co-wives. Because women in 99.5% of cultures around the world marry only one man at once, it is fair to conclude that monandry, one spouse, is the overwhelmingly predominant marriage pattern for the human female.

This is not to suggest that women never have a harem of men. Polyandry is rare; only 0.5% of all societies permit a woman to take several husbands simultaneously.[35] But it does occur under peculiar circumstances—such as when the women are very rich.

The Tlingit Indians of southern Alaska were wealthy before the Europeans arrived. They lived, as they do today, along the coast of one of the most abundant fishing grounds in the world, the Alaskan archipelago. During the summer months Tlingit men fished for salmon and trapped myriad animals in the woods along the shore. Women joined their husbands at summer fishing and hunting camps, collected berries and wild plants, and converted the catch into dried fish, rich oils, smoked meats, pelts, and valuable trade items of wood and shell. Then, in the autumn, men and women went on trading expeditions along the coast.

But commerce among the Tlingit was fundamentally different from that of Europeans. Women were the traders. Women set the prices; women did the bargaining; women finalized transactions; and women pocketed the gains. Women were often high-ranking.[36] And it was not uncommon for a wealthy woman to have two husbands.

Polyandry also occurred traditionally in the Himalayas, for a different ecological reason. Well-to-do Tibetan families in the highlands of Limi, Nepal, were determined to keep their estates together; if they divided their landholdings among their heirs, the precious property would lose its value. Besides, parents needed several sons to work the soil, herd the cattle, yaks, and goats, and work for overlords. So if a couple bore several sons, they coaxed these boys to share a wife. From the woman's perspective, this is polyandry.

Not surprisingly, these co-husbands had problems with one another. Brothers were often of different ages, and a wife of twenty-two might find her fifteen-year-old husband immature and her twenty-seven-year-old spouse sexually exciting. Younger brothers endured the sexual favoritism in order to remain on the family land, however, surrounded by the jewels, the rugs, the horses—the good life. But resentments festered.

⁀

Polyandry is rare in people as well as in other creatures, for a good biological reason.[37] Female birds and mammals can bear only a limited number of offspring during their lives. Gestation takes time. The young often require additional care before weaning. And females have distinct intervals between successive births. Women, for example, cannot regularly bear more than about twenty-five children during a lifetime. The record is held by a Russian woman who had sixty-nine babies, mostly multiple births, during the course of twenty-seven pregnancies. But this is phenomenal. Most women in gathering–hunting cultures bear no more than about five infants.[38] Polyandry may help a woman's young survive, but it does not help a woman bear more than a limited number of infants.

And for men, polyandry can spell genetic suicide. Male mammals do not go through pregnancy, nor do they lactate. So, like the ancient Chinese emperors, all men can have thousands of offspring—if they can get a parade of cooperative partners and withstand sexual exhaustion. Hence, if a man joins the harem of a single woman, much of his sperm is wasted.

## Horde Living

Even rarer than polyandry is "group marriage," polygynandry, from the Greek meaning "many females males." This sexual tactic deserves mention not because of its frequency but because it reveals the single most important point about human bonding.

You can count on the fingers of one hand the number of peoples that practice group marriage. Among them were the traditional Pahari, a tribe in northern India. There, wives were so expensive that two brothers sometimes had to pool their money to pay the "bride price" to a girl's father. She married both at once. Then, if the brothers became prosperous, they purchased a second bride. Apparently both wives made love to both husbands.[39]

Group wedlock also occurs in the United States in sex communes that crop up decade after decade.[40] The classic example was the Oneida community. What went on at this colony illustrates the most essential point about our human mating game.

This avant-garde colony was started in the 1830s by a religious zealot, John Humphrey Noyes, a daring and sexually energetic man who wished to create a Christian, communist utopia.[41] In 1847 his community settled in Oneida, New York, where it functioned until 1881. In its heyday over five hundred women, men, and children worked the communal lands and manufactured the steel traps they sold to the outside world. Everyone lived in one building, Mansion House, which still stands. Each adult had his or her own room. But everything else was shared, including the children they brought into the commune, their clothes, and their sex partners.

Noyes ruled. Romantic love for a particular person was considered selfish, shameful. Men were forbidden to ejaculate unless their partners had passed menopause. No children were to be born. And everybody was supposed to copulate with everybody else.

In 1868 Noyes lifted the ban on reproducing, and, by special permission, several women conceived. Noyes and his son sired twelve of the sixty-two children born within the next few years. But there was growing friction among community members. The younger men were expected to have sex with the older women, while Noyes had first claim to the pubescent girls. In 1879 the men revolted and accused Noyes of raping several young women. He fled. Within months the community disbanded.

Most interesting about the Oneida sexual experiment is this: despite his dictatorial regulations Noyes was never able to keep men and women from falling in love and forming clandestine pair-bonds with one another. Attraction between people was more powerful than his decrees. In fact, no Western experiment in group marriage has managed to thrive for more than a few years. As Margaret Mead put it, "No matter how many communes anybody invents, the family always creeps back."[42]

The human animal seems to be psychologically built to form a pair-bond with a single mate.

Is monogamy natural?

Yes.

There certainly are exceptions. Given the opportunity, men often opt for multiple spouses to unconsciously further their genetic lines. Polygyny is also natural. But co-wives fight. Women join harems when the resources they can garner outweigh the disadvantages. Polyandry is also natural. But co-husbands argue too. In short, both men and women have to be cajoled by riches to share a spouse. Whereas gorillas, horses, and animals of many other species *always* form harems, among human beings polygyny and polyandry seem to be optional, opportunistic exceptions.

Monogamy is the rule.[43] Human beings almost never have to be cajoled into pairing. Instead, we do this naturally. We flirt. We court. We fall in love. We marry. And the vast majority of us marry only one person at a time. Pair-bonding is a trademark of the human animal.

## Arranged Love

This is not to suggest that all wives and husbands are infatuated with each other when they wed. In many traditional societies the first marriage of a son or daughter is arranged.[44] Where marriage has been a family's means of making alliances—for example, among many traditional peoples who farmed in Europe and North Africa, as well as in preindustrial India, China, and Japan—a young couple might not even meet until their wedding night. But where arranged marriages are still prevalent today, the views of both the boy and girl are sought before wedding plans proceed.

Modern Egyptians provide a good example. Parents of potential spouses design a meeting between the youths. If the two like each other, parents begin to plan the marriage. Even in New York City, traditional Chinese, Korean, Russian-Jewish, West Indian, and Arab parents often introduce their sons or daughters to appropriate partners and encourage them to wed.

Interestingly, many of these young people fall in love. This is well documented in India. Hindu children are taught that marital love is the essence of life. So men and women often enter married life enthusiastically, *expecting* a romance to blossom. Indeed, romance often does. As the

Hindus explain it, "First we marry, then we fall in love."[45] I am not surprised. Since love can be triggered by a single glance in a single moment, no wonder some of these arranged courtships rapidly turn into romantic attachments.

〜

So where are we? The basic human reproductive strategy is monogamy, one spouse. Moreover, even where men and women live with several spouses simultaneously, individuals generally have one partner whom they prefer. In free sex communes, men and women tend to pair. Even where marriages are strictly arranged, love blossoms—as the novel *The Family*, by Pa Chin, powerfully illustrates.

Chin wrote about life in a traditional Chinese household in the 1930s. Teetering between the ancient Chinese concept of filial piety and modern values of individualism, the young sons of a tyrannical old man struggle to make life meaningful. The eldest accepts his fate and his arranged marriage. But daily he pines for his beloved, a sweetheart who dies of unrequited love for him. The family's chambermaid hurls herself into a lake and drowns; she is of the wrong station to marry the son she loves and wants to avoid an arranged marriage with a hideous old man. The youngest son steals out of the family compound by moonlight to seek fulfillment in one of the freer cities of Westernizing China. All the while, the patriarch dines with his concubine, a woman he fell in love with years before.

For hundreds of years Chinese tradition tried to curb romantic love. Fate, resignation, and obedience were drummed into the young. And the most painful of all the world's fashions—the thousand-year-old practice of footbinding—kept a young wife at her loom, preventing her from fleeing her husband's house. Today, however, the Chinese have shed their custom of arranged marriages. They are buying pulpy romance novels, playing sentimental tunes, dating, divorcing partners they never loved, and choosing spouses for themselves. They call their convention "free love."

To court, to fall in love, to form a pair-bond is human. Nevertheless, many seem to practice a dual reproductive strategy: monogamy *and* adultery. Why are some of us sexually unfaithful to our vows?

# 4

## Why Adultery?

### The Nature of Philandering

That we can call these delicate creatures ours,
And not their appetites. I had rather be a toad,
And live upon the vapor of a dungeon,
Than keep a corner in the thing I love
For others' uses.

—WILLIAM SHAKESPEARE, *OTHELLO*

Along the southern Adriatic coast, the flat Italian beaches are broken by rocky hills that descend into the sea. Here, behind the boulders, in secluded caverns with shallow pools and sandy shoals, young Italian men of the mid-1900s seduced foreign women they picked up in the resort hotels, on the beaches, and in the bars and discos. Here the boys lost their virginity in their late teens, and here they honed their sexual skills, counted their conquests, and built their reputations as dexterous, passionate Italian lovers, personas they would cultivate throughout their lives.

Because local Italian girls were too supervised to be enticed, and because prostitution was not practiced in these villages, young men were dependent on the seasonal tourist trade for their sexual education until they wed. But by middle age, these men entered a new network of sexual liaisons, an elaborate quasi-institutionalized system of extramarital affairs with local village women. With time each philanderer learned to exercise discretion and follow strict rules that everybody understood.

As psychologist Lewis Diana reported, adultery was the rule rather than the exception in these towns that dotted the central and southern Adriatic coast; almost every man had a lover he visited regularly on week-days, either late in the morning or in the early evening while husbands were still at work in the vineyards, on fishing boats, in their retail shops, or off on their own clandestine business.

Generally middle- and upper-class men had long affairs with married women of the same or lower social standing. Sometimes younger male servants visited the wives of landowners, while prestigious men occasionally had trysts with their maids or cooks. But the most enduring relationships were those between men and women who were married to others; many of these affairs lasted for several years or even life.

The only dalliances that were taboo were those between older, unattached women and young, unmarried men—largely because young men boast. Gossip was intolerable. In these villages, family was the warp and weft of social life, and whispering threatened to expose the network of extramarital relationships, seriously disrupting community cohesion and destroying family life. So although infidelity was commonplace among adults—and known to most because of the lack of privacy—a code of absolute silence prevailed. Family life must not be undermined.

One breach of this collective complicity occurred when a retired Italian businessman who had lived in America since childhood made a comment in a men's club about a woman he hoped to lure into a sexual rendezvous. All listeners immediately fell silent. Then, one by one, each man rose and walked out. As Diana reports, "The man had pulled a monumental blunder. No married man ever speaks of his interest in other women. The taboo is stringent and unbreakable. Life is difficult enough not to jeopardize one of its rare diversions."[1]

An ocean away, in Amazonia, extramarital affairs were equally coveted—but much more complex. Among the traditional Kuikuru, a group of about 160 people who lived in a single village along the Xingu River in the jungles of Brazil, men and women often married shortly after puberty.

But sometimes, within months of matrimony, both spouses began to take lovers, known as *ajois*.[2]

*Ajois* got their friends to arrange their assignations. Then they strolled out of the communal compound at the planned moment under the pretense of fetching water, bathing, fishing, or going to tend the garden. The sweethearts met and snuck off to a distant clearing in the forest where they talked, exchanged small gifts, and had sex. Even the oldest Kuikuru man and woman in the village regularly slipped away for an afternoon rendezvous, says anthropologist Robert Carneiro. Most villagers had between four and twelve lovers at a time.

Unlike the men of coastal Italy, however, the Kuikuru enjoyed discussing these affairs. Even small children could rattle off the lattice of *ajois* relationships, much as American youngsters recite their ABCs. Only husband and wife refrained from speaking with each other about their outside sexual adventures, largely because, once faced with the facts, a spouse might feel obliged to confront the offending party publicly, a disruption and embarrassment that all wished to avoid. If a woman flaunted her friendship with a paramour, however, or spent so much time outside the village that she neglected her daily chores, a husband sometimes did get irritated. Then a public argument would erupt. But the Kuikuru considered sexual freedom normal; retribution for adultery was rare.

Dozens of ethnographic studies, not to mention countless works of history and fiction, have testified to the prevalence of extramarital sexual activities among men and women around the world.[3] Although we flirt, fall in love, and marry, human beings also tend to be sexually unfaithful to a spouse. So this chapter explores this second aspect of our dual human reproductive strategy—how clandestine relationships vary; why the predisposition for adultery evolved.

## The Many Faces of Adultery

The Turu of Tanzania traditionally enjoyed sexual license during the puberty ceremony of their teenage boys. On the first day's festivities, extramarital lovers danced to imitate intercourse and sang songs extolling the penis, vagina, and copulation. If these dances were not "hot," or full of sexual passion, as the Turu said, the celebration would be a failure. That evening sweethearts consummated what they had suggested all day.[4]

Wife lending, known as wife hospitality, was customary among several Inuit (Eskimo) peoples. This form of adultery stemmed from their concept of kinship. If a husband was eager to cement his ties with a hunting companion, he could offer the sexual services of his wife—but only with her permission. If all agreed, she had sex with this business partner for several days or even weeks. Women also offered sex to visitors and strangers. But Inuit women saw these extramarital couplings as precious offerings of everlasting kinship, not as social indiscretions.[5]

The most curious custom prescribing overt adultery may come from Western heritage. In several European societies, a feudal lord was said to have had the right to deflower the bride of a vassal on his wedding night—a custom known as the *jus primae noctis*, or "right of the first night." Historians question whether this rite was widely exercised, if at all; but there seems to be some evidence that medieval Scottish nobles did indeed bed their subjects' brides.[6]

Which raises the question: What constitutes adultery?

Definitions vary. The Lozi of Africa do not associate adultery only with intercourse. The Lozi say that if a man accompanies a married woman he is not related to as she walks along a path, or if he gives her a beer or some snuff, he has committed adultery. This sounds farfetched. But Americans do not always associate adultery just with sexual intercourse either. If an American businessman finds himself in a foreign city buying dinner for an attractive colleague and then performing every sexual act with her except coitus, he might think that he has been adulterous—despite the lack of intercourse. In fact, in a poll taken by *People* magazine, some 74% of the 750 respondents believed that one does not actually need to engage in intercourse to be unfaithful.[7]

Among the Kofyar of Nigeria, people define adultery quite differently. A woman who is dissatisfied with her husband but does not wish to divorce can take a legitimate extra lover who lives openly with her in her husband's homestead. Kofyar men are permitted the same privilege. And no one regards these extramarital relationships as adultery.

The *Oxford English Dictionary* defines adultery as sexual intercourse by a married person with someone other than the person's spouse. Today American psychologists have broadened this definition to include sexual infidelity (sexual exchanges with no romantic involvement), romantic infidelity (romantic exchanges with no sexual interaction), and sexual plus romantic involvement.[8]

## The Double Standard for Adultery

Those living in all preindustrial agricultural societies, where people used the plow (rather than the hoe) to grow crops such as the traditional Japanese, Chinese, Hindu, and preindustrial Europeans, would not have agreed. In these patriarchal societies, adultery was not a term regularly applied to men; it was considered largely a female vice.

The sexual double standard for adultery arose in farming cultures in tandem with the belief that the male was the bearer of the family "seed." It was his duty to reproduce and pass on his lineage. Throughout much of Asia, husbands were encouraged to have concubines.[9] In China, where a man could have only a single legal wife, concubines were often taken into the family compound and given private apartments, luxuries, and attention. Moreover, these women were treated with much more respect than is a mistress in the West today—largely because concubines served an important purpose, to bear sons. And because their children contained the blood of the patrilineage, all infants born out of wedlock in China were considered legitimate.

A traditional Chinese or Japanese man could be branded as adulterous only if he slept with the wife of another man. This was taboo. Illicit sex with a married woman was a violation against the woman's husband and his entire ancestry. In China these lawbreakers were burned to death. If a man seduced the wife of his guru in India, he might be made to sit on an iron plate that was glowing hot, then chop off his own penis. A Japanese man's only honorable course was suicide. In traditional Asian agricultural societies, only geishas, prostitutes, slaves, and concubines were fair game. Sex with them was not considered adultery.

A woman's sexual rights in traditional India, China, and Japan were an entirely different matter. A woman's worth was measured in two ways: her ability to increase her husband's property and prestige with the dowry she brought into the marriage, and her womb's capacity to nurture her husband's seed. Because a woman's responsibility in life was to produce descendants for her mate, she had to be chaste at marriage and sexually faithful to her husband all her life. Paternity had to be secure so as not to jeopardize her husband's family line. As a result, a respectable girl was often married off by age fourteen, before she succumbed to clandestine suitors. Then she was tethered to her husband's home under lifelong surveillance by his kin.

And extramarital sex was strictly forbidden to women. An unfaithful wife was not fit to live. A Hindu man could kill an adulterous spouse. In China and Japan a guilty woman was expected to kill herself instead. In these traditional patriarchal societies, a promiscuous wife threatened a man's land, his wealth, his name, his status. Both his ancestors and his descendants were at risk.

⁓

This same double standard for adultery was first recorded among the forebears of Western civilization in several law codes written in Semitic dialects between 1800 and 1100 B.C. in towns in ancient Mesopotamia.[10] Surviving portions deal with the legal position and rights and duties of women.

Like those of other agrarian communities, these early peoples of the Tigris–Euphrates valley felt that a woman had to "maintain her virtue." A wife who was adulterous could be executed or have her nose chopped off. Meanwhile, a husband had license to fornicate with prostitutes whenever he chose; philandering was a transgression only if he coupled with another man's wife or took the virginity of a peer's eligible daughter. Only for these crimes could he receive a stiff fine, castration, or death.

As in America today, however, more than one sexual code operated simultaneously. Some ancients engaged in fertility celebrations in which extramarital coitus was expected. For them sex had an aura of sanctity; the sex act brought fertility and power. But for the most part, stricter codes prevailed in the cradle of Western civilization. Only women, however, were expected to be faithful to a spouse. Among most historical agricultural Asian peoples, male adultery was essentially a trespass against another's property. Moreover, as in other ancient agrarian societies, adultery was not considered sinful, an offense against God.

This would change.

## "Thou Shalt Not Commit Adultery"

Adultery first became allied with sin in Western history, according to historian Vern Bullough, among the ancient Hebrews. Prior to the Babylonian exile, earliest Judaism had a simple code of sexual conduct; few sexual practices were equated with immorality. But in the post-exile period, from roughly 516 B.C. until the Romans destroyed Jerusalem in 70 A.D., Jewish sexual mores became increasingly identified with God. By Mosaic law a woman had to be a virgin on her wedding night, then remain permanently faithful to her husband's bed. But prostitutes, concubines, widows, and maidservants were permitted to men. Only intercourse with a married woman was banned.[11] God had spoken: "Thou shalt not commit adultery."

In the following Talmudic period, during the first few centuries of the Christian era, Hebrew attitudes toward sex became more explicit.

God, it was said, decreed that husband and wife engage in the marital act on the eve of the Sabbath. Lists were drawn up prescribing the minimal sexual obligations of different social classes. Gentlemen of leisure were to copulate with their wives nightly; laborers who resided in the same city where they worked should engage in intercourse two times a week; businessmen who traveled to other cities should indulge once a week; camel drivers were obliged to have marital sex every thirty days. And scholars should perform their marital duties on Friday night.[12] Sex within marriage became blessed, celebrated, holy.

"Awake, O north wind, and come, O south wind! Blow upon my garden, let its fragrance be wafted abroad. Let my beloved come to his garden, and eat its choicest fruits." This was but a part of the Song of Solomon, the extravagant and joyous ode to love between husband and wife that the Jews included in the Hebrew Bible in about 100 A.D. A wife's hair, her teeth, her lips, her cheeks, her neck, her breasts were all cause for celebration before the Lord.[13] The Jews likened the adoration between husband and wife to the love between the peoples of Israel and the Lord. But homosexuality, bestiality, transvestitism, masturbation, and adultery by a wife or by a man with another married woman were condemned by God.

This Hebraic attitude toward adultery would greatly influence Western mores, as would some curious customs of the ancient Greeks.

Often called the first people in history to devote themselves to play, the classical Greeks reveled in their games. As Greek gods indulged their concupiscence, so would Greek mortals. By the fifth century B.C. sexual frolic was among the favorite pastimes—for men. Greek men considered themselves superior to women. Well-bred girls were married off in their early teens to men twice their age, then treated more like wards than wives, cloistered in the house to bear sons. A husband's only heinous sexual misdeed was coitus with another man's wife, a transgression for which he could be put to death.

But these life-threatening liaisons seem not to have occurred with any frequency. Instead, most married gentlemen in classical Athens and Sparta amused themselves with a host of legitimate extramarital pursuits. Concubines looked after their daily needs. Educated courtesans, known as *hetaerae*, entertained them outside the home. And some men, particularly among the upper classes, partook regularly of homosexual rendezvous with teenage boys.

Early Christians would react violently to these appetites, but they would cherish other Greek ideals. Although the Greeks generally celebrated sex, some of them also harbored a deep misgiving that sex was contaminating, defiling, impure.[14] Heavenly celibacy. As early as 600 B.C. cultists had even begun to espouse asceticism and celibacy, concepts that would be adopted by fringe groups within the Hebraic tradition, then seep from generation to generation to influence early Christian leaders and eventually saturate the mores of Western men and women.[15]

Asceticism and celibacy remained alive—yet peripheral to daily life—in classical Rome. The ancient Romans were well known for their libertinism.[16] By 100 B.C. many Romans apparently regarded adultery the way some Americans feel about cheating on taxes—justified.

But the Romans also had their stoic side. Many liked to hark back to the good old days when Rome, they maintained, was a village of high moral integrity and everybody displayed *gravitas*, a sense of dignity and responsibility. An undercurrent of morality, continence, and abstinence was common in the Roman character.[17] And despite the sexual excesses of emperors and ordinary citizens—women as well as men—during Rome's glory days, some philosophers and teachers in these centuries continued to nurture and spread the little-known Greek philosophy of self-denial of all carnal pleasures.

⟳

This strain of Greco-Roman asceticism, commingled with the Hebrew concept that certain forms of sexual activity, including adultery, were sinful in the eyes of God, appealed to early Christian leaders.

Interpretations of Jesus's teachings on the subject of sexual conduct vary widely. Perhaps Jesus held sex within marriage in high esteem. But Mark 10:11 has Jesus speak as follows on adultery: "Whoever divorces his wife and marries another, commits adultery against her; and if she divorces her husband and marries another, she commits adultery." Even divorce and remarriage were now seen as licentious actions.

Then in the centuries after Jesus, some influential leaders of the Christian faith became more and more hostile to sex of any kind. Although some suggest that Paul may have been a sex-affirming Jew of the Hebraic tradition, he certainly had a fondness for celibacy too. As he wrote in 1 Corinthians 7:8–9, "To the unmarried and the widows I say that it is well for them to remain single as I do. But if they cannot exercise self-control, they should marry. For it is better to marry than to be aflame with passion."[18]

Sex begone. Celibacy was not officially imposed on all Christian clergy until the eleventh century. But as the generations passed in early Christendom, sexual abstinence was becoming increasingly allied with God, adultery with sin—for both men and women.

Saint Augustine, who lived from 354 to 430 A.D., would spread these teachings across the Christian world. As a young man, Augustine was eager to convert to Christianity, but he could not overcome his lust for his mistress and his devotion to their son. As he wrote in his *Confessions*, a classic book of Christian mysticism and the story of his conversion, he prayed regularly to God, saying, "Give me chastity and continency, but do not give it yet."[19]

At the behest of his strong-willed mother, Monica, Augustine eventually cast out his concubine in order to take a legal wife of the correct social standing. But this wedding never came to pass. During the two years he waited to marry, he took a temporary mistress. And this led him to a watershed. Suffering a stricken conscience, he abandoned his marriage plans, converted to Christianity, and adopted a life of continence instead. It was not much later that Augustine came to see coitus as vile, lust as shameful, all acts surrounding intercourse as unnatural.[20] Celibacy he called the highest good. Intercourse between husband and wife should be for procreation only. And adultery, by men as well as women, was the devil incarnate.

This attitude that adultery is a moral transgression *for both sexes* has dominated Western mores ever since.

## Unfaithfully Yours in America

This moral code has not deterred Western men and women—or people in any other society—from cheating on their mates, however. Americans are no exception. Despite our attitude that philandering is immoral, regardless of our sense of guilt when we engage in trysts, in spite of the risks to family, friends, and livelihood that adultery inevitably entails, we indulge in extramarital affairs with avid regularity. As George Burns once summed it up, "Happiness is having a large, loving, caring, close-knit family in another city."[21]

How many Americans are adulterous we will never know. In the 1920s psychiatrist Gilbert Hamilton, a pioneer in sex research, reported that 28 of 100 men and 24 of 100 women interviewed had strayed.[22] The famous Kinsey reports in the late forties and early fifties found that a little over a third of husbands in a sample of 6,427 men were unfaithful; and 26% of the 6,972 married, divorced, and widowed American women sampled had engaged in extramarital coitus by age forty.[23]

Decades later these figures had not changed significantly—despite enormous changes in American attitudes toward sex during the sixties and seventies, the pinnacle of the "sexual revolution." A survey by Morton Hunt in the seventies reported that 41% of the 691 men and about 25% of the 740 married white middle-class women had philandered.[24] Two new trends stood out, however: both sexes started their trysts earlier than in former decades; and the double standard was eroding. Whereas only 9% of the wives under age twenty-five in the 1950s had taken a paramour, about 25% of young wives in the 1970s had done so.

Adultery continued to start earlier in the 1980s. In a poll of 12,000 married individuals, about 25% of the men and women under age twenty-five had cheated on a spouse.[25]

Today there is little change in these statistics. The National Opinion Research Center in Chicago reports that some 25% of American men and 15% of American women philander at some point during marriage.[26] Other studies of American married couples indicate that 20–40% of heterosexual married men and 20–25% of heterosexual married women have had an extramarital affair during their lifetime.[27] Still others indicate that some 30–50% of American married men and women are adulterous.[28] And in a series of recent studies, 50% of the participating Americans said that they had tried to "poach" a member of another partnership; 80% had had someone try to seduce them away from their partnership, and 25% had lost a partner to someone who engaged in "mate poaching."[29]

⁂

"Who's been sleeping in my bed?" asks Papa Bear in one of America's folk tales. No one knows the extent of adulterous sex in the United States—either today or in yesteryear. After all, unlike Hawthorne's Hester Prynne, adulterers do not display their trysts by wearing the letter *A*. And sexual transgressions rarely reach the courts or census takers.

But of one thing I am sure: despite our cultural taboos against infidelity, Americans are adulterous. Societal mores, religious teachings, and friends and relatives urge us to invest all of our sexual and romantic energy on one person—a husband or a wife. But in practice a sizable percentage of both men and women actually spread their time, their vigor, and their love among multiple partners.

And we are hardly extraordinary.

I have read forty-two ethnographies describing different peoples past and present; adultery occurred in every one. Some of these men and women lived in tenements, others in row houses or thatched huts. Some raised rice; some raised money. Some were rich, some poor. Some espoused Christianity, Islam or Buddhism; others worshiped gods embodied in the sun, the wind, the rocks and trees. Regardless of their traditions of marriage, despite their customs of divorce, irrespective of any of their cultural mores about sex, all of these societies had some adulterers—even where adultery was punished by death. There exists no culture in which adultery is unknown; no cultural device or code that extinguishes philandering. Indeed, in one study of fifty-three societies (as in America), mate poaching—actively trying to seduce someone who is already in a partnership—occurred in nearly every one.[30]

"Friendship is constant in all other things, save the office and affairs of love," Shakespeare wrote. Like the stereotypic flirt, the smile, the brain physiology for romantic love, and our drive to form a pair-bond to rear our young, philandering seems to be part of our ancient reproductive game.

## Why Do Men and Women Philander?

"The chains of marriage are heavy and it takes two to carry them—sometimes three," Oscar Wilde once said. Public whipping, branding, beating, ostracism, mutilation of genitals, chopping off the nose and ears, slashing feet, chopping at one's hips and thighs, divorce, desertion, death by stoning, burning, drowning, choking, shooting, stabbing: cruelties are meted out to people around the world for philandering. Given these punishments, it is astonishing that humans engage in extramarital affairs at all. Yet we do.

When asked why they had an extramarital affair, adulterers regularly say, "for lust," "for love," or "I don't know." Some want to get caught in order to patch up a marriage. Others use their dalliance to improve their marriage by satisfying some of their needs outside the home. Still others use their escapade as an excuse to leave a spouse. Some seek attention. Some want autonomy. Some want to feel special, desired, more masculine or feminine, more attractive or better understood. Some want more communication, more intimacy, or just more sex. Some want to solve a sex problem. Others crave drama, excitement, or danger. A few seek revenge. Some men put their wives on a pedestal, but like to sleep with women from "the gutter." A few like a triangle, a tug-of-war. Others get high on secrecy. Some philanderers want to prove to themselves that they are still young, the "last-chance" affair. Some want to find the "perfect" love. Some are caught in an arranged marriage they did not choose. Some want the accessories that philandering can bring—including fancy food, lavish presents, and travel. And some just fall in love with someone new.

## Anatomy of Adultery

Psychologists can also rattle off a host of psychological, sociological and economic forces that contribute to infidelity.[31]

Foremost is the degree to which one is satisfied with one's primary relationship. When you believe your needs are not being fulfilled, feel no love or support from your partner, and regard your sex life as insufficient, you are more likely to stray. Boredom makes one susceptible to adultery. Poor communication with a spouse, including fewer positive and more negative interactions, leads to sexual betrayal.[32] One's perceived ability to live happily without one's partner also elevates one's risk of infidelity; while one's concern over losing valuable possessions, friends and connections reduces the tendency to philander.

The desire for self-expansion also plays a role. People are drawn to a partner who expands their interests, goals and self-worth.[33] This self-expansion starts as new lovers begin to spend time together, telling secrets, revealing hopes and dreams, and melding their partner's resources, perspectives, and identities with their own. But as one's self-expansion declines, one may become restless for new adventures of the mind or body, leading to adultery.

Men and women who were securely attached to their parents during childhood tend to build more stable partnerships and engage in less infidelity, whereas those who were insecurely attached to parental figures are more likely to philander.[34]

Individuals who are more open to new experiences tend to be more adulterous, as well as those who are less conscientious, less agreeable, and more neurotic.[35] Individuals whose spouses are less agreeable or conscientious are also more likely to be unfaithful.[36] And where partners are equally open, conscientious, agreeable, and neurotic, individuals are more likely to be faithful.[37] These correlations are found among peoples of North and South America, Western, Eastern and Southern Europe, the Middle East, Africa, Oceania, South Asia, and East Asia.[38]

An imbalance of social power has been associated with infidelity. Wives who report that they "get their way" more often during disagreements are more likely to have extramarital affairs. Men and women who regard themselves as more socially desirable than their spouses have more sexual peccadillos and cheat sooner after wedding. Alcoholics and those who are clinically depressed tend to have a higher incidence of infidelity. And some women and men are narcissistic; they need multiple lovers to show off their glitzy façade.

American women who are more educated than their husbands are more likely to be unfaithful. Individuals with a higher income also tend to have more affairs, while those who are financially dependent on their partner tend not to cheat. Individuals who work outside the home are more likely to seek sexual adventures. The likelihood of extramarital involvement is also greater among individuals whose jobs involve physically touching clients, discussing personal concerns with colleagues or clients, or working alone with a coworker.

The chronic illness of a spouse, the frigidity of the wife, or constant travel by one's mate also affect one's susceptibility to adultery.[39] A pregnancy and the months following the birth of a child are high-risk times for male infidelity as well. And despite what you might expect, religious beliefs do not stop one from philandering—and one's religious denomination plays no part in one's frequency of unfaithfulness.

Kinsey and his colleagues found that young blue-collar men indulged in a great deal of cheating, but decreased their sexual pursuits by their forties, whereas white-collar, college-educated men tended to philander less in their twenties, then increase their dalliances to almost once a week by age fifty. Women, on the other hand, reached the peak of their adultery in their mid-thirties and early forties. Today philandering is still particularly prevalent among married women aged forty to forty-five and married men aged fifty-five to sixty-five, while individuals outside of these age ranges are less likely to be unfaithful.

There are some gender differences too. Women tend to have a greater emotional connection with their extra lovers, and they seek more intimacy and self-esteem from their coquetries. Among women, the intensity and frequency of affairs are also often correlated with the degree of dissatisfaction they feel for their spouse. Among men, however, infidelity is less dependent on the state of their core relationship.

Of all the myriad data on promiscuity, perhaps the most revealing statistic was reported by Glass and Wright in 1985: *Among individuals engaging in infidelity, 56% of men and 34% of women rated their marriage as "happy" or "very happy."*

Why do men and women around the world engage in infidelity when they are *happy* with their primary partnership—and may jeopardize all they have, including their marriage, children, social standing, financial well-being, and health, when they cheat?

## Biology of Adultery

Data from genetics and neuroscience offer clues to some underlying biological mechanisms that most likely contribute to the worldwide frequency and persistence of adultery.

Please recall the prairie vole. These individuals form lifelong pair-bonds soon after puberty and raise several litters as a team. And this pairing has been directly correlated with neurochemical activities in the brain. When prairie voles first engage in sex, copulation triggers activity in oxytocin receptors (in the nucleus accumbens) among females and vasopressin receptors (in the ventral pallidum) among males. This stimulates dopamine release in several brain regions—producing feelings of wanting, seeking, focus, energy, pleasure, and motivation—driving these furry little creatures to prefer a particular mate, initiate a pair-bond, and express enduring attachment behaviors.[40]

But specific variations in a particular gene in the vasopressin system contribute to *variability* in the strength of a male prairie vole's pair-bond,[41] including the degree to which a male expresses sexual fidelity to his partner.[42]

A gene linked with adultery in prairie voles? What does this have to do with people? A lot. Humans have similar genes in the vasopressin system. And recently scientists investigated whether one of these genes affects pair-bonding behavior in 552 Swedish men.[43] All were either married or had been living with a partner for at least five years.

The results were remarkable. Men who inherited this gene scored significantly lower on the Partner Bonding Scale, a questionnaire that measures one's degree of attachment to a mate. Moreover, scores were dose-dependent. Men carrying two copies of this gene showed the lowest scores on the Partner Bonding Scale; those carrying one copy expressed more feelings of attachment; and men who had no copies of this gene were the most attached to their partner. Men carrying this vasopressin gene had also experienced more marital crises during the previous year, including threats of divorce. Once again, these results were dose-dependent. Last, the spouses of men with one or two copies of this gene scored significantly lower on questionnaires measuring marital satisfaction. This study did not measure infidelity directly, but it suggests one of the biological systems likely to contribute to cheating.

But other genes are most likely also involved. In a recent study of 181 young men and women, biologist Justin Garcia and his colleagues found a direct link between specific genes in the dopamine system and a greater frequency of uncommitted sexual intercourse, largely one-night stands, as well as a higher frequency of sexual infidelity.[44]

# The Sweaty T-Shirt Experiment

Another biological system may contribute to philandering. In the now classic "sweaty T-shirt" experiment, women sniffed the T-shirts of several anonymous men and selected the T-shirts of those they felt were the sexiest. Interestingly, they selected the T-shirts of men with genes that were different from their own in a specific region of the immune system, the major histocompatibility complex.[45] Perhaps these women were unconsciously attracted to men with different genes because similarity between partners in this part of the immune system can lead to complications of fertility and pregnancy.[46]

Tellingly, in a subsequent investigation, women married to men who shared *similar* genes in this part of the immune system were also more adulterous. And the more of these genes a woman shared with her spouse, the more extra partners she engaged.[47]

⌒

Brain architecture may also contribute to infidelity.

I have maintained that humankind has evolved three primary brain systems that guide mating and reproduction: the sex drive; romantic love; and the feelings of deep attachment.[48] These three basic neural systems interact with one another (and many other brain systems) in myriad flexible combinations to provide the range of motivations, emotions and behaviors necessary to orchestrate our complex human reproductive strategy.

However, these three brain systems are not always well connected. So it is biologically possible to express deep feelings of attachment for a primary partner *while* one feels intense romantic love for another individual, *while* one feels the sex drive for even more extra partners.[49] The relative biological independence of these three neural systems enable us to engage in social monogamy and clandestine infidelity *simultaneously*.[50] Our brain architecture easily accommodates infidelity.

Because philandering is so prevalent worldwide, because it is associated with a wide range of psychological, sociological, and economic factors, and because it is correlated with a growing number of biological systems, it is likely that our human predisposition toward infidelity evolved during our long prehistory.

# Why Adultery?

From a Darwinian perspective, it is easy to explain why men are—by nature—interested in sexual variety. If an ancestral man bore children with one woman, he had, genetically speaking, "reproduced" himself. But if he also engaged in dalliances with another woman and, by chance, sired another child, he doubled his contribution to the next generation.[51] So those men who sought sexual variety throughout deep history also tended to have more children. These young survived and passed to subsequent generations whatever it is in the male genetic makeup that seeks what poet Lord Byron called "fresh features."

But why would women have evolved a roving eye? A woman can't bear another child each time she sneaks into bed with an extra lover; she can get pregnant only at certain times of her menstrual cycle. Also, it takes a woman nine months to bear a child, and she will not conceive again for several months or years. Moreover, ancestral women most likely needed a partner to protect and provision them as they reared their helpless young (as I will maintain in subsequent chapters). So anthropologists have long reasoned that our female forebears were more inclined to be sexually faithful to a partner—passing to modern women the propensity for fidelity.

Man the natural playboy; woman the doting spouse? I suspect that evolution has bred women to be just as adulterous as men—albeit for different reasons. I can think of four.

The most obvious of these was elegantly put by Nisa, a !Kung woman who may still live in the Kalahari Desert in southern Africa. When anthropologist Marjorie Shostak met Nisa in 1970, Nisa was living in a hunting-gathering band with her fifth husband. Nisa had engaged a lot of extra lovers though. And when Shostak asked Nisa why she had taken on so many paramours, Nisa replied, "There are many kinds of work a woman has to do, and she should have lovers wherever she goes. If she goes somewhere to visit and is alone, then someone there will give her beads, someone else will give her meat, and someone else will give her other food. When she returns to her village, she will have been well taken care of."[52] Nisa summed up in a few sentences a fine adaptive explanation for female interest in sexual variety—supplementary subsistence, ultimately enabling her young to disproportionately survive.

Second, adultery probably served ancestral females as an insurance policy. If a "husband" died or deserted her, she had other males she might be able to enlist to help with parental chores.

Third, if an ancestral woman was "married" to a poor hunter with bad eyesight and an angry, unsupportive temperament, she might upgrade her genetic line by having healthier and more attractive offspring with another man—Mr. Good Genes.

Fourth, if an ancestral woman had offspring with an array of fathers, each child would be somewhat different. This genetic variability increased the likelihood that some from among her young would survive unpredictable fluctuations in the environment.

As long as prehistoric females were secretive about their extramarital affairs, they could garner extra resources, life insurance, better genes, and more varied DNA for their future lineage.[53] Hence those who engaged several lovers lived on—passing through the centuries whatever it is in the female brain that motivates contemporary women to philander.

## Evolution of Female *Clandestine* Adultery

Perhaps female secretive philandering began with more open sexuality.

Women are sexy: At orgasm, the blood vessels of a man's genitals eject the blood and other fluids back into the body cavity; the penis goes limp; and sex is over. Most men must start from the beginning to achieve orgasm again. For a woman, sex may have just begun. A woman's genitals have not expelled all the fluids. If she knows how, she can climax again soon, and again and again if she wants to. Sometimes orgasms occur in such rapid succession that one is indistinguishable from the next—continual orgasm.

This high female sexual capacity, in conjunction with data on other primates, led anthropologist Sarah Hrdy to a novel hypothesis about the primitive beginnings of human female philandering.[54] Hrdy pointed out that female apes and monkeys engage in a great deal of nonreproductive coitus. During estrus, for example, a female chimp will copulate with every male in the vicinity except her sons. This is not necessary to conceive a child. So Hrdy proposed that the female chimp's pursuit of sexual variety has two Darwinian purposes: to befriend males who may try to kill a female's coming newborn; and to confuse paternity so that each male in the community will act paternally toward her forthcoming child.

Hrdy then applied this reasoning to women, attributing the high female sexual capacity to an ancient evolutionary tactic to copulate with multiple partners, thereby obtaining supplementary paternal investment and insurance against infanticide from all of them.

Perhaps our first female ancestors living in the trees pursued sex with a variety of males to make and keep friends. Then, when our forebears were driven into the woodlands and spreading grass of Africa over four million years ago and pair-bonding evolved to raise the young, females turned from open promiscuity to clandestine copulations, reaping the benefits of extra resources and better or more varied genes from extra lovers.

For millions of years, adultery most likely had genetic payoffs for both sexes. And although the wife who climbs into bed with an acquaintance while on a business trip is certainly not thinking of her genetic future as she draws down the bedcovers, and the last thing a husband wants is to impregnate the coworker he seduces after the Christmas party, it is the millennia of sneaking off with extra lovers—and the genetic payoffs these dalliances accrued—that have produced the human predisposition for adultery seen around the world today.

## Which Sex Philanders More: Men or Women?

Decades of research have shown that men have more one-night stands, as well as more short or long-term affairs, leading many contemporary researchers to believe that men are more adulterous than women.[55]

But who are all these men are sleeping with?

Many in the world would not even agree with the largely Western view that men are all Don Juans, whereas women are the shy, retiring recipients of sex. Certainly most living in the Middle East would not. The custom of the veil evolved in Muslim societies partly because Islamic people believed that women are highly seductive. Clitoridectomy, the excising of the clitoris (and often much of the surrounding genital tissue), is traditionally done in several African cultures, in part to curb the high female libido. Talmudic writers in the early Christian era stipulated that it was a husband's duty to copulate with his wife regularly, largely because they thought women had a higher sex drive than men. The traditional Cayapa Indians of western Ecuador thought women were lechers. And traditionally, the Spanish men who strutted, preened, and philandered in the small towns of Andalusia were convinced that women were dangerous, potent, and promiscuous.

In fact, had you asked Clellan Ford and Frank Beach, sex researchers of the 1950s, which sex was more interested in sexual variety, they would have replied, "In those societies which have no double standard in sexual matters and in which a variety of liaisons are permitted, the women avail themselves as eagerly of their opportunity as do the men."[56]

## The Oldest Profession

In fact, women have long embarked on more than one sexual career, engaging either in clandestine adultery or open promiscuity. Among the Mehinaku of Amazonia, the most sexually active person in the jungle village was a woman who received fish, meat, or trinkets in payment for her trysts with a variety of partners.[57] Some traditional Navajo women chose not to marry; instead, they lived alone and entertained a variety of male visitors for a fee.[58] Women in many other American Indian tribes traditionally accompanied men on their hunting expeditions, returning home with meat in exchange for satisfying the sexual needs of *several* of these hunters.[59] An unmarried Canela girl of central Brazil who wished to earn food or services selected a would-be lover and asked her brother to arrange a date. Many of these trysts became long-term business relationships.[60] Madams flourished among the traditional Sierra Tarascans of Mexico. These older women had a string of girls they could summon at a moment's notice.[61] Nupe women of sub-Saharan Africa came to the marketplace at night dressed in their finery and jewels; here they sold kola nuts, but buyers could also purchase the woman for the night.[62]

There is no question that desperately poor women in many countries engage in prostitution purely for the money. But many of the middle-class "sex workers" I have interviewed in New York said they also liked the freedom and sexual variety.

And women who pursue this vocation are not alone. The animal kingdom is rife with loose females. Female chimpanzees, other mammals, and many female birds, bugs, and reptiles solicit males and copulate in return for food. Among Australian bush crickets and other insects, the male's offering is called the "nuptial gift." Prostitution deserves its venerable title, "the oldest profession in the world."

All these data lead one to suspect that some women avail themselves of "extra" lovers with relish, perhaps as avidly as men. Indeed, along with the decline of the sexual double standard today, male and female rates of infidelity are becoming increasingly similar among people under age forty in developed countries.[63]

## A Modest Proposal

"Thou shalt commit adultery." Because of a printer's error in the 1805 edition of the Bible, this commandment suddenly dictated philandering. It soon became known as the wicked Bible.[64] But the human animal seems cursed with a contradiction of the spirit. We search for true love, find him or her, and settle in. Then, if the spell begins to fade, the mind begins to wander. And there is little evidence that women shun clandestine (and sometimes open) sexual adventures. Instead, both men and women seem to exhibit a *mixed* reproductive strategy. Monogamy *and* adultery are our fare. Oscar Wilde summed up this plight, saying "There are two great tragedies in life, losing the one you love and winning the one you love."

Alas, winning often leads to another part of our human reproductive strategy, our tendency to divorce.

# Blueprint for Divorce

## The Three- to Four-Year Itch

She was a worthy womman al hir lyve,
Housbondes at chirche dore she hadde fyve.

—GEOFFREY CHAUCER, "THE WIFE OF BATH'S TALE"

"Oh eyes be strong, you cherish people and then they're gone." Safia, a middle-aged Bedouin woman of Egypt's Western Desert, held back her tears as she recited this sad poem to anthropologist Lila Abu-Lughod.[1] A year earlier her spouse of almost twenty years had come to her while she was baking and said, "You're divorced." At the time Safia had acted aloof, nonchalant. She still feigned indifference, saying to the anthropologist, "I didn't care when he divorced me. I never liked him." But Safia was concealing her despair. Only in a little poem could she reveal her vulnerability, longing, and attachment.

Although their songs and stories express passion between women and men, traditionally the Bedouins believed that romantic love was shameful. Individuals in their society were supposed to marry according to their family's bidding. One should feel deep love only for parents, brothers, sisters, and children—not necessarily for a spouse. So the Bedouins were horrified by public displays of affection between husband and wife. And although they believed spouses could fall deeply in love, honorable people maintained *hasham*—sexual modesty and propriety. Unveiled passions appeared only in short verse.[2]

Today these nomads have settled down to herd sheep, tend fig and olive groves, smuggle, or pursue other business ventures. But they carry with them an ancient love of love.

Before the railroad, before the Toyota truck, their ancestors traversed the deserts of North Africa, moving caravans of dates and other goods from oases in the sand to markets in the Nile valley. With them they brought their Arabian tribal mores—a love for independence, honor, courage, gallantry, and hospitality, a penchant for vendettas, and, above all, a taste for women, wine, and song.[3] Safia's short poem, like all Bedouin verse on the exhilaration of romance and the despair of love, was a remembrance of desert song masters long deceased.

"I divorce thee; I divorce thee; I divorce thee." These words, too, come from pre-Islamic times. In those days women were honored and respected. They were also prized goods. Girls were wards of the family; after marriage, women became the property of a spouse and could be dismissed if unsatisfactory. As al-Ghazali, the outstanding eleventh-century intellectual and author, described divorce in ancient Arabian society, it was easy to obtain.[4] One merely had to pronounce a statement of divorce three times.

In the sixth century A.D. the Prophet Muhammad built on this tribal custom. Unlike early Christian fathers who venerated celibacy, Muhammad believed that coitus was one of the great joys of life and that marriage guarded men and women from the irreligious world of promiscuity. So he insisted that his followers wed. As he declared, "I fast and I eat, I keep vigil and I sleep, and I am married. And whoever is not willing to follow my Sunna [tradition] does not belong to me."[5] There would be no celibacy in Islam.

To this day Muhammad's influence has produced what scientists call a sex-positive Islamic culture, a society that venerates man/woman love, sex, and marriage. Western society, on the other hand, is sometimes called sex-negative, because our historical religious precepts extolled the virtues of celibacy and monasticism.

Muhammad sealed other traditions. Although he saw women as subordinate to men, a belief inherited from pre-Islamic peoples, he introduced a host of social, moral, and legal codes to protect women, as well as a list of explicit rights and duties of each spouse. Among these guidelines: a man should have no more than four wives, and he must circulate among them on consecutive nights. Above all, a husband must provide for each without favoritism.

A wife had responsibilities too, particularly to bear and raise children, to cook, and to obey her husband. In Islam, marriage rested on a legal contract. And unlike Christian matrimony, which became a sacrament and hence indissoluble, the Muslim wedding pledge could be broken. The Prophet's bidding was from God.

Today these traditional divorce procedures still exist in much of the Islamic world, although in some places divorce has become harder to obtain. The most acceptable means of divorce is still Talaqus-Sunna, in conformity with the dictates of the Prophet. This form of *talaq*, or divorce, can be done in either of two slightly varied, approved ways. One of them, *talaq ahsan*, consists of a single pronouncement, "I divorce thee; I divorce thee; I divorce thee," made while the wife is not menstruating, along with sexual abstinence for three months. The divorce is revoked if the husband withdraws his words or if the couple resume intercourse during this three-month waiting period.

Islamic law gives a host of other stipulations about divorce—when it is appropriate for a wife to leave a husband and how either spouse can negotiate their separation with grace—for Muhammad savored harmony between men and women, be they together or apart. As the Koran enjoined, "Then, when they have reached their term, take them back in kindness or part from them in kindness." [6]

Still, Safia felt sorrow when her husband went away.

## Parting

We all have our share of troubles. But probably one of the hardest things we do is leave a spouse. Is there any way to do this well?

I doubt it. But people have devised many formal ways to end a marriage. In some societies special courts or councils negotiate divorces. Sometimes the village headman hears divorce cases. Most often divorce is considered a private matter to be handled by the parties and their families.[7] This can be as easy as moving a hammock from one fireplace to the next, or it can disrupt an entire community—as occurred in India.

The *New York Times* reported the divorce case of a young Hindu girl, Ganga, who fled her husband of five years after he beat her severely.[8] The next day over five hundred people met in a field near the village to hear the couple and their kin answer questions posed by respected elders of their caste. But when Ganga accused her husband's father and uncle of trying to assault her sexually, an argument erupted. Insults soon led to combat with long sticks, and in no time several men lay in the field, clubbed and bleeding. The ruckus stopped only when word spread that the police were coming. Divorce proceedings no doubt continued with bitter words behind mud walls.

Whether done in anger or dispassion, with full state regalia, or with a minimum of fuss, divorce is indisputably a part of the human condition. Almost everywhere in the world people permit divorce. The ancient Incas did not. The Roman Catholic Church does not allow remarriage after a divorce. And in some cultures divorces are difficult to obtain.[9]

But from the tundra of Siberia to the jungles of Amazonia, people accept divorce as regrettable, though sometimes necessary. They have specific social or legal procedures for divorce. And they do divorce. Moreover, unlike many Westerners, traditional peoples do not make divorce a moral issue. The Mongols of Siberia sum up a common worldwide attitude: "If two individuals cannot get along harmoniously together, they had better live apart."[10]

I am often asked, "Which sex more often leaves the other?"

We will never know. Laws and customs often dictate which spouse begins divorce proceedings. But which individual actually initiates the emotional, physical, and legal separation is not measurable. After all the arguing and tears are over, sometimes even the parties involved are not sure who left whom.

## Why Do People Divorce?

Bitter quarrels, insensitive remarks, lack of humor, watching too much television, inability to listen, drunkenness, sexual rejection—the reasons men or women give for why they leave a marriage are as varied as their motives for having wedded in the first place. But there are some common circumstances under which people around the globe choose to abandon a relationship.

Overt adultery heads the list. In a study of 160 societies, anthropologist Laura Betzig established that blatant philandering, particularly by the wife, is the most commonly offered rationale for seeking to dissolve a marriage. Sterility and barrenness come next. Cruelty, particularly by the husband, ranks third among worldwide reasons for divorce. Then come an array of charges about a spouse's personality and conduct. Bad temper, jealousy, talkativeness, nagging, disrespect, laziness by the wife, nonsupport by the husband, sexual neglect, quarrelsomeness, absence, and running off with a lover are among the many explanations.[11]

I am not surprised that adultery and infertility are paramount. Darwin theorized that people marry primarily to breed. Unquestionably, many people wed to gain an economically valuable spouse or to accumulate children to support them as they age; still others marry to cement ties with relatives, friends, or enemies; and today many marry to seal a love relationship. But as Betzig has proven, Darwin was correct: the main reasons given for divorce are closely linked to sex and reproduction.[12]

It should also follow that most divorced persons of reproductive age remarry or form a new pair-bond with someone else.[13] Indeed, the majority still do.

Today many men and women opt to live together or make some other kind of formal partnership rather than remarrying after a divorce. However, Rose Kreider of the U.S. Census Bureau reports that "most people remarry following a divorce from a first marriage."[14] A host of studies indicate that divorce and remarriage are also common cross-culturally.

Despite dashed dreams, with full memory of the vicious quarrels, regardless of the inevitable realization that marriage or a live-in relationship can be irritating, dull, and painful, the majority of people who divorce fall in love again and either remarry or build a new life with a new partner. We seem to have an eternal optimism about our next sweetheart.

Samuel Johnson defined remarriage as the triumph of hope over experience. Americans joke about the "seven-year itch." Anthropologists call this human habit "serial monogamy." Call it what you will, the human penchant to divorce and form a new bond with another is worldwide. And it displays several striking patterns.

## Money Talks

First of all, divorce *rates* are high in societies where women and men *both* own land, animals, currency, information, and/or other valued goods or resources, and where *both* partners have the right to distribute or exchange their personal riches beyond the immediate family circle. If you own a bank in New York City, if you possess the rights to the only local water hole in the Australian outback, or if you take your grain to market in Nigeria and come home with wealth that you can keep, invest, sell, barter, or give away, you are rich.

*Where men and women are not dependent on each other to survive economically, bad marriages can end*—and often do.

A vivid example of the power of economic autonomy is seen among the !Kung Bushmen of the Kalahari Desert. Here, men and women often marry more than once.[15] And it is no coincidence, I think, that !Kung women are economically and socially powerful.

Although the !Kung are rapidly adopting Western values and twenty-first-century technology, their high divorce rate is not a new development. When anthropologists recorded their lifeways in the 1960s, these people lived in small groups of some ten to thirty individuals during the rainy season. Then, as the weather turned and the blistering October sun sucked up the surface water, they assembled in larger communities around permanent water holes. But even when the !Kung were scattered across the bush, men and women traveled regularly between communities, connecting a fluid network of several hundred kin.

!Kung women commuted to work. Not every morning—but every two to three days, when staples waned, a wife went collecting. Carrying her nursing infant in her shawl and leaving her older youngsters in the "day care" of friends and relatives, she joined a group of women and marched off through the chaparral.

Each foraging expedition was novel. Sometimes a woman returned with baobab fruit, wild onions, tsama melons, and sweet mongongo nuts. On other days she gathered sour plums, tsin beans, leafy greens, and water roots. Honey, caterpillars, tortoises, and birds' eggs were groceries too. And regularly a woman returned with valuable information as well. From the animal tracks she discovered as she walked, she could tell which beasts had passed by, when, how many were in the herd, and where the group was headed.

!Kung men went hunting two to three days a week, in quest of a dove or sand grouse, a springhare, a porcupine, an antelope, even a giraffe. Sometimes a husband came home with just enough meat to feed his wife and children; sometimes a group of men felled a beast large enough to divide with hunting companions, relatives, and friends. Meat was a delicacy. And good hunters were honored. But men brought home meat only one day in four.

Consequently women provided at least 50% of dinner (if not a lot more) almost every night. Women also shared the rights to water sites in the desert—a situation not unlike owning the local bank. During their reproductive years women held high status as childbearers. Older women often became shamans and leaders in community affairs as well.

So !Kung women were powerful.

And when a husband and wife found themselves in a desperate marriage, either one or the other generally packed up a few belongings and departed for another camp.

Why? Because they could. !Kung spouses often argued for months before breaking up. Cruel words and bitter tears spilled onto the desert sand. Neighbors invariably got involved. But eventually most unhappy relationships ended. Of the 331 marriages !Kung women reported to sociologist Nancy Howell in the 1970s, 134 ended in divorce.[16] Then men and women wed again. Some !Kung women had as many as five consecutive spouses. Wealth spells power.

~

This correlation between economic independence and divorce rate is seen in a host of cultures.[17] Among the Yoruba of West Africa, for example, women traditionally controlled the complex marketing system. They grew the crops, then took their produce to a weekly market—a market run entirely by women. As a result Yoruba women brought home not only staples but also money and luxuries, independent wealth. Up to 46% of all Yoruba marriages ended in divorce.[18]

The Hadza live on the grasslands around Olduvai Gorge, Tanzania. Although the gorge area is dry and rocky, it abounds with roots, berries, and small game, and during the rainy season spouses regularly leave camp separately in the morning to forage. Then in the dry season, bands assemble around permanent water holes, men hunt large game, and all dance, gamble, gossip, and share the meat. But Hadza men and women are not dependent on one another to provide the evening meal. And their marriages reflect this independent spirit. In the 1960s their divorce rate was roughly five times higher than that in the United States.[19]

Personal economic autonomy spells freedom to depart. And, for me, the most vivid illustration of this correlation are the Navajo of the American Southwest—undoubtedly because I lived with them for several months in 1968.

To get there, I took the old Route 66 west out of Gallup, New Mexico, drove some forty-five minutes, swung north on a broad dirt road through the chaparral and sage, kept going past the Pine Springs trading post and on beyond an abandoned hogan (a seven-sided log house) and the big pine tree, then up the hill of wildflowers. There was our wooden house—with a potbellied stove for heat, a gas range for cooking fry bread, coffee, and mutton soup, two big brass beds, a beat-up kitchen table, and three kerosene lamps we used to sit around at night and talk. A usually jolly little home, with a front door looking east, two big tanks of precious water nestled in a nearby grove of pines, and an orange canyon ribboning through our vast front yard.

My Navajo "mother" orchestrated daily life. She collected Indian paintbrush and other wildflowers, carded and dyed wool, and wove Navajo blankets to support a family of five. She also owned the land around her. The Navajo are matrilineal; children trace their descent through their mother's lineage, so women owned a great deal of property. Women were also medical diagnosticians who played a vital role in Navajo ritual life. They analyzed the sick, identified physical illnesses, and prescribed the appropriate Navajo curing. So women enjoyed a lot of prestige; they participated in all community affairs. And about one out of three divorced.[20]

"One shouldn't marry only to be unhappy the remainder of one's days," the Micmac of eastern Canada say.[21] Much of the world agrees. Where women and men *can* leave each other, unhappy people often do. Then traditionally they wed again.

Divorce rates are much lower where spouses are dependent on each other to make ends meet.

The most notable correlation between economic dependence and a low divorce rate is seen in preindustrial Europe and in all other societies that still use the plow for agriculture, such as parts of India and China.[22] Some people trace this low divorce rate among historical Christian Europeans to religious causes—for understandable reasons. Jesus forbade divorce.[23] And as I have mentioned, by the eleventh century A.D. Christian marriage had become a sacrament; divorce was impossible for most Christians.

But culture often complements nature's laws, and the low divorce rates seen in preindustrial European societies were also due to an inescapable ecological reality: farming couples needed each other to survive.[24] A woman living on a farm depended on her husband to move the rocks, fell the trees, and plow the land. Her husband needed her to sow, weed, pick, prepare, and store the vegetables. Together they worked the land.

More important, whoever elected to leave the marriage left empty-handed. Neither spouse could dig up half the wheat and relocate. Farming women and men were tied to the soil, to each other, and to an elaborate network of stationary kin. Under these ecological circumstances, divorce was not practical.

No wonder divorce was rare throughout preindustrial Europe, across the breadbasket of the Caucasus, and among many agrarian peoples stretching to the Pacific Rim.

## Working Women

The Industrial Revolution changed this economic relationship between men and women and divorce rates increased (see chapter 16).

The United States is a good example. When factories appeared beyond the barns of agricultural America, women and men began to leave the farm for work, and what did they bring home but money—movable, divisible property. During much of the 1800s most women still ran the house. But in the early decades of the twentieth century American middle-class women began to join the labor force in greater numbers, giving them economic autonomy.

Not coincidentally, the American divorce rate, which started to rise with the advent of the Industrial Revolution, continued its slow but steady climb. For an unhappy husband will leave a wife who brings home a paycheck long before he will desert the woman who weeds his garden and milks his cows. And a woman with a salary is often less tolerant of marital despair than one dependent on her spouse to provide the evening meal.

Today nearly half of all marriages in the U.S. end in divorce.[25] And many observers have identified women's employment outside the home—and their control over their own money—as a prime factor in this rising frequency of divorce.[26]

A rise in the divorce rate in tandem with female economic autonomy has been seen before in Western history. When the Romans won several foreign wars in the centuries preceding Christ, trade monopolies brought unprecedented wealth to Rome. An urban upper class emerged. Rich Roman patricians were now less eager to let massive dowries pass into the hands of sons-in-law. So with a series of new marriage regulations in the first century B.C., upper-class women came to control more of their fortunes—and their futures. And as a class of increasingly financially independent women rose in ancient Rome, divorce became epidemic.[27]

## Ties That Bind

"All you need is love," the Beatles sang. Not so. Many other cultural factors besides economic autonomy contribute to the stability or instability of a marriage.

For example, in the past divorce rates were higher in the United States among partners who came from different socioeconomic, ethnic, and religious backgrounds.[28] This is changing, though.

In a study of 459 women in Detroit, sociologist Martin Whyte discovered that these factors had little effect on the fate of a relationship. Instead, similar personality traits, shared habits, parallel interests, common values, joint leisure activities, and mutual friends were the best predictors of marital stability. Interestingly, Whyte also concluded, "It helps if you marry at a mature age, if you are very much in love, if you are white and come from a close and loving home."[29] People without these attributes are at greater risk.

Psychologists report that inflexible people make unstable marriages. Therapists say that where the ties holding a couple together outweigh the forces pulling them apart, individuals tend to stay together. How spouses adjust to one another, how they bargain, how they fight, and how they listen and persuade make a difference too. Where there is little compromise, marriages are more likely to dissolve. Demographers have shown that when there is an excess of men or a dearth of women, wives become scarce commodities and people are less likely to separate.[30] And couples that marry very young tend to divorce.[31]

Anthropologists have added a cross-cultural perspective to our understanding of divorce.[32] Divorce is common in matrilineal cultures like that of the Navajo, probably because a wife has resources, her children are members of her clan, and her husband has more responsibilities for his sister's offspring than for his own. Hence spouses are companions, not vital economic partners.

Where a husband must pay a "bride price" to the family of his intended for the privilege of marrying her, divorce rates are often lower because at divorce these goods must be returned. Endogamy, marrying within one's own community, is associated with longer-lasting relationships because common relatives, friends, and obligations tend to bind the pair into a common network.[33]

Polygyny has a curious effect on divorce. When a man has several wives, the women tend to fight for the attention and resources of their single husband. Jealousies lead to showdowns and divorce. More important, a man with several women can spare the services of one, while a man with a single wife will think hard before he deserts the only woman who cooks for him. As a matter of fact, divorce rates have *declined* in Muslim societies since contact with Western mores;[34] our tradition of monogamy is affecting Islamic family life.

～

"There is no society in the world where people have stayed married without enormous community pressure to do so," anthropologist Margaret Mead once said.[35] She was right. Divorce rates are just as high in many traditional societies as in the United States.[36]

This seems curious. After all the smiles and gazes, the dizzying sensations of adoration, the shared secrets and private jokes, the lovely times in bed, the days and nights with family and friends, the children they have borne, the property they have collected, the colorful experiences they have amassed through all the hours, months, and years they laughed and loved and struggled as a team, why do men and women leave rich relationships behind?

Perhaps this restlessness is driven by currents buried in our human psyche, profound reproductive forces that evolved across eons of daily mating throughout our shadowed past.

## The Divorce Itch

Hoping to get some insight into the nature of divorce, I turned to the Demographic Yearbooks of the United Nations. These volumes were begun in 1947 when census-takers in countries as culturally diverse as Finland, Russia, Egypt, South Africa, Brunei, Venezuela, and the United States started to ask their inhabitants about divorce.

From these data, collected largely every decade up to 2012 by the Statistical Office of the United Nations on dozens of societies, I culled the answers to three questions: How many years were you married when you divorced? How old were you when you divorced? How many children did you have at the time of your divorce?

Three remarkable patterns emerged.

And they ring of evolutionary forces.

Most striking, divorce generally occurs early in marriage—peaking between three and four years after wedding—followed by a gradual decline in divorce as more years of marriage go by.[37]

When I put these divorce peaks (modes to statisticians) for all years available between 1947 and 1989 (188 cases in sixty-two societies) on a master chart for the first edition of this book, it became evident that there was no seven-year itch: a three- to four-year itch emerged instead. For this revised edition, I analyzed the most recent data on divorce collected by the United Nations in over eighty societies between 2003 and 2011. This broad pattern remained the same.[38] (See appendix C.)

This three- to four-year divorce peak has not substantially altered over the past six decades, despite massive societal changes. Indeed, even Shakespeare left his wife, Anne, in Stratford, to pursue his career in London some three to four years after wedding.[39]

There certainly are variations from this three- to four-year divorce peak, however. In Egypt and other Muslim countries, for example, divorces occurred most frequently during the first few months of marriage—nowhere near the three- to four-year mark. And this basic Muslim pattern remained the same even in the most recent data collected between 2003 and 2011.[40]

These variations are not surprising, though. In many Muslim cultures the groom's family is expected to return their new daughter-in-law to her parents if she is not fitting into her new home—something in-laws do rapidly when they do it. Moreover, the Koran exempts a Muslim husband from paying half of the wedding fee if he dissolves the union before consummating it.[41] Thus social pressure and economic incentive both spur unhappily married Egyptians and other Muslim men and women to divorce fast. Last, these United Nations data include "revocable divorces," provisional decrees that require few financial reparations. Revocable divorces make the process of separation quick and easy and the duration of marriage short.[42]

In the past few decades, the American divorce peak has hovered somewhat below the common three- to four-year peak, and it is interesting to speculate on this variation too. In some years, such as 1977, divorces peaked around the fourth year of marriage.[43] But other years divorces peaked earlier—between the second and third year after wedding.[44] Why?

This American divorce peak has nothing to do with the rising divorce *rate* in the United States. The divorce rate doubled between 1960 and 1980, yet couples divorced in or around the second year of marriage throughout this time.

American fast divorce cannot be explained by the growing number of couples who live together either. The numbers of men and women who took up residence together without marrying almost tripled in the 1970s—but the number of years that individuals remained together did not budge.[45]

Perhaps this early divorce peak occurs because many young Americans are dedicated to the concept of partnering with a soul mate—someone in perfect harmony with themselves. So if partners are not satisfied with the match, they bail out soon after the infatuation high wears off.

These United Nations data have other problems—due to the fact that people vary dramatically regarding when they wed and when they untie the knot.[46]

In some societies, partners court for months; in others they marry quickly. The time involved in preparing for the wedding, the months or years a person will endure an awful marriage, the ease or difficulty of obtaining a divorce, and the length of time needed to get the divorce decree also vary from one person and one culture to the next.

In actuality, then, human relationships begin before they are legally recorded and founder before they become legally defunct.

There is no way to measure all the variables that skew these data collected by the United Nations. *But here is a focal point of this book*: given the vast number of cultural factors and individual variations involved in marriage and divorce, one would expect even fairly significant divorce patterns to disappear. In short, it is remarkable that *any* pattern appears at all.

Yet, despite the varying traditions for marrying, the myriad worldwide opinions about divorce, and the diverse procedures for parting, men and women desert each other in a roughly common pattern.

Some of these people are bankers; others garden, herd cattle, fish, or trade to make a living. Some have a college education; some neither read or write. Among these millions of men and women from over eighty different cultures, individuals speak different languages, ply different trades, wear different clothes, carry different currencies, whisper different prayers, fear different devils, and harbor different hopes and different dreams. Nevertheless, their divorces regularly cluster around a three- to four-year mark.

And this cross-cultural divorce pattern is unrelated to the divorce rate. It occurs in societies where the divorce rate is high and in cultures where divorce is rare.

⮎

"Curiouser and curiouser," as Lewis Carroll wrote in *Alice in Wonderland*. Marriage has a cross-cultural pattern of decay.

This pattern of human bonding is even embedded in Western mythology. During the twelfth century traveling European minstrels called together lords and ladies, knights and commoners, to hear the fatal epic saga of Tristan and Iseult—the first modern Western romance. "My lords," a bard began, "if you would hear a high tale of love and of death, here is that of Tristan and Queen Iseult; how to their full joy, but to their sorrow also, they loved each other, and how at last, they died of that love together upon one day; she by him and he by her." [47]

As the French writer Denis de Rougemont has said of this tale, it is "a kind of archetype of our most complex feelings of unrest." His observation is more astute than he may have known. The story begins when a young knight and a beautiful queen share an elixir known to induce love for *about three years*.

Are we predisposed to break up after a few years of love and bonding?

Perhaps this divorce itch after three to four years of wedding is a human blueprint, a primordial design.

There are other patterns to human divorce.

## Divorce Is for the Young

Between 1946 and 1964 some 76 million Americans were born. Hail the baby boom, a mass production following World War II. Today these people range from age fifty-one to sixty-nine. And because they see divorce among their peers, they assume that marital dissolution is most prevalent in middle age.

It is not. American divorces occur among the young far more often than among middle aged or older people.[48] Today, 10% of American women have had three or more husbands by age forty.[49] Moreover, 80% of women who divorced before age twenty-five remarried before turning thirty-five; and 44% of women and 55% of men who divorced after age twenty-five remarried before age forty. Equally interesting, after their breeding years were over, only one in three of today's Americans divorced.[50]

In sixty-eight societies for which age-at-divorce data are available in the United Nations yearbooks, divorce is also for the young. Divorces peak between ages 25–29 for women and 30–34 for men. Divorce then becomes less and less frequent as people age.

This seems strange. Why wouldn't partners become bored or sated with each other as they get older, or after their children have left home for work or college? They don't. Instead, men and women divorce with impressive regularity when they are in their late twenties and early thirties—*during the height of their reproductive and parenting years*.

## Divorcing with Young Children

A third pattern to emerge from the United Nations data regards "divorce with dependent children."[51] Among the millions of people recorded in sixty-seven societies between 1998 and 2007, 43% of all divorces occurred among couples with no dependent children; 29% among those with one dependent child; 18% among couples with two children; and 5% among those with three children. Couples with four or more young rarely split. Hence, the more children a couple bear, the less likely they are to divorce.

I can understand, from a Darwinian perspective, why couples with no children break up: both individuals will mate again and probably go on to bear young—ensuring their genetic futures. Moreover, I can understand why couples with three or more children remain married: it's genetically logical to remain together to raise their flock. Besides, perhaps they have a lot of children because they are happily wed and dedicated to their family life.

But why do over one-quarter of all divorces involve one dependent child; and almost 20% occur among couples with two offspring? This is remarkable: a lot of men and women apparently abandon a mateship after having one or two children to find new love and bond again.

Americans fit this global pattern almost perfectly. Rose Kreider of the U.S. Census Bureau reported in 2006 that the median duration of remarriage following divorce from a first marriage is about three to four years, and has remained "consistent over time" since 1950. Further, approximately 60% of men and women who remarried were aged 25–44. And 50% of the women and 47% of the men had already had one or two children when they wed again.[52]

## Blueprint for Divorce

In short, marriage shows several general patterns of decay. Divorce rates peak among couples married three to four years. Divorce risk is greatest among spouses in their late twenties and early thirties—the height of their reproductive years. A great many divorces occur among partners with one or two children. Divorced men and women find new partners while they are still young—often in another three to four years.[53] Then they remarry or make some other kind of live-in stable partnership, and often have more young. In fact, today 28% of U.S. mothers with two or more offspring have produced children by more than one man.[54]

Serial monogamy—and bearing young with more than one partner—is also common in cultures where the United Nations has not gathered data.

Along the headwaters of the Amazon, on coral atolls in the Pacific, in the Arctic tundra, in the Australian outback, and in other remote parts of the world, men and women leave each other too. Yet few scientists or census-takers have asked these out-of-the-way peoples how long their marriages lasted, how old they were when they divorced, or how many children were involved. But the scant data show much of the same patterns.

Among the traditional jungle-living Yanomamo of Venezuela, nearly 100% of all infants live with their natural mother; the majority also have their natural father living with them. But the co-residence of the biological parents declines sharply after the child reaches the age of five—not just because a parent dies but because spouses divorce.[55]

Among the Fort Jameson Ngoni of southern Africa divorces peak between the fourth and fifth year of marriage too.[56]

People around the world will tell you that a marriage strengthens when a child is born.[57] For example, in traditional rural Japan a marriage was often not even noted by village record-keepers until a child was produced.[58] Andaman Islanders did not consider a marriage fully consummated until spouses become parents.[59] And the Tiv of Nigeria called a union a "trial marriage" until an infant cemented the pair.[60]

But the birth of a child does not necessarily produce *lifelong* marriage.[61] I suspect the Aweikoma of eastern Brazil best illustrate trends in traditional societies. Here typically "a couple with several children stays together til death. . . . But separations before many children are born are legion."[62] This is exactly the pattern seen in the United Nations data.

There are exceptions, of course. Among the Kanuri Muslims of Nigeria divorce peaks prior to the first full year of marriage. Anthropologist Ronald Cohen thinks this early divorce peak occurs because "young girls tend not to stay with first husbands whom they are forced to marry by parents."[63] Interestingly, the !Kung Bushmen also divorce within months of wedding, and they also have arranged first marriages.[64]

Even this is consistent with the United Nations sample, although it is the exception, not the rule. As you recall, Egypt and other Muslim countries all exhibit a divorce peak before the first full year of marriage. And these countries have high incidences of arranged first marriages. An arranged marriage appears to provoke one to bail out fast.

All sorts of cultural mores skew patterns of human bonding. The economic autonomy of women, urbanism, secularism, and arranged marriages make up but a fraction. Despite these influences, human mating has some general patterns: Women and men from western Siberia to the southern tip of South America marry. Many leave each other. Many depart between the third and fourth year after wedding. Many leave at the height of their reproductive years. Many divorce with a single child. And many find a new partner, fall in love again, and have more young—all during their reproductive years.

Planned obsolescence of the pair-bond? Perhaps.

We are not puppets on a string of DNA. We have evolved a huge cerebral cortex with which we weigh our options, make decisions, and direct our behavior. Yet, year upon decade upon century upon millennium almost all of us still play these ancient scripts—strutting, preening, flirting, courting, dazzling, then capturing one another. Then nesting. Then breeding. Then some philander; some depart. Then, drunk on hope, most court anew, fall in love, and start again. Eternal optimist, the human animal seems restless during the reproductive years, then settles in as he or she matures. Why?

The answer lies, I think, in the vagaries of our past, "when wild in woods the noble savage ran."

# "When Wild in Woods the Noble Savage Ran"

## Life in the Trees

> I am as free as Nature first made man
> Ere the base laws of servitude began
> When wild in woods the noble savage ran.
>
> —JOHN DRYDEN, "THE CONQUEST OF GRANADA"

Mahogany trees, tropical evergreens, laurels, wild pear trees, litchi fruit trees, mango trees, rubber trees, myrrh trees, ebony trees—trees, trees, and more trees stretched from Africa's eastern shores to the Atlantic Ocean.[1] Twenty-one million years ago equatorial Africa was a curtain of impenetrable green. Glades, pools, swamps, and streams, even more open woodlands and grassy plains occasionally interrupted these forests. But fossilized seeds, fruits, and nuts dug up at Rusinga Island in Lake Victoria and nearby sites suggest that East Africa was largely windless woods.[2]

Butterflies danced in the dim light that filtered through the sky of leaves. Flying squirrels glided from bough to bough and bats hung in darkened crevices. Ancient relatives of rhinos, elephants, hippos, warthogs, okapi, tusked deer, and other forest creatures fed among the ferns. And golden moles, elephant shrews, hamsters, hedgehogs, mice, gerbils, and many other small creatures gathered insect larvae, earthworms, herbs, and berries on the damp forest floor. The temperature was slightly higher than it is today, and almost every afternoon rain poured onto the steamy jungles, feeding the lakes and streams with fresh water, pelting the upper stories of the thick forest canopy.

Ancient relatives of ours roamed among these trees.

They have an array of scientific names, but they are often referred to collectively as the prehominoids—the ancestors of the Old World monkeys, apes, and humans. The earliest lived from twenty-two million to seventeen million years ago in East Africa. Hundreds of their fossil teeth and bones have been found. They had a mixture of ape-like and monkeylike features, although some looked more like monkeys while others had more characteristics of apes.[3] Moreover, some were about the size of a modern house cat, whereas others were as big as modern chimps.

None resembled human beings. But from among these kin both our ancestors and the living great apes would one day emerge.

How these males and females spent their days and nights is difficult to say. Perhaps some ran along tree limbs the way many monkeys do, leaping from branch to branch and climbing to follow adjacent highways above the ground. Some may have hung from tree limbs and swung beneath them instead.

This distinction is actually important to human evolution, for these are quite different ways to move around.

When the precursors of apes and humans abandoned life atop the stronger central limbs to hang below smaller branches, they evolved the basic structures of our human frame. To begin with, our ancestors lost their tails. These graceful appendages served their predecessors as the balancing pole serves the acrobat—a righting device perfectly designed to provide added stability as they scurried along sturdy boughs.

But as the forebears of the apes and man began to hang below the branches, tails became baggage that nature could discard.

Other streamlining features were adopted for swinging below the branches, particularly adjustments of the shoulder, arm, and torso. Gently pick up the family kitten by its forelimbs and watch its head dangle behind its paws; the cat can't see between its limbs. Then find a jungle gym in a playground and hang by your arms. Notice how your shoulders do not collapse before your face; you can see between your elbows as you suspend. The human collarbone, the position of our shoulder blades across our backs, our broad breastbone (or sternum), our wide, shallow ribcage, and our reduced lumbar vertebrae all evolved for hanging the body from above rather than supporting it from underneath.

Equally distinctive, humans and all the apes can rotate their wrists 180 degrees. Hence you and I can swing across a jungle gym palm up or palm away. Our ancestors acquired all of these anatomical features of the arms and upper body long ago—in order to dangle from tree limbs, swing below them, and feed on fruit and flowers.

Exactly when these changes occurred has been debated for decades. But these prehominoids lived among the leaves. And from the dozens of jaws and teeth they left behind, it is obvious that these creatures spent much of their day collecting fruit.[4] With their projecting snouts, shearing fangs, and bucked front teeth, they plucked, stripped, husked, and shelled their daily fare. They must have drunk from tulip-shaped bromeliads, from other plants, and from crannies that cupped water from the daily rains. And certainly they chattered with their companions, jockeyed for rank and food, and tucked into the crotches of sturdy limbs to sleep.

## Jungle Love

No doubt the prehominoids had sex too. Perhaps they even felt mild infatuation as they sniffed and stroked and groomed one another prior to copulation. But it is unlikely that sex was daily fare for these early relatives.

Why? Because all female primates—except women—have a period of heat, or estrus. Female monkeys of some species come into heat seasonally; other monkeys and all the apes have a monthly menstrual cycle. But in the middle of each rotation, which can last from about twenty-eight days to more than forty-five, they come into heat for a period of one to about twenty days, depending on the species and the individual.

Baboons illustrate a common primate pattern of sexuality, and their sex lives may say several things about coitus among our prehominoid relatives twenty-one million years ago.

With the beginning of estrus a female baboon's odor changes, and the "sex skin" around her genitals swells, announcing her fertility like a flag. She begins to "present," tipping her buttocks, looking over her shoulder, crouching, and backing toward males to invite copulation. When her period of heat wanes, however, a female baboon regularly refuses coitus—until next month. Females do not normally copulate when they are pregnant. And after parturition they do not resume estrus or regular sexual activity until they have weaned their infant—a period of about five to twenty-one months. Hence female baboons are available for sex only about one twenty-fifth of their adult lives.[5]

Our primitive ancestors may have been no more sexually active.

The sex lives of several apes confirm this. Female "common" chimps have a period of heat that lasts some ten to fourteen days; female gorillas come into heat for one to four days; and orangutans display estrus about five to six days of their monthly menstrual cycles.[6] Among these wild relatives, the vast majority of copulations occur during this period of heat although they do have sex at other times as well.[7] But at pregnancy these apes cease cycling and stop regular sexual activity. And estrus does not resume until a mother has weaned her young—a period of postpartum sexual quiescence that lasts three to four years among common chimps and gorillas, much longer among orangutans.[8] Only pygmy chimps (known as bonobos) copulate more regularly. But because these creatures exhibit an unusual pattern of sexuality, they probably do not qualify as a useful model for life as it was some twenty-one million years ago.[9]

Indeed, our ancestors in the trees were probably like ordinary primates—and sex was periodic. Some females were sexier than others, just as some apes and women are today. Some had longer periods of heat; some were more popular with the males. But coupling was generally confined to estrus. Placid days may have become orgiastic as females came into heat and males struggled among the branches for the privilege of coitus. But females must have resumed sexual quiescence during pregnancy too, then abstained until they weaned their young.

Even ordinary primates make exceptions, however, and that leads me to offer a few more speculations about sex among our furry forebears. Because social upheaval stimulates females of many species to copulate at times other than mid-cycle estrus, it is likely that a new leader, a new member in the group, or some special food item like meat provoked some females to copulate when they were not in heat.[10] Females probably used sex to obtain delicacies and make friends.

Females probably occasionally stole a little sex while pregnant or nursing too. Rhesus monkeys, as well as common chimps and gorillas, sometimes copulate during the first few months of pregnancy or before they have weaned an infant.[11] So it is reasonable to suggest that these ancestors also did. Sometimes they may have masturbated, as gorillas do.[12] Since homosexuality is known among female gorillas, chimps, and many other species, our female forebears must have mounted or rubbed against one another for stimulation.[13] Last, males may have occasionally forced females into coitus when they were not receptive.[14]

We can say nothing more about the sexuality or mating system of these early relatives except that profound changes in the environment would push some of them imperceptibly toward humanity—and our worldwide penchant to flirt, to fall in love, to marry, and, in some, a predisposition to be unfaithful, to divorce, and to pair again.

It all began with churning molten currents in the inner earth.

## Commotion in the Ocean

More than thirty million years ago Africa and the Arabian Peninsula formed a single island continent that lay slightly south of its position today.[15] To the north lay a sea, the Tethys Ocean, that stretched from the Atlantic in the west to the Pacific in the east, connecting the waters of the world. This sluice was the earth's radiator. Hot bottom waters from the Tethys swept around the globe, heating tides and winds that bathed the world's beaches with warm waves and its forests with warm rain.[16]

This furnace would disappear.

Pulled by fiery currents beneath the land, the African–Arabian plate of the earth's crust moved north. By some twenty-one million years ago, it was pressing into the Middle East to make the Zagros, the Taurus, and Caucasus mountain ranges. Soon an immense land corridor stretched from Africa into Eurasia, connecting the vast forests of the ancient world.[17]

Now the Tethys was squeezed in half. From its western portion, what would become the Mediterranean Sea, warm salty water still spilled into the Atlantic Ocean. But the eastern Tethys, what later evolved into the Indian Ocean, no longer received tropical currents. The Atlantic and the Indo-Pacific oceans were disconnected. Warm tides no longer swept around the globe, warming the jungles of the ancient world.[18]

Since the dawn of the Cenozoic era, when the mammals replaced the dinosaurs over sixty-five million years ago, world temperatures had begun to drop. Now they plunged again. In Antarctica ice caps formed on mountaintops. Along the equator the land began to dry.

The earth was cooling down.

Further climatic upheavals struck East Africa. Earlier jostling of the earth's crust had left two yawning gashes, parallel rifts that stretched five thousand kilometers from today's northern Ethiopia south through Malawi. But as the African–Arabian continent drifted north, these rifts continued to spread apart. Between them the ground sank, forming the East African landscape we know today—a series of low valleys nestled between mountainous highlands on either side.[19]

Clouds from equatorial Africa now dumped warm moisture before they rose over the western shoulder of the Western Rift, while trade winds from the Indian Ocean dumped their rain before rising over the Eastern Rift. The Rift Valley region came into "rain shadow." Where mists had veiled the morning sun, now days were clear and parched.

Seasons soon marked the ceaseless round of births and deaths. Monsoons still swept off the Indian Ocean between October and April twenty-one million years ago, but by May many of the tropical plants were dormant. Fig trees, acacia trees, and mango and wild pear trees no longer bore their fruit or flowers all year long; tender buds, new leaves, and shoots burgeoned only in the rainy season.[20]

Hot rains that had soaked East Africa every afternoon were becoming a thing of the past.

Even worse, volcanoes began to spray forth molten rock. Some had begun to spout as early as twenty-one million years ago. But by sixteen million years ago, Tinderet, Yelele, Napak, Moroto, Kadam, Elgon, and

Kisingeri threw off streams of lava and clouds of ash on the animals and plants below.[21]

With the cooling of the earth, the effects of rain shadow, and the active volcanoes in the region, the tropical forests of East Africa began to shrink—as jungles were thinning around the world.

Replacing all these trees were two expanding ecological niches: the woodlands and the savannas.[22] Along lakes and riverbanks, trees still packed together. But where the ground rose and streams turned into rivulets, woodlands spread. Here single-story trees stretched out, barely touching one another with their boughs. Beneath them wove boulevards of grass. And where water was even scarcer, herbs and grasses that had struggled to survive below a dome of branches began to spread into miles and miles of thinly wooded savanna plains.[23]

By sixteen to fourteen million years ago the lush, protective world of the prehominoids was coming to an end.

Havoc reigned.

So did opportunity.

Around this time many forest animals died out. The tiny ancient relatives of the horse and other creatures migrated into Africa from the dwindling forests of Eurasia. And many other species emerged from forest glades to congregate in larger groups and evolve into novel species in the woodlands and on the grass. Among these immigrants were the forerunners of the modern rhino and giraffe, the ostrich, myriad kinds of antelopes, and other browsing and grazing herbivores that swarm the Serengeti Plains today. Evolving with them were their predators, the predecessors of the lions, cheetahs, and other carnivores, as well as jackals and hyenas—the garbage collectors of the ancient world.[24]

Turmoil in the ocean, the new land bridge to Eurasia, seasonality, the thinning forest canopy, and the expanding woodlands and grassy plains would enormously affect our ancestors. Due undoubtedly to the new highway out of Africa, for example, many trickled into France, Spain, Italy, Hungary, Greece, and Slovakia, then on to Turkey, India, China, and other parts of Asia, while the African stay-at-homes remained in the dwindling forests, the more open woodlands, and the spreading grass.

Equally important, many of these early explorers showed distinctive physical features of the living apes, and even a few traits of our first true ancestors—those in the line toward you and me.[25]

They were known as the hominoids, the precursors of humans and the great apes: the orangutan, gorilla, and the two species of chimpanzee, the common chimp and the bonobo. From within this general stock, our first forebears would emerge.[26]

Friends you pick; relatives you are stuck with. So although today's African apes have certainly evolved over the past several million years (and these hominoids had several characteristics of the monkeys as well as apes), the modern African apes' close biological ties to humankind make them the most appropriate models for reconstructing life as it may have been between fourteen and eight million years ago—just before the first ancestors in the human line appeared in the forests and woodlands of East Africa; just before our primordial patterns of pair-bonding, adultery, divorce, and remarriage probably began to evolve.

## Gorilla Tactics

Gorillas live in harems. Today these shy, beguiling creatures still roam the dormant Virunga volcanoes of Zaire, Uganda, and Rwanda. Until her murder in the jungle in 1985, anthropologist Dian Fossey studied thirty-five of these gorilla bands, recording their daily lives for some eighteen years.

Each gorilla harem is led by a single adult silverback male (so-called because of the saddle of silvery hair that spreads across his back) and at least two "wives." Often a black-backed (subadult) or a younger fully adult male occupies a lesser position at the flank of a gorilla band, accompanied by his younger wives. The leader, the younger males, their wives, and a gaggle of sundry young wander together among the moss-laden hagenia trees, foraging for thistle and wild celery in the mist and underbrush, deep in the heart of Africa.

Female gorillas begin to copulate by age nine to eleven. As her monthly one- to four-day estrous period starts, a female begins to court the group's highest-ranking male that is not her father or full sibling.[27] She tips her buttocks toward him, looks into his brown eyes, and backs assertively toward him, rubbing her genitals rhythmically against him or sitting on his lap to copulate face to face. All the while she makes soft, high, fluttering calls.[28]

If no eligible "husband" is available, however, she leaves her natal band to join another group where a suitable male resides. And if no partner is present there either, she joins a solitary bachelor and travels independently with him. If her mate cannot entice a second female to join them within a few months, however, a female will desert her lover and travel with a harem. Female gorillas do not tolerate monogamy; they want harem life.

Young males are also mobile. If a black-backed male reaches puberty in a band where one or more young adult females reside, he often remains in his natal group to breed with them. But if no females have reached puberty or if all are full siblings, he either transfers to another group or wanders as a solitary bachelor in order to attract young females for a harem of his own.

This mobility inhibits incest. In fact, on only one occasion did Fossey witness incest: a silverback mated with his daughter. Curiously, months after she gave birth, the infant was killed by family members. Bone splinters in their feces indicated that the baby was partially eaten too.[29]

Once a harem is established, the husband and his co-wives settle down; normally they mate for life—sunbathing when the sun breaks through, moving in their rhythmic round of work and play. Occasionally a female leaves her spouse to join a different mate—serial monandry.[30] But this is rare.

Mates are not necessarily sexually faithful to their partners, though. An estrous female mates only with her husband, who interrupts her sexual overtures to other males. Once pregnant, however, a female often begins to copulate with lower-ranking males—directly under her husband's nose. And unless sex becomes too vigorous, her spouse does not interrupt these rendezvous. Gorillas philander and tolerate adultery.

Did our arboreal ancestors living eight million years ago travel in harems as gorillas do? Did males and females mate for life, then copulate occasionally with other members of the band? Perhaps.

There are major differences between human sexual tastes and the reproductive habits of gorillas, however. Gorillas always copulate in public, whereas a hallmark of human coupling is privacy. More important, male gorillas *always* form harems. Not so men. As you know, the vast majority of human males have only a single wife at once. Female gorillas and human females have even less in common. Although women do join harems, they usually bicker with their co-wives; sometimes they even kill one another's children. Jealousy is rampant in human polygynous marriages.

Women are not temperamentally built for harem life.

What most distinguishes human beings from gorillas, though, is the length of our "relationships." Gorillas almost always mate for life. People, on the other hand, tend to switch partners—sometimes several times. For us, long marriages often take some work.

## The Primal Horde

Darwin, Freud, Engels, and many other thinkers have postulated that our earliest ancestors lived in a "primal horde"—that men and women copulated with whom they liked, when they liked.[31] As Lucretius, the Roman philosopher, wrote in the first century A.D., "The human beings that lived in those days in the fields were a tougher sort of people, as the tough earth had made them. . . . They lived for many revolutions of the sun, roaming far and wide in the manner of wild beasts. And Venus joined the bodies of lovers in the forest; for they were brought together by mutual desire, or by the frenzied force and violent lust of the man, or by a bribe of acorns, pears, or arbute-berries."[32]

Lucretius may have been correct. Common chimps and bonobos live in hordes and sexual bribery is commonplace. Moreover, genetic data indicate that these African apes are our closest relatives; indeed, we are as genetically similar to them as the domesticated dog is to the wolf. And we shared a common heritage until our forebears split off some eight to five million years ago.[33] So we can surmise some basic things about our past from examining their lives.

Today bonobos (*Pan paniscus*) remain in a few swampy jungles that hug the Zaire (Congo) River. Here they display feats of acrobatics—arm swinging, leaping, diving, and walking on two limbs like tightrope artists—often a hundred feet above the ground. They spend most of their time moving on the forest floor, however, strolling through the woods on all four limbs, looking for juicy fruits, seeds, shoots, leaves, honey, worms, and caterpillars, digging holes to excavate mushrooms, or stealing sugarcane and pineapples from farmers.[34]

They eat meat too. On several occasions anthropologists saw males stalk flying squirrels—unsuccessfully. In other instances males silently caught and killed a small forest antelope, a duiker, and shared its meat. And bonobos dig in the mud beside streams to collect fish and scatter termite mounds to eat the milling residents.[35] Perhaps our hominoid ancestors hunted animals and collected other proteins to supplement their diet of fruit and nuts.

Bonobos travel in mixed groups of males, females, and young. Some parties are small; two to eight individuals often stroll in a relatively stable band. Yet fifteen to thirty, even a hundred individuals sometimes assemble to eat, relax or sleep near one another. Individuals come and go between groups, depending on the food supply—thus connecting a cohesive community of several dozen animals. Here is a primal horde.

Sex is almost a daily pastime. Female bonobos have an extended monthly period of heat, stretching through almost three-quarters of their menstrual cycle. But sex, as mentioned earlier, is not confined to estrus. Females copulate during most of their menstrual cycles—a pattern of coitus approaching that of women.[36]

And females bribe their male friends with sex quite regularly. A female will walk up to a male who is eating sugarcane, sit beside him and beg (palm up) as people do; then she looks plaintively at the delicacy and back at him. He feels her gaze. When he gives her the treat, she tips her buttocks and copulates; then she ambles off with the cane in hand. A female is not beyond soliciting another female either, sauntering up to a comrade, climbing into her arms face to face, wrapping her legs around her waist, and rubbing her genitals on those of her partner before accepting sticks of cane. Male–male homosexuality, fellatio, also occurs.[37]

Bonobos engage in sex to ease tension, to stimulate sharing during meals, to reduce stress while traveling, and to reaffirm friendships during anxious reunions. "Make love, not war" is clearly a bonobo scheme.

Did our ancestors do the same?

Bonobos display many of the sexual habits that people exhibit on the streets, in the bars and restaurants, and behind apartment doors in New York, Paris, Moscow, and Hong Kong. Prior to coitus bonobos often stare deeply into each other's eyes. As I have mentioned, this copulatory gaze is a central component of human courtship too. And bonobos walk arm in arm, kiss each other's hands and feet, and embrace with long, deep, tongue-inserting French kisses.[38]

Bonobos in the San Diego Zoo also copulate in the missionary position (face to face with the male on top) 70% of the time, although this may be because they have access to a flat dry surface.[39] In the African forest 40 of 106 observed copulations were face to face; the balance were in the rear-entry pose instead.[40] But bonobos like variety. A female will sit on a male's lap to copulate, couple face to face from on top of him, crouch while her partner stands, have intercourse while both are standing, or couple while hanging in a tree. Sometimes the two manipulate each other's genitals while mating. And they tend to gaze at each other as they "make love."

Our last tree-dwelling ancestors probably kissed and hugged prior to coitus too; maybe they even had sex *en face* while looking deep into each other's eyes.[41]

Because bonobos appear to be the smartest of the apes, because they have many physical traits quite similar to those of people, and because these chimps copulate with flair and frequency, some anthropologists conjecture that bonobos are much like the African hominoid prototype, our last common tree-dwelling ancestor.[42]

Nevertheless, bonobos display some fundamental differences in their sexual behavior. For one thing, bonobos do not form long-term pair-bonds the way humans do. Nor do they raise their young as husband and wife.

Males do care for infant siblings.[43] But monogamy is no life for them. Promiscuity is their fare.

Human philandering is, most likely, a prehuman behavior pattern.

## Chimpanzee Days

Just as promiscuous are common chimpanzees, *Pan troglodytes*, named after Pan, the spirit of Mother Nature and a god to the ancient Greeks. In 1960 Jane Goodall began to watch these creatures at the Gombe Stream Reserve, Tanzania, and she has observed some remarkable behaviors that help to visualize life as it may have been among our tree-dwelling ancestors some eight million years ago.

These chimps live in communities of fifteen to eighty individuals in ranges of five to twelve square kilometers along the eastern shore of Lake Tanganyika. "Home" varies from thick forests to more open woodlands to stretches of savanna grass with scattered trees. Because the food supply is dispersed and uneven, individuals are obliged to travel in small, temporary groups.

Males move along the ground in parties of about four or five. Two or more mothers with infants sometimes join one another for a few hours as a "nursery" party. And individuals often amble by themselves or with one or more friends in a small mixed-sex group. Parties are flexible; individuals come and go. But if members of one party find a particularly lush supply of figs, new buds, or some other delicacy, they hoot through the forest or drum on trees with their fists. Then all assemble for the meal.

Female common chimps have a mid-cycle estrus that often lasts ten to sixteen days, and their patterns of sexuality are another model for life as it may have been for our ancestors long ago.[44]

As a female comes into heat, the sex skin around her genitals balloons like a huge pink flower—a passport to male activities. She often joins an all-male party and proceeds to seduce all except her sons and brothers. As many as eight males may line up and wait their turn, in what is known as "opportunistic mating." Males copulate within two minutes of one another; intromission, thrusting, and ejaculation normally take only ten to fifteen seconds.[45]

More dominant courtiers may attempt to monopolize an estrous female instead, what is called "possessive mating." A male will stare intently to get a female's attention, sit with his legs open to display an erect penis, flick it, rock from side to side, beckon her with outstretched arms, swagger in front of her, or follow a female doggedly.[46] One male slept on the ground in the rain all night waiting for a nesting estrous female to arise. When a male succeeds in attracting a female to his side, he sticks close to her and tries to prevent copulations with other males. Sometimes males even chase, charge, or attack other suitors.

But confrontations of this sort take precious time—minutes the female sometimes uses to copulate with as many as three other admirers.

Female chimps are sexually aggressive. On one occasion Flo, the sexiest of the chimps at Gombe, copulated several dozen times during the course of a single day. Adolescent females are sometimes insatiable, even tweaking the flaccid penises of uninterested companions. Some females appear to masturbate as well. Moreover, female chimps can be picky. They prefer the males who groom them and give them food—not necessarily the most dominant individuals in the male hierarchy.[47] Some courtiers they flatly refuse. With others they have long-standing friendships and copulate more regularly. And both sexes avoid coitus with close relatives, such as mother or siblings.[48]

Moreover, female chimps like sexual adventure. Adolescent females at Gombe often leave their natal group for the duration of their estrus to seek males in a nearby community, a habit many continue as adults. When neighboring males see the unfamiliar female coming, they inspect the enlarged, pink sex skin around her vulva that signals estrus. Then they copulate rather than attack the stranger. Like human teenagers, female common chimps regularly leave home to mate. Some return; others transfer permanently instead.

Were ancestral hominoid women sexually aggressive? Did they join all-male parties during estrus, copulate with these bachelors, masturbate at times, and make friends with specific males? Probably.

They may have made longer partnerships as well.

## Making Dates

Sometimes an estrous female common chimp and a single male vanish to copulate out of sight and earshot—what is known as "going on safari."[49] These trysts are often initiated by the male. With hair and penis erect, he beckons, rocks from side to side, waves branches, and gazes intently at his potential paramour. When she moves toward him, he turns and walks away, hoping she will follow. These gestures become more intense until she does his bidding. Sometimes a male even attacks a female until she acquiesces.

Here, then, are traces of monogamy—complete with coitus in private. These clandestine consortships often last several days; a few last several weeks. And "going on safari" has reproductive payoffs. At least half of the fourteen pregnancies recorded at Gombe in the 1970s occurred while a female was traveling with a single partner.[50]

Perhaps our ancestors in the trees occasionally made similar short-term pair-bonds, vanished into the leaves to copulate face to face, hugged, stroked, kissed each other's faces, hands, and bodies, fed each other bits of fruit, and bore young from these "affairs."

But, once again, these chimps differ in a vital respect from you and me. When a female common chimp becomes noticeably pregnant, she begins to roam alone or joins a group of mothers and infants. And as she nears parturition, she settles in a small "home" range. Some females pick a spot in the center of a community; some make home at the periphery of the neighborhood. On this turf she bears her infant and raises it *alone*.

Chimpanzees do not form pair-bonds to rear their young. To chimps, fathering is unknown.

⤳

Common chimps display many other social habits, however, that would germinate among our forebears, then flourish in humankind. Among them is war.

The males at Gombe guard the borders of their turf. Three or more adult males set off together. Sometimes they call loudly, perhaps to scare off outsiders; usually they scout in silence. They stop to stand and peer over tall grass or climb trees to scan adjacent property. Some inspect discarded food, examine strange nests, or listen for intruding chimps as they steal along. When they encounter neighbors, they urinate or defecate out of nervousness and touch one another for reassurance; then they call aggressively and perform mock charges. Some wave branches. Some slap the ground. Some hurl or roll stones. Then both groups retreat.[51]

And in a now-classic event in 1974, a chimpanzee war erupted. In the early 1970s a splinter group of seven males and three females had begun to travel chiefly in the southern portion of the Kasakela community's real estate, and by 1972 these emigrants had established themselves as a separate community, known to observers as Kahama, after the river valley to the south. Intermittently Kasakela males met Kahama males at their new border and called, drummed on trees, and dragged branches in unfriendly displays before mutually retreating.

In 1974, however, five Kasakela males penetrated deep into southern territory, surprised a Kahama male, and beat him up. As Goodall described the incident, one Kasakela male held the victim down while others bit him, kicked him, pummeled him with their fists, and jumped on him. Finally one male rose onto his hind legs, screamed above the melee, and hurled a rock at the enemy. It fell short. After ten more minutes of mayhem, the warriors abandoned the Kahama male with bleeding wounds and broken bones.[52]

Over the next three years five more Kahama males and one female met the same fate. By 1977, Kasakela males had exterminated most of their neighbors; the rest vanished. The Kasakela community soon extended its range south along the shores of Lake Tanganyika.[53]

Had our tree-dwelling ancestors begun to wage war on one another some eight million years ago? It's plausible.

≈

They probably had begun to hunt for meat as well.[54] Chimpanzee hunters are always adults, almost always males. The victims are normally juvenile baboons, monkeys, bushbuck, or bushpigs. Sometimes a male simply seizes an unsuspecting monkey feeding nearby in a tree and tears it to shreds, "opportunistic hunting." But planned, cooperative group hunting expeditions are also common. The hunt is always silent. Only the direction of the hunter's gaze, his ruffled hair, his cocked head, the determination of his gait, or exchanged glances alert others that the chase is on. Then a group of males surround their victim together.

As soon as one chimp grabs the prey, a tug-of-war begins. Each hunter hollers and retreats with pieces, and minutes later all in earshot assemble to form "sharing clusters" around possessors of the spoils. Some chimps beg, palm up; others stare at the possessor or the meat; still others retrieve dropped morsels from the foliage below. Then everyone sits to eat, leisurely adding leaves to supplement the protein—the original steak-and-salad dinner. Sometimes it takes a dozen chimps all day to consume a carcass weighing less than twenty pounds, an event not unlike an American holiday dinner.

Chimps do fight over meat. Tempers sometimes flare, but rank does not guarantee a larger portion. In this one aspect of chimpanzee social life, subordinates do not defer to leaders. Instead, age has clout. So does sex appeal. An estrous female often receives extra pieces.[55]

Forethought, group hunting, cooperation, sharing—these hunting skills would be greatly improved by our ancestors. But one key element of human hunting is often missing among chimps: the use of weapons. It does occur occasionally, however.

In one instance, a group of Gombe males surrounded four adult bushpigs, and the hunters tried to extricate a piglet from their midst. Finally one aged male hurled a melon-sized rock, striking an adult pig. The bushpigs fled, leaving the piglet behind. Immediately the chimp hunters captured, disassembled, and devoured the youngster.[56] Male chimps have also fashioned spearlike projectiles to hurl at unsuspecting prey.

But chimps use weapons more often when confronting one another.[57] They drop tree limbs on those beneath them, whip their enemies with saplings, rise onto their hind legs to brandish sticks, hurl rocks and branches, and drag logs or roll stones as they charge their adversaries.

Perhaps when our tree-dwelling ancestors were not courting estrous females, they were making war, hunting, or attacking one another with sticks and stones. Most likely they also spent a great deal of time just trying to keep the peace.[58]

⁓

While male chimps make more weapons, females make and use more tools—particularly when they gather insects.[59] Female chimps "dip" for ants, opening a subterranean ant nest with their fingers and inserting a slender twig. As the ants stream up the pole, the hunter picks off the tiny, milling creatures with her lips, sweeps them into her mouth, then chews frantically to devour the ants before they bite her tongue. They "fish" in the tunnels of termite compounds with long grass stems as well. Chimps also use rocks to open nuts and tough-skinned fruits, leaves to wipe dirt from their bodies, sticks to pick their teeth, foliage to fan away flies, chewed leaves to sop water from a tree crotch, and sticks and stones to hurl at cats and snakes and hostile chimpanzees.[60]

Our last tree-dwelling relatives may have used tools regularly as well.

Dentistry and doctoring probably also came from our tree-dwelling predecessors. At Gombe the budding chimp "dentist," Belle, used twigs to clean the teeth of a young male as he held his mouth wide open. On one occasion she made a successful extraction too—pulling out an infected tooth as her patient lay still, head back, mouth gaping.[61] At the Primate Research Center at Central Washington University a young male used a twig to clean a foot sore on one of his companions.[62] Chimps also pick away scabs when they groom one another.

Chimps do not always desert their dying either. After a female chimp at Gombe was attacked by a group of males, her daughter sat beside her crushed body for hours, brushing off the flies until her mother passed away. But the juvenile did not leave a leaf, a branch, or stone to commemorate her mother's death. Only elephants "bury" their companions, placing branches over the head and shoulders of their deceased.[63]

Our last tree-dwelling ancestors probably had a rich world of etiquette as well. Chimps today give gifts of leaves and twigs to their chimp superiors. They bow to high-ranking companions. They keep "friends" and travel with these companions. They shake hands, stroke one another reassuringly, and pat each other's fannies the way football players do. They clench their teeth and draw back their lips into the "human" nervous social smile. They pout, sulk, and stage tantrums. And they groom each other regularly, picking grass and dirt from each other's hair—much as we pick lint from someone's sweater.

## Noble Savages

Did our last tree-dwelling relatives live in communities like chimpanzees?[64] Did they gang up on one another, protect their boundaries, and war on neighbors—a consuming passion of humanity today? Did they use sticks to dip for ants, cooperate to hunt for meat, and share the spoils? It seems reasonable.

Some may have been early doctors; others, warriors. They probably played practical jokes like dumping water or foliage on an unsuspecting comrade—because chimps love to be buffoons and play pranks on one another today. Some of our forebears must have been serious, some inventive, some shy, some courageous, some sweet, some self-centered, some patient, some sneaky, some curious, some stubborn, some petty—as people and all the apes can be.

They must have had a sense of family too. Chimpanzees, gorillas, and all the higher primates associate regularly with mother, sisters, and brothers. And they probably were scared of most strangers, had tiffs with peers, bowed to superiors, kissed their sex partners, walked arm in arm, and held hands and feet. They undoubtedly communicated their fondness, amusement, irritation, and many other emotions with facial expressions, giggles, pants, and hoots. And surely they spent a great deal of time sitting on the forest floor, patting, stroking, hugging, picking dirt and leaves from one another, playing with their infants, friends, and lovers.

Maybe they also vanished into the forest with a consort for a few days or weeks of private sex. Perhaps some even felt some infatuation for this temporary mate or sadness when the safari ended. But most likely sex was a casual affair. Eight million years ago children grew up under the tutelage of mother and her female friends.

The "father," the "husband," and the "wife" had not yet evolved.

# Our Gang

By six million years ago, however, someone new had emerged in Africa. Some of these creatures wandered the broad corridors of grass that wove between the woodland trees of Kenya.[65] Some lived in the woods of Chad. And by some 4.4 million years ago, more than thirty-five individuals lived and died in the forests that hugged the sluggish rivers of today's Ethiopia.

They may be what laymen would consider the "missing link"— the first to split off from the forebears of our closest cousins, the chimpanzees, to begin their march toward humanity. We have their bones. They've been given several scientific names. But most belong to the species *Ardipithecus ramidus*.

Please meet Ardi, one of these ancient kin.

*Ardi* means "ground" or "floor" in the local Ethiopian language of the Afar tribesmen; *ramid* means "root." Ardi left much of her skeleton in what is now Aramis, in the Middle Awash (after the Awash River), in the Rift Valley of Ethiopia.[66] She stood four feet tall, weighed about 110 pounds and, from the architecture of her teeth, she ate a lot of plants, nuts, and small mammals. She traveled in the hackberry, fig, and palm trees that spread across the area, sharing her days with monkeys, antelopes, rhinos, bears, otters, bats, squirrels, hyenas, peafowl, insects, and different kinds of plants—all of which left more than 150,000 bits of their fossilized remains.

But Ardi was a special woman. Her opposable big toe splayed out, enabling her to grasp tree limbs. This apelike feature is vastly different from the aligned toes of all later hominins—those in the line closer to you and me. Yet other aspects of her feet enabled her to walk upright, bipedally, on two feet instead of four.

This was a huge step toward humanity. Her upper pelvis had also changed. She didn't lurch from side to side (as chimps do) as she strolled bipedally along the ground. Yet her lower pelvis was apelike, built to attach massive muscles for climbing trees. She even had aspects of a monkeylike hand, with long fingers and short, flexible palms. And although aspects of her skull and spine had modified for walking on two legs, her brain was no larger than that of chimps.

But Ardi and her male and female friends also had an outstanding *human* trait: reduced canine teeth. Moreover, the skeletal remains of *Ardipithecus ramidis* show no evidence of substantial body size variations between the sexes.[67] These traits are the first indications that human romantic love and pair-bonding had emerged.[68]

Or so reasons anthropologist Owen Lovejoy. Lovejoy bases his hypothesis for the early evolution of monogamy, or pair-bonding, on the long-accepted fact that male primates living in hordes use their huge, sharp, daggerlike canine teeth to fight other males for breeding opportunities. So he proposes that because *Ardipithecus* males had reduced canines, they no longer had to fight with one another for female favors. Instead *they had begun to pair to rear their young*: monogamy—a hallmark of our lineage. Lovejoy maintains that the evolution of monogamy occurred along with the evolution of primitive bipedalism.

Ardi was a complex girl. Not everyone agrees that she and her companions had split off from the ancestors of the chimps;[69] nor do all believe that Ardi formed a pair-bond with a lover to rear her tiny young. But Ardi and her chums must have spent a good deal of time on the forest floor, even cautiously walking through the more open woodland trees. Perhaps the bravest of her comrades even huddled at the fringe of the expanding grass, then dashed into this sea of danger to collect the leftovers of a lion's kill and quickly retreated to the forest or woodland trees to eat unmolested by predators.

Our forebears had begun to spend more time on the ground.

Ardi's thoughts are lost in time and rock. But the stage was set, the players in the wings. From Ardi's general stock our first clearly humanlike relatives would soon emerge—and develop a dual craving for devotion and philandering that would plague their descendants to this day.

# 7

## Out of Eden

### On the Origin of Monogamy and Desertion

The beast and bird their common charge attend,
The mothers nurse it, and the sires defend;
The young dismiss'd to wander earth or air,
There stops the Instinct, and there ends the care;
The link dissolves, each seeks a fresh embrace,
Another love succeeds, another race.
A longer care Man's helpless kind demands;
That longer care contracts more lasting bands.

—ALEXANDER POPE, "ESSAY ON MAN"

It was the beginning of the wet season in East Africa some 3.6 million years ago. For weeks the volcano Sadiman had periodically belched forth clouds of gray volcanic ash, daily spreading a blanket of dust on the woodlands and plains below. Every afternoon showers moistened the ash; then during the cool evenings it hardened—engraving raindrops, acacia leaf prints, and the tracks of passing antelopes, giraffes, rhinos, elephants, pigs, guinea fowl, baboons, hares, insects, hyenas, a saber-toothed cat, and some ancient relatives of ours.[1]

Three primitive hominins—individuals who are clearly on some branch of the human tree—had picked their way through the volcanic muck, leaving their footprints for posterity. The largest had walked across the ash, sinking about five centimeters with every step. Beside these prints were those of a smaller hominin, perhaps a female, who stood a little over four feet tall. And because a third pair of tracks were superimposed on those of the largest creature, anthropologists deduce that a somewhat smaller hominin had followed, stepping carefully in the footsteps of the leader. All three were heading north to a small gorge, perhaps to camp in the trees beside the stream, because the tracks proceed seventy-seven feet to the canyon's edge. Then abruptly they disappear.

In 1978 Mary Leakey, the well-known archaeologist and wife of Louis Leakey, the grand old man of African paleoanthropology (both now deceased), and her team discovered these footprints eroding out of an ancient geologic stratum.[2] Since the mid-1970s Leakey had been excavating a site called Laetoli, an area in northern Tanzania named by the local Masai tribesmen for a red lily that carpets the area today. Within weeks of the 1978 field season she found these signatures of our past.

Whether these creatures strolled, strode, or picked their way, even whether they walked together or at different times, is not clear from the many analyses of these tracks. But that they lived and died near the gorge is beyond doubt. In other field seasons Leakey unearthed a host of other hominin fossils—skull and jaw fragments and the isolated teeth of more than twenty-two individuals who wandered through these woodlands below Mount Sadiman between 3.5 and 3.8 million years ago.[3]

## Lucy in the Sky with Diamonds

They were not alone. To the north, along the Hadar River of the Afar region of Ethiopia, lived Lucy. Anthropologist Donald Johanson and teammates unearthed much of Lucy in 1974.

Named after the Beatles song "Lucy in the Sky with Diamonds," Lucy had stood some three and a half feet tall, weighed about sixty pounds, and had dined along the edge of a shallow lake in what was then the rolling wooded and grassy countryside of Ethiopia. She suffered from arthritis and died in her early twenties, around 3.2 million years ago.[4]

Johanson's team recovered about 40% of Lucy's skeleton. And although her toes and fingers were curved and somewhat longer than ours, suggesting that Lucy spent time in the trees, the remains of her hip, knee, ankle, and foot confirm that she walked on two feet instead of four.[5] The following year Johanson unearthed what could have been Lucy's friends, the partial remains of at least thirteen more individuals who strode through the woodlands of Ethiopia so long ago. Since then even more have been unearthed.

Exactly who these "people" at Laetoli and Hadar were, we do not know. Those who study hominin footprints are known as ichnologists, and they, as well as many other anthropologists, think a foot like Lucy's could have left the prints at Laetoli. So they place all these individuals in the same early species, *Australopithecus afarensis*, a branch of hominins that all anthropologists believe split from the ancestors of the apes, and lies somewhere near the beginning of our human family tree.

These creatures probably looked something like modern chimps, with brains that were slightly larger (but no more than a third the size of ours), heavy ridges on their brows, dark eyes and skin, thin lips, no chins, and protruding jaws with bucked front teeth. Many details of their skulls, jaws, and skeletons are reminiscent of apes. And males were considerably larger and more robust than females.[6] Moreover, the shape of a recovered hyoid bone, a component of the voice box, indicates that they spoke with hoos and roars and barks—like chimps.[7] These people did not speak with human language.

———————————

(OVERLEAF) *A moment in our human ancestry: The scene depicted on the following pages shows members of the species* Australopithecus afarensis, *early humanlike forebears living in the woodlands and plains of East Africa 3.2 million years ago. These "people" had long (and somewhat curved) fingers and toes, short legs, long arms, small brains, projecting jaws, and other anatomical details that vividly distinguish them from contemporary people. But they walked erect and were likely early members of the human family tree. Individuals such as these probably traveled in bands of twelve to twenty-five friends and relatives, formed temporary pair-bonds shortly after puberty, shared food with a mate, remained paired for at least the infancy of a single child (about three to four years), and often parted after the child stopped suckling and joined a multi-age playgroup where it could be cared for by many additional members of the band. Then typically each parent formed a new pair-bond with a new lover and bore more young. Illustration by John Gurche.*

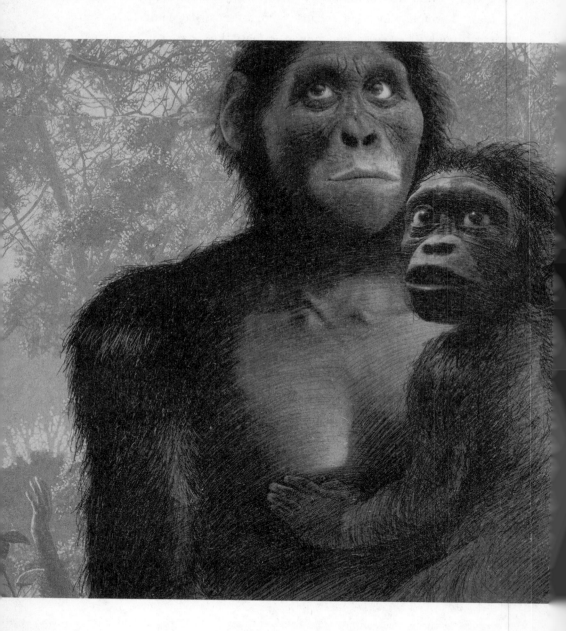

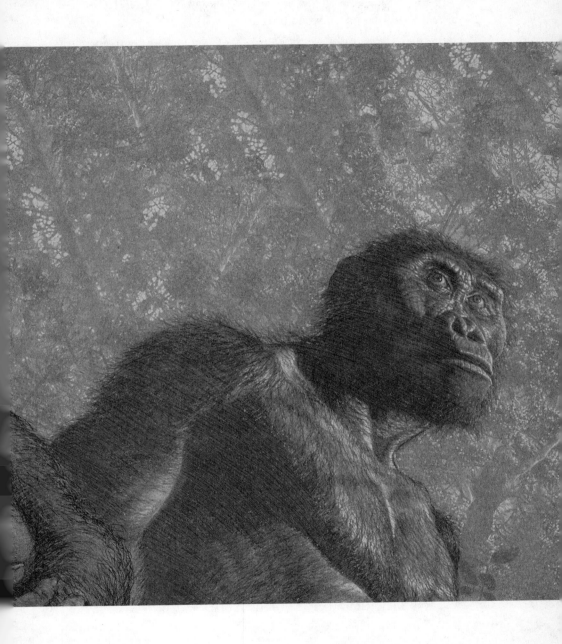

But their bodies had many human qualities. Most important, they walked erect, on two feet instead of four.

Where had these individuals come from? How had their ancestors turned down the road toward humanity?

## The Crucible

"Two roads diverged in a wood, and I—I took the one less traveled by, and that has made all the difference." Robert Frost captured that moment in life that irrevocably changes everything that follows. Such a time occurred in human evolution, an era when our first ancestors stepped irreversibly away from their tree-dwelling relatives and began along the path that led to modern human social life.

Silent is the fossil record of this nativity.

Yet through the centuries, theologians, philosophers, and scientists have woven, from threads of knowledge, theories of our genesis. The following is my version. It stems from scientific data in a variety of disciplines, including what we know of the animals and plants that flourished across ancient Africa, the lifeways of modern apes and monkeys, the mating habits of other monogamous species, such as foxes and robins, the lifestyles of modern hunting-gathering peoples, and human patterns of romantic love, attachment, and abandonment that I have presented in this book.

Here, then, is a hypothesis for the origin of the human predisposition for *serial* monogamy—the human predisposition to fall in love, form a pair-bond, leave this relationship after three to four years (often after bearing a single child), and then fall in love anew and bond again.

⁓

The time was somewhere between four and six million years ago; let's make it four million—just after Ardi roamed the woods some 4.4 million years ago and just before Lucy's contemporaries left their bones and footprints below Mount Sadiman about 3.6 million years ago.

Beside the shallow blue-green lakes and lazy rivers, forest trees and climbing vines cloaked the shore. But farther from the water's edge, mahoganies and evergreens thinned out. Here stretched the woodlands—where trees barely touched one another with their boughs and grass wove between their trunks. And beyond the woodlands, across the rolling hills of East Africa, stretched fields of grass.

Ancient varieties of elephants, ostriches, okapi, gazelles, zebras, wildebeests, bushbuck, elands, buffalo, even primitive horses (immigrants from Asia) strode across these open plazas. Their enemies—ancestral lions, cheetahs, and feral dogs—followed. At dawn, at dusk, through the day and night, these carnivores stole the weak from among the herds. Then vultures, hyenas, jackals, and other scavengers picked the fallen bare.[8]

It was into this more open landscape that our first ancestors were being pushed by the shrinking of the forests. At first they probably ventured into the woodlands only in the dry season, when forest fruits and buds were hard to find. But hunger and competition must have pushed them on. Perhaps whole communities, as many as thirty individuals—the old, the young, the adventurous, and the fearful—congregated beneath these boughs when the branches of the thicker forest were picked clean.

Perhaps three or four related females roamed together to look for termite mounds or ants. When they came upon a cashew grove or field of seeds, they hooted, calling the less courageous onto the more open land. Most likely small groups of males combed the woodlands for fresh meat, grabbing nestling birds, shrews, baby antelopes, even unsuspecting baboons—anything that looked edible, even dead animals.

Man the scavenger. Anthropologists now believe that our ancestors descended to the ground to collect and scavenge for a living.[9]

## Meat Pirates

Anthropologist Gary Tunnell tested this hypothesis; he used bushcraft to see whether our ancestors could have survived by opportunistic hunting and scavenging millions of years ago.[10] Tunnell set up his tent on the Serengeti Plains of East Africa, choosing an area of six square kilometers in southwestern Kenya. He shared his turf with nine lions. The trick would be to scavenge from their dinner rather than becoming part of it.

At night Tunnell slept below two high cliffs amid the sleeping-trees of the local baboon troop. These neighbors alerted him when the largest lion made his nightly visit to smell Tunnell and mark the pride's range beside his tent. Through the night, again at dawn, Tunnell listened. This way he established where the lions made their nightly kill. Then, at 9 A.M., after the lions were asleep, he set out on a specific route in search of meat.

Tunnell always found edible protein—an unwary warthog, a crippled topi, three sleeping bats, several glutted vultures, ten catfish in a dying pool, a three-foot lizard in a tiny canyon, or the carcass of a buffalo, wildebeest, or Grant's gazelle killed by lions or cheetahs hours earlier. Tunnell did not eat any of his discoveries. But he concluded that with no more than a sharpened rock and a pointed stick just one human scavenger and a comrade to help butcher flesh could easily feed a group of ten—as long as they stayed out of the territories of hyenas, humankind's major competitor for meat.

Like Tunnell, the modern Hadza of Tanzania sometimes scavenge in the dry season. They listen to the night calls of the lions and watch the vultures fly. The next morning they find the kill, move in, drive away the carnivores, and collect the meat with expert tools.

Our first ground-dwelling ancestors certainly did not use sophisticated tools the way the Hadza do. But chimps in captivity have sharpened sticks into spears; some have even whacked off an edge of rock to produce a cutting edge. So perhaps the smartest of the band occasionally felled a small mammal with a sharpened stick, then disarticulated it with a sharpened rock.[11]

And they could have scavenged quite a haul. Lions and cheetahs often leave their meals unfinished. Leopards park their kills unattended, hanging in a tree.[12] Perhaps our ancestors waited until the last of the cats had staggered off to sleep, then crept back to the carcass to smash the skull, collect the brains, pull off skin and tendons, and harvest scraps of flesh. Sometimes they may have thrown stones instead, terrifying the feeding carnivores just long enough to dart in, grab bits of meat, and flee.

Our first ancestors undoubtedly lived largely on fruits and vegetables, however, as well as seeds, roots, corms, and rhizomes.[13] Sedges, water lilies, and cattails—a veritable supermarket of carbohydrates—must have been easy to collect at the edge of lakes and rivers.[14] With just a stick and a stone, our first forebears could have eaten a rich variety of fruits, nuts, and berries too.

Their dinners must have been interrupted frequently, however. In the more open countryside it is impossible to eat unnoticed. Eating takes time. The big cats, primordial enemies of the primates, were at eye level. And gone was the safety of the forest branches.

So, like Tunnell, our first hominin ancestors probably stayed in the short grass where they could see, kept trees and cliffs in sight, and avoided tall grass, thickets, and the forest fringe where lions snooze. They probably also kept an eye on the local baboon troop. When these creatures got nervous, they became even more vigilant. Then, if a lion surprised them, our ancestors bunched up back to back, rose onto their hind legs, waved their arms and branches, hurled rocks, and screamed.

## Evolution of Bipedalism

They made one last adjustment to ground living—an adaptation that would irrevocably change the course of human history and eventually life on earth. At some point our ancestors began to pick up and *carry* in their arms what food they could collect and scavenge and cart it to a clump of trees or cliff—a place where they could eat unmolested by predators. Tunnell is convinced they never lingered at a kill or carted food to where they slept; instead, they collected, carried, and "dined out."

*And to carry regularly with your hands, you have to walk erect—on two feet instead of four.*

↝

"Man alone has become a biped," Darwin wrote in 1871.[15] Today anthropologists believe that the first hominins adapted bipedalism to collect, scavenge, and carry their meals to safe spots where they could eat in peace. Moreover, carrying a simple sharpened stick, they could pry roots and tubers from the soil. Carrying stones, they could stun a warthog, a baby antelope, or a baboon. Carrying branches, they could scare a jackal or a vulture from its meal. With carrying, they could tote meat *and* vegetables to a safe spot atop a cliff or in the trees.

With bipedalism, they also evolved a metabolically more efficient gait for moving long distances slowly—the natural human stride. Now the head is elevated, good for seeing food and predators. And when these early forebears began to use their hands to carry, they could also begin to use their mouths to make more complex sounds, to warn a friend or signal plans.

What a transformation our ancestors underwent.

With walking, they evolved big toes that rotated to lie parallel to the others. They developed an arch from heel to toe and a second arch across the ball of the foot that together acted as a trampoline, stretching, then springing with each step to propel the body forward. With strong new muscles in the buttocks, a pelvis that had became broad and flat, knees aligned below their hips, and sturdy anklebones, they no longer waddled when they walked. Instead, they almost effortlessly caught themselves as they fell forward—striding much as we do today.

With walking, collecting, and carrying, Lucy's grandmother's grandmother's grandmother's ancestors had found their woodlands and savanna niche.

But bipedalism, I propose, would start a sexual revolution.

## The Monogamy Threshold

When our forebears lived continually in the trees and females walked exclusively on all four limbs, the newborn clung to mother's abdomen. Then, as the infant aged, it rode on mother's back as the female ambled along—unimpeded by her child.

But as they adapted to life largely on the ground, females began to regularly walk erect. Now they had to carry the infant in their arms instead of on their backs.

How could an ancient female carry sticks and stones, jump to catch a hare, dart after a lizard, or hurl stones at lions to drive them from a kill—and carry an infant too? How could a female sit on the dangerous, open ground to dig for roots, collect vegetables, or dip for ants—and protect her child? In the forest, children played among the trees. In the woodlands, on the ground, children had to be carried and watched constantly or they would end up in a lion's belly.

To make matters worse, a mother's load was not symmetrical. She was obliged to carry her infant on one hip. And Johanna Watson has shown that carrying an asymmetric weight, such as a child, uses much more energy than carrying evenly spread cargo.[16]

So I propose that as our forebears began to walk bipedally on a regular basis, mothers went over what is called the monogamy threshold. They began to need extra protection and extra food *while they carried their infants*—or they and their offspring would not survive.

The time was ripe for the evolution of the husband and the father.[17]

## Fatherhood

Pair-bonding is rare in nature. The Nile crocodile, American toad, damsel fish, starfish-eating shrimp, wood roach, dung beetle, horned beetle, and some desert wood lice are all monogamous. Among birds, 90% form pair-bonds.

But only about 3% of mammals form a long-term relationship with a single mate. Among them are some muskrats, some bats, Asiatic clawless otters, beavers, deer mice, dwarf mongooses, the klipspringer, the reedbuck, the dik-dik and a few other antelopes, gibbons and siamangs, some seals, a few South American monkeys, and all of the wild dogs: foxes, wolves, coyotes, jackals, the maned wolf of South America, and the raccoon dog of Japan all form pair-bonds and raise their young as "husband" and "wife."[18]

Monogamy is rare in mammals because it is not normally to a male's genetic advantage to remain with one female when he can copulate with several and pass more of his genes onto posterity. So males of most species, like gorillas, try to accumulate a harem.

They do this in several ways. If a male can defend an asset, such as the best place to eat or breed, several females will simply gather on his real estate; male impalas, for example, compete to win rich grazing pastures where roaming herds of females linger. If resources are so evenly distributed across the landscape that land is not defensible, a male may try to attach himself to a group of females traveling together and guard his entourage against intruding males—as lions do. And when a male cannot sequester a harem one way or another, he may establish a large territory and scramble to mate with several females spread across his range—rather like the milkman who visits house to house. Male orangutans do this.

So it takes very special circumstances before a male will travel with a *single* mate and help her defend her young.

From a feminine perspective, pair-bonding is not normally adaptive either. A male can be more trouble than he is worth. Females of many species prefer to live with female relatives and copulate with visitors; female elephants do this. And if a female needs a male for protection, why not travel in a mixed group and copulate with several males—the common tactic of female chimps.

A host of ecological and biological conditions must be present in the right proportions before perquisites exceed expenses, making monogamy the best—or only—alternative for both males and females of a species.

A proper mixture of these conditions occurs in the lives of monogamous red foxes and eastern robins. And studying the sex lives of these creatures gave me my first important clue to the evolution of monogamy, divorce, and remarriage (serial monogamy) in humankind.[19]

## Fox Love

Female red foxes bear exceedingly helpless, immature babies, a trait known as altriciality.[20] Kits are born blind and deaf. Not only does the vixen bear infantile young, but she often delivers as many as five of them. Moreover, unlike mice that have rich milk and can leave their altricial newborns sleeping in a nest while they forage elsewhere, the female fox has milk that is low in fat and protein, so she must feed her kits constantly for several weeks. She cannot leave her pups to feed herself.

What an ecological conundrum. The female fox will starve to death if she does not have a mate to bring her food while she attends to her helpless kits.

Monogamy is suitable to the male fox, however. These animals live in territories where the resources are spread out. Under normal conditions a male is not able to acquire a piece of property so rich in food and breeding sites that two females are willing to reside on his land and share one mate. But a male can travel with a female and guard her from other males during her peak of estrus (assuring paternity for the litter), then help her raise their altricial young in a small home range.[21]

Monogamy is thus the best alternative for both sexes, and red foxes form pair-bonds to raise their young. But here's the clue: foxes do not bond for life.

In February the vixen begins her mating dance. Typically several suitors dog her heels. At the peak of estrus one becomes her mate. They lick each other's faces, walk side by side, mark their territory, and build several dens as winter wanes. Then, after giving birth in spring, the vixen nurses her pups for almost three weeks while her "husband" returns nightly to feed her a mouse, a fish, or some other delicacy. Through the vibrant summer days and nights, both parents guard the den, train the kits, and hunt for the voracious family. But as summer dies, father returns to the den less and less. In August mother's maternal temper changes too; she drives her kits from the lair and departs herself.

Among foxes the pair-bond lasts only through the breeding season.[22]

Monogamy for the length of the breeding season is also common among birds.

Most birds form a pair-bond for the same reasons foxes do. Because territories generally vary little in their quality of food and breeding sites, a male eastern robin, for example, can rarely acquire a particularly elegant homestead and attract several females to his real estate. But he can defend a small territory and help a single mate rear her (and his) young. Female eastern robins need this help. They deliver several eggs that need incubating, then chicks that need feeding and protecting. Someone must remain with these infants constantly. And since baby eastern robins do not suckle from a teat, males are just as qualified to parent.

As a result of these and other circumstances, eastern robins form pair-bonds to raise their broods.[23]

But here's the clue again: like red foxes, eastern robins do not mate for life. They pair up in the spring and raise one or more broods through the torpid summer months. But when the last of the fledglings fly in August, mates split up to join a flock. Ornithologist Eugene Morton has estimated that in at least 50% of all monogamous avian species, males and females pair *only through a breeding season*—just long enough to raise their young through infancy.[24] The next year a couple may return to the same spot and pair again; more often one dies or disappears, and individuals change mates.

## A Theory on the Evolution of Monogamy and Desertion

Our first hominin ancestors had several things in common with red foxes and eastern robins. In the cradle of humanity our forebears survived by walking, collecting, scavenging, and moving on; nuts, berries, fruit, and meat were spread across the grass. A male nomad could not collect or defend enough resources to attract a harem. Nor could he monopolize the best place to breed because our ancestors had coitus when they rested, then moved along; there was no best place to breed. And even if a male could attract a group of females to follow him, how could he protect them? When lions were not stalking his herd of "wives," bachelors would have lurked behind to steal them. Under normal circumstances polygyny could not work.

But a male could walk beside a single female (within the larger multi-male/multi-female group), guard her during estrus from other males, and help her raise her young—monogamy.

The female's plight was even more compelling. It is unlikely that our first female ancestors bore highly infantile, altricial babies the way women do today, or that they delivered litters. None of the apes bear litters, babies that would tumble from the branches. But, as mentioned above, when our ancestors rose onto two legs from four, females became burdened by their young. They needed help—provisions and protection—at least until they weaned the child.

So as pair-bonding became the *only* alternative for females, and a viable option for males, the brain circuitry for intense romantic attraction and a sense of attachment to a partner evolved.

## The Three- to Four-Year Itch

But why did these early pair-bonds need to be permanent? Perhaps like foxes and robins, once the mother no longer had to carry her infant continually at her side or nurse her baby day and night, her urgent dependency on a protector-provider was reduced.

Her incipient "husband" was less dependent too. To safeguard his genetic future, he had been obliged to protect his offspring until others in the band could begin to help him with the task. As the child grew out of infancy, however, he could depart. *Ancient lovers probably did not need to remain pair-bonded past the infancy of a child, unless a second dependent baby was born.*

And here's a central point of this book: in hunting-gathering societies, human birth intervals tend to be every three to four years.[25]

Among the traditional !Kung, mothers hold their infants near their skin, breast-feed regularly through the day and night, nurse on demand, and offer their breasts as pacifiers. As a result of this constant body contact and nipple stimulation, as well as high levels of exercise and a low-fat diet, ovulation is suppressed and the ability to become pregnant is postponed for about three years. Hence !Kung births are about four years apart. Four years was the usual period between successive births among continually breast-feeding traditional Australian aborigines[26] and the Gainj of New Guinea.[27] Infants were generally also weaned around the third to fourth year among the traditional Yanomamo of Amazonia,[28] the Netsilik Eskimos,[29] the Lepcha of Sikkim,[30] and the Dani of New Guinea.[31]

Much affects birth intervals. But these data suggest that a four-year pattern of birth spacing—caused by frequent exercise, low body weight, and the habit of continual nursing through the day and night—was the regular pattern of birth spacing during our long evolutionary past.[32] Thus the modern worldwide divorce peak—after three to four years of marriage—conforms to the traditional period between human successive births—*three to four years.*

～

So here is my theory. Like pair-bonding in foxes, robins, and many other species that mate only through a breeding season, human pair-bonds originally evolved to last only long enough to raise a single dependent child through infancy—the first three to four years—unless a second infant was conceived.

There certainly must have been variations to this pattern. Some couples did not conceive for months or years after mating. Often a baby must have died in infancy, triggering a return to female cycling, extending the relationship. Some couples probably remained together regardless of infertility because they liked one another or because no other mates were available. A host of factors must have affected the length of primitive pair-bonds.

But as decades turned into centuries and then millennia, those first hominin forebears who remained together *at least long enough* to rear a single child through infancy—about three to four years—enabled this infant to survive the most vulnerable period of its life, selecting for the beginnings of monogamy—and desertion.

The seven-year itch, recast as a three- to four-year human reproductive cycle, may be a biological phenomenon.

## Nature Red in Tooth and Claw

Serial bonding was probably adaptive too.

When asked why all of her marriages failed, Margaret Mead replied, "I have been married three times, and not one of them was a failure." Mead was what my father would have called a rugged individual. But many people idealize lifelong marriage. From a Darwinian perspective, however, there were advantages to serial pairing millions of years ago.

Foremost, genetic variety. When ancestral males and females bred with several partners, they produced more varied young—with more varied talents and abilities. In a climate of unremitting danger, more might survive nature's constant drive to weed out poor strains.

Equally important, the second time around, an ancestral male could pick a younger female more capable of bearing healthy babies;[33] and a female had the opportunity to choose a mate who could provide better protection and support.[34]

Today these patterns still prevail. Men and women often have a child with one mate and then more with a second partner. Men still remarry younger women, and women still remarry with men they think are more caring, more supportive. Although all this recycling can lead to painful social tangles, from a Darwinian perspective having children with more than one individual makes genetic sense.

But was it to a male's genetic advantage to abandon his biological offspring to mate again and possibly acquire responsibilities for stepchildren? Likewise, was it reproductively logical for an ancestral female to subject her children to the whims of a "stepfather"? Darwinian wisdom says it's not adaptive to desert one's own DNA to nurture the protoplasm of another.

The answers to these questions, I think, are simple. The vicissitudes of step-parenting have dramatically increased in modern times. Today Western parents raise their children largely by themselves, and the costs of education and entertainment are high. Children want iPhones, computers, and college educations. Hence step-parenting has considerable economic disadvantages.

But in our prehistoric past, a child joined a multi-age playgroup soon after being weaned, and older siblings, grandparents, and other community members helped nurture them all. The *isolated* nuclear family did not exist. Day care was free. And the costs of education and entertainment were low. So step-parenting (after the infancy of the offspring) was considerably less taxing in the past. In fact, stepparenting is common in traditional societies today, probably for these reasons.

Ancestral children probably did not suffer severely from primitive divorce either, as long as a stepfather appeared after the child had entered a playgroup and had joined the community at large. If a stepfather appeared while the infant was still suckling, however, the consequences for the infant may have been disastrous—due to another harsh reality of nature best illustrated by lions.

When male lions overtake a pride and drive out its former male leader(s), they kill all new infants. From the Darwinian perspective it is not to their advantage to raise offspring they have not sired. The females of the pride quickly return into estrus after their infants die, the new leaders mate with them, and thus these male lions raise cubs with their own DNA.[35]

This pattern of infanticide has its ghastly counterpart in modern people. Today in the United States and Canada some male stepparents kill infant stepchildren. After the stepchild is past age four, however, the rate of infanticide reduces.[36] Here, then, was another reason an ancestral female probably felt freer to switch partners after her child had learned to walk and join community affairs.

## Bonding with the Neighbors

There also may have been cultural advantages to primitive "divorce" and "remarriage." Edward Tylor, a founding father of anthropology, observed in 1889, "Among tribes of low culture there is but one means known of keeping up alliances, and that means is inter-marriage."[37] As he put it, "Marry-out or be killed-out."

Today many gardening peoples of New Guinea, Africa, Amazonia, and elsewhere marry off their children in order to make or keep friends. But these first marriages tend not to last very long.[38] Apparently nobody gets very upset about these divorces either. The marriage agreement has been honored. The alliance between adults has been reinforced. The offspring have returned undamaged. No grandchildren have been produced. And parents are delighted to see their young again.

If the faintest inklings of these attitudes prevailed some four million years ago, why not "marry" more than once? With each new pair-bond social ties would be extended to a band nearby.

Undoubtedly our first forebears were not thinking of their DNA when they deserted one another; people are still largely oblivious of the genetic consequences of their sexual and reproductive lives. But those ancestral males and females who practiced serial bonding some four million years ago in Lucy's day bore more offspring who survived—passing our human penchant for serial pairing across the eons to you and me.

## Caveats

I am not suggesting that our first forebears abandoned each other casually. "Divorce" must have caused chaos, just as it does today. Around the world people argue before they separate. Some commit homicide or suicide. Children get confused, frightened, and displaced. Relatives battle. Sometimes whole communities get involved. Even among other primates, rearrangements in the social order often lead to vicious fights.

Nor am I suggesting that primitive children were independent by age three or four, either nutritionally or emotionally. But children in contemporary hunting-gathering communities begin to join multi-age playgroups at about this age. Older siblings, relatives, friends, and just about everyone else in the community take a greater role in caring for the child as well. In other species these older siblings are called "helpers at the nest," whereas in humans, the mother's adult relatives and friends who help with childcare duties are known as alloparents. Undoubtedly these extra mothers and fathers, seen in a host of other species and all human tribal cultures, existed in prehistoric bands.

Finally, I am not suggesting that *all* males and females in our early prehistory abandoned each other as soon as their offspring began to toddle out of infancy. In fact, modern divorce data show several striking circumstances under which lifelong monogamy occurs—circumstances that undoubtedly led some of our forebears to stick together too.

One circumstance associated with stable, long-term human pair-bonds is increasing chronological age. As you recall, around the world divorce continues to decline after age thirty-four. Perhaps, four million years ago, aging couples remained together in order to support each other and grandparent their children's young—selecting for these modern human tendencies.

Second, lifelong monogamy is most common today among couples in the United Nations sample who have three or more dependent children—a pattern that is also common in traditional societies.[39] Hence the more children you bear with a mate, the more likely you are to stay together. This tendency may also stem from the early days of humankind when parents with several offspring could not desert a large family. Why should they? If parents were compatible—and the mateship was conducive to raising several young—it was genetically advantageous to both partners to mate for life.

Third, lifelong monogamy occurs for an ecological reason. You may remember that divorce is less common in societies where men and women are economically dependent on one another—most notably in societies that use the plow for agriculture. Divorce is also low in herding cultures and other societies where men do the majority of the heavy labor and control important resources that women depend on to survive.

So if either gender was totally dependent on the resources of the other in these early days of humanity, lifelong monogamy was probably the norm.

I doubt this was the general case, however. Our first ancestors most likely traveled in small nomadic groups of four or five mated pairs, their offspring, and sundry single relatives and friends. Meat was a shared luxury. And females were efficient gatherers. The double-income family was the norm, and ancient females were just as economically successful as males. So when partners became caught in a quarrelsome "marriage," either she or he strode off to join another band.

Serial monogamy was probably the most common reproductive strategy during our long prehistoric past.

## Special Friendships

How serial monogamy evolved can only be surmised. Our earliest ancestors probably lived in communities much like those of modern chimps.[40]

Everybody copulated with just about everybody else, except with mother and close siblings. Then gradually monogamy emerged. The lifestyles of olive baboons provide a fascinating model for how pair-bonding could have evolved in these primal hordes.[41]

Olive baboons travel in troops of about sixty animals through the grass of East Africa. Each troop is composed of several female-centered families, each headed by a matriarch surrounded by her children and often her sisters and their young. Like human families in many small towns, one baboon matriline dominates local social life, another family holds second rank, and so forth. And everyone knows who is who.

But most sons leave home at puberty to join a nearby group. And male baboons often enter a new troop by making a "special friendship" with a specific female.

Ray, for example, was a young, healthy, handsome male who appeared at the periphery of one baboon troop, the Pumphouse Gang, soon after anthropologist Shirley Strum began to hunker at the edge herself. Ray remained on the fringe of group activities for several months, a loner. But gradually he made friends with Naomi, a low-ranking female. Every day Ray came closer to Naomi until finally they sat side by side to eat and slept near each other every night. Through Naomi, Ray made friends with other females and eventually he became welcome in the troop.

These "special friendships" have other payoffs.[42] At the height of her monthly estrus, a female baboon forms a consort with a single partner— often with a "special friend." Other males follow the pair, harass them, and try to distract the male and steal the "bride." But if consort partners are also special friends, the female tends to stick close to her "lover," making it difficult for other males to interrupt them. If her "special friend" catches a baby gazelle hidden in the grass, she is the first to get a bite. His vigilance also provides a "buffer zone"—space where she can relax, play with her offspring, and eat undisturbed.

A male in a "special friendship" gets payoffs too. Often this companion becomes the social father of a female's young. He carries, grooms, cuddles, and protects them. But he uses these infants too. If another male threatens him, a male grabs an infant and holds it to his chest. This instantly stops attack. Among baboons, "special friends" are teammates that exchange favors, tit for tat.

Our ancestors probably made "special friendships" long before they descended from the trees. As you recall, chimpanzees sometimes go "on safari" with a consort. But when bipedalism obliged females to carry young through the dangerous open land, thus requiring male protection and provisioning, these friendships could well have turned into deeper, longer-term relationships—the primitive beginnings of human pair-bonding.

How our ancestral relatives met a "spouse" or "mate" is relatively easy to explain. Parties of four or five females, their "special friends," and their children, a group large enough to protect itself yet small enough to move quickly, probably traveled together.[43] Most likely the territories of these bands overlapped. This way a meal missed by one group of these first ancestors was collected by the next to wander by.

In many primate species either males or females leave their natal group at puberty, so it seems probable that when groups met, adolescents occasionally switched residence. In the woodlands of Africa four million years ago, individuals probably grew up within a large, loosely connected network of several different communities. From among these individuals the young made "special friends" and then developed pair-bonds.

Females were probably attracted to males who were friendly, attentive, and willing to share their food, while males may have been drawn to sexy females from high-status families. During a female's estrus, her mate undoubtedly tried to guard her from the advances of other males, perhaps not always effectively. Males and females probably sneaked off with other lovers when they could. But together a mated pair roamed the grass beneath the woodland trees. Together they collected and shared their food. Together they protected and raised their child *at least through infancy*.

Then one morning, if the partnership had become boring or stressful, either he or she left the band to travel with a new "special friend" in a different group.

## The Mixed Human Reproductive Strategy

Evolved obsolescence of the attachment system in the brain? The serially monogamous lifestyles of some birds and mammals, the conduct of nonhuman primates, the daily lives of people in hunter-gatherer societies, and modern patterns of marriage and divorce around the world all lead me to suspect that by 3.2 million years ago, Lucy had already adopted our basic human mixed reproductive strategy: serial social monogamy and, for some, clandestine adultery.

This reproductive strategy had several parts. Young and childless couples tended to form short-term pair-bonds, desert each other, and bond again. Couples with one or two children tended to remain together at least long enough to raise their young through infancy; then many "divorced"; then they picked new mates. Couples with three or more children tended to bond long-term. Aging couples tended to stay together. And some males and females were adulterous along the way.

Not everyone followed this reproductive script; many still do not. But because these patterns appear across the continents, they probably evolved with genesis.

⁓

In the movie *The African Queen*, Katharine Hepburn remarks to Humphrey Bogart, "Nature, Mr. Allnut, is what we were put on this earth to rise above." Can we rise above this natural heritage?

Of course we can. Our contemporary marriage patterns are a testament to the triumph of culture and personality over natural human predispositions. Over half of all American marriages last for life; many marital partners are faithful to their spouses. The world is full of people who marry once and forgo adultery. Some men have harems; some women have harems. Some of us even choose celibacy or childlessness—genetic death. So malleable an animal is Man.

But we have whisperings within.

And with the evolution of serial monogamy and clandestine adultery would emerge powerful feelings of attachment, abandonment, and love addiction. Love—in all its myriad forms—would take possession of our lives.

8
_____

# The Tyranny of Love

## Evolution of Attachment and Love Addictions

We are never so defenseless against suffering as
when we love.

—SIGMUND FREUD

To see her smile, to hear his voice, to watch her walk, to recall a charming moment or witty remark—the slightest perception of one's sweetheart sends a tidal wave of exhilaration through the brain. "This whirlwind, this delirium of Eros," wrote poet Robert Lowell, one of millions, if not billions, of people who have experienced the engulfing storm of romantic love. What a great equalizer this passion is—reducing poets and presidents, academics and technicians, to the same stuttering state of anticipation, hope, agony, and bliss.

Yet, the brain cannot sustain this revved-up state forever. Some people maintain that smitten feeling for only weeks or months. If a couple has a real barrier to their relationship, such as an ocean or a spouse, they can sometimes maintain this ecstasy for several years. And in our brain scanning study of people married an average of twenty-one years, we have proven that romantic love can sometimes last for decades.

But that intense euphoria of early romance often begins to wane. And as the excitement and novelty subside, calmer feelings of deep union begin to flourish. Psychologist Elaine Hatfield calls this "companionate love," which she defines as "a feeling of happy togetherness with someone whose life has become deeply entwined with yours."[1] I believe this companionate love is generated by a distinct brain system—that of attachment.

Romantic love; attachment: these two types of loving are easily distinguished by men and women around the world. The Taita of Kenya say that love comes in two forms: an irresistible longing, a "kind of sickness"; and a deep, enduring affection for another.[2] Brazilians say, "Love is born in a glance and matures in a smile."[3] For the Koreans, *sarang* is a word close to the Western concept of romantic love, while *chong* is more like feelings of long-term attachment.

&#8766;

The progression of love is also well noted around the world. Abigail Adams, the wife of America's second president, wrote to her husband, John, in 1793, "Years subdue the ardor of passion, but in lieu thereof friendship and affection deep-rooted subsists."[4] Nisa, the !Kung woman of the Kalahari Desert whom I mentioned earlier, also explained this arc vividly, saying, "When two people are first together, their hearts are on fire and their passion is very great. After a while, the fire cools and that's how it stays. They continue to love each other, but it's in a different way—warm and dependable."[5]

In spite of this common course of love, the three basic brain systems for mating that I have elsewhere proposed—lust, romantic love, and attachment—can actually ignite in any order. Some people have sex first, then fall in love. Some fall madly in love with someone they just met, then have sex several weeks down the road. Some even build a deep attachment to a friend at work or in their social circle, then later fall madly in love and have sex with him or her.

Yet, generally, feelings of lust and passionate romantic love are triggered first, followed by feelings of deep attachment—what psychologist Theodor Reik called the warm "afterglow."

&#8766;

Westerners love romantic love. Our movies, plays, operas, ballets, songs, and poems all celebrate this passion, what the ancient Greeks called "madness from the gods." We revel in the sex drive too. But I think attachment—that sense of contentment, sharing, and cosmic oneness with another—is the most elegant of these three basic drives. As you walk together holding hands, as you sit next to one another reading or watching TV in the evening, as you laugh together at a movie or stroll arm-in-arm through a park or on the beach, your souls feel merged. All the world's your paradise.

Perhaps Lucy felt this calm, this paradise, as she lay in the arms of a longtime "special friend" beside a shallow, blue-green lake in today's Ethiopia some 3.2 million years ago. I say this because feelings of partner attachment are deeply woven into the mammalian brain. This brain system probably evolved along with human pair-bonding long ago.

## Companionate Love

The contemporary psychological investigation of human attachment began with a British psychiatrist, John Bowlby,[6] and an American psychologist, Mary Ainsworth,[7] who proposed that, to promote the survival of their young, primates have evolved an innate attachment system designed to motivate infants to seek comfort and safety from their primary caregiver, generally mother.

Since then extensive research has been done on the behaviors, feelings, and biological mechanisms associated with this attachment system in human adults and other creaturess.[8] Moreover, researchers have proposed that these attachment circuits remain active throughout the life course—serving as a foundation for emotional commitment between pair-bonded partners for the purpose of raising offspring.[9]

Today we know some of the neural foundations of this "companionate love." But to grasp how this brain system generates the sensation of attachment to a sweetheart, I must reintroduce you to some American Midwesterners: prairie voles.

## Satisfaction Hormones

As you may recall from chapter 2 on romantic love, these brown-gray, mouse-like rodents become attracted to specific partners—an animal magnetism now linked foremost with the dopamine system in the mammalian brain.

Unlike most mammals, however, prairie voles then form a pair-bond to rear their young; some 90% mate for life. And today scientists have pinpointed a primary cause of this attachment behavior in male prairie voles. As the male ejaculates in a female, the activity of vasopressin increases in specific brain regions, triggering a cascade of responses including his spousal and parenting zeal.[10]

Is vasopressin nature's cocktail for male attachment?

Probably. When scientists injected vasopressin into the brains of *virgin* male prairie voles reared in the lab, these males immediately began to defend their mating and parenting territory from other males. And when each was introduced to a female, he became instantaneously possessive of her.[11] Moreover, when these scientists blocked the production of vasopressin in the brain, male prairie voles acted like rakes instead—copulating with a female, then abandoning her to mate with another.

More remarkable, when neuroscientist Larry Young and colleagues modified a harmless virus to carry the genetic code for vasopressin receptors and injected the virus into males of another species, meadow voles (creatures that do not form pair-bonds), these animals also began to make solid attachments to their current sexual partners.[12] And most important to this book: men with related genes for vasopressin transmission also tend to make more stable partnerships.[13]

The paternal instinct, it appears, has at least one biological ingredient: vasopressin. I suspect this neural circuitry had evolved in hominins by the time that Lucy and her "special friend" were cradling one another 3.2 million years ago.

⌒

"I love thee to the level of every days / Most quiet need by sun and candlelight," wrote poet Elizabeth Barrett Browning. Few poets write about attachment, perhaps because this sense of cosmic union rarely propels one from the warmth of bed to write ecstatic verse in the dead of night. Barrett Browning's lines are an exception. They ring of deep attachment. And as she was writing them, she may have been flooded by another chemical now associated with feelings of attachment: oxytocin—a neurochemical closely related to vasopressin and equally ubiquitous in nature.[14]

Like vasopressin, oxytocin is made in the hypothalamus. Unlike vasopressin, oxytocin is released in all female mammals (including women) during the birthing process. It initiates contractions of the uterus and stimulates the mammary glands to produce milk. But oxytocin also stimulates bonding between a mother and her infant. And more and more data now indicate that oxytocin can also produce feelings of attachment to a preferred mating partner.[15]

You have undoubtedly felt the power of these "cuddle chemicals," as vasopressin and oxytocin are sometimes called. At orgasm, the activities of oxytocin spike in men and women.[16] These "satisfaction hormones" undoubtedly contribute to your sense of fusion, closeness, and attachment after sweet sex with a beloved.

## The Web of Love

So I believe we have evolved these three powerful brain systems to orchestrate our social and reproductive lives. The *sex drive* motivates us to seek a range of mating partners. *Romantic love* drives us to focus our mating energy on a single individual at a time. And feelings of deep *attachment* enable us to remain with this special other at least long enough to rear a single child through infancy together.

Each of these basic drives produces different behaviors, feelings, hopes, and dreams. And each is associated primarily with different neurochemical systems. Lust is associated primarily with the hormone testosterone, in both men and women. Romantic love is linked with the natural stimulant, dopamine, and perhaps also with norepinephrine and low activity of serotonin. While feelings of deep attachment are produced principally by the neuropeptides, oxytocin and vasopressin.

And all are *survival mechanisms* that run along primitive circuits of the human mind.

So I shall propose that these brain systems for lust, romantic love and attachment began to take their human forms soon after our forebears descended from the fast-disappearing trees of Africa to walk on two feet instead of four and form pair-bonds to rear their helpless young at least through infancy as a team.

Lucy loved, some 3.2 million years ago. She felt sexual craving, passionate rapture, and deep feelings of attachment toward her mate—a symphony, sometimes even a cacophony of joyous, exciting, and calming sensations.

~

But the evolution of these brain systems most likely also caused havoc in Lucy's life—as they do today—due to one of nature's tricks: these three brain systems are not always well connected. Indeed, you can feel profound attachment for a long-term spouse *while* you feel romantic passion for someone in the office or your social circle, *while* you feel the sex drive for yet others. You can even lie in bed at night and swing from one feeling to the next. There is a committee meeting in session in your head as you swing from one feeling to another.

Indeed, we seem emotionally unfinished, crippled by the complications this wiring can cause—leading to feelings of possessiveness, jealousy, abandonment, rage, and love addiction. All, I suspect, are primitive, ubiquitous, and enduring legacies that have come across the eons from Ardi's and then Lucy's days.

## Jealousy

"The green-eyed monster which doth mock the meat it feeds on." So colorfully did Shakespeare describe jealousy—this intense human affliction, a combination of possessiveness and suspicion of a partner. Jealousy can arise at any time in a relationship. When you are head over heels in love, when you are snugly attached, while you are philandering yourself, after you have been rejected, even after you have walked away from a partnership, the green-eyed monster can come calling.

Psychological tests of American men and women show that neither gender is routinely more jealous than the other—although the sexes handle their jealousy differently. Women are generally more willing to pretend indifference to patch up a sullied partnership; women are also more inclined to try to seduce or struggle to understand and discuss the situation. Men try to challenge their rival, or look more important, or shower their sweetheart with gifts and compliments. Men are also more inclined to leave a mate when they feel jealous. And those of either sex who feel inadequate, insecure, or overly dependent tend to be more suspicious and possessive.

The green-eyed monster can be dangerous too. In records collected in sixty-six cultures, Jankowiak and Hardgrave found that 88% of men and 64% of women have turned to physical violence when they felt betrayed; indeed, male jealousy is a leading cause of spousal homicide in the United States today.[17]

Jealousy is not unique to Westerners, either.[18] An aboriginal man of Arnhem Land, Australia, expressed this vividly: "We Yolngu are a jealous people and always have been since the days we lived in the bush in clans. We are jealous of our wife or husband, for fear she or he is looking at another. If a husband has several wives he is all the more jealous, and the wives are jealous of each other. . . . Make no mistake, the big J is part of our nature."[19]

Jealousy appears to have animal antecedents too, because male and female animals of many species behave in proprietary ways. In fact, this possessiveness is so common in birds and mammals that ethologists refer to it as "mate guarding."[20]

## Mate Guarding

Male gibbons, for example, drive other males from the family territory, while female gibbons drive off other females. On one occasion Passion, a female chimp at the Gombe Stream Reserve, Tanzania, solicited a young male. He ignored her sexy gestures and began to copulate with her daughter, Pom. Appearing incensed, Passion rushed up and slapped him hard.[21]

A more compelling example of this possessiveness has been documented in bluebirds. In a test of "cuckoldry-tolerance," anthropologist David Barash interrupted the annual mating ritual of a pair of mountain bluebirds that had just begun to build their nest. While the cock was out foraging, Barash placed a stuffed male bluebird about a meter from their home. The resident male returned and began to squawk, hover, and snap his bill at the dummy. But he also attacked his "wife," pulling some primary feathers from her wing. She fled. Two days later a new "wife" moved in.[22]

Wife-beating by a jealous male bluebird?

Alas, this possessiveness has genetic logic. Jealous males of any species will guard their partners more assiduously; thus jealous males are more likely to sire young and pass on their DNA. Jealous females who drive off other females, on the other hand, acquire more protection and resources from their mates—additional assets for themselves and their offspring. Jealousy helps curb philandering in females and desertion by males—selecting for whatever it is in the human brain that produces a jealous rage. Most likely vasopressin is involved, because vasopressin stimulates male prairie voles to guard their mates.[23]

Our human craving for sex; our appetite for romance; our sense of merging attachment with a mate; our possessive jealousy; our restlessness during long relationships; our perennial optimism about our next sweetheart: these passions drag us like a kite upon the wind as we soar and plunge unpredictably from one feeling to another. But of all the kaleidoscopic emotions linked with our ancestral disposition for *serial* monogamy, perhaps none is more painful than dismissal by a lover: abandonment—leading to love addiction.

## Love Addicts

"When we want to read of the deeds of love, whither do we turn? To the murder column." George Bernard Shaw knew the power of romantic love and attachment. Both, I will maintain, are addictions—wonderful addictions when the relationship is going well; horribly negative addictions when the partnership breaks down. Moreover, these love addictions evolved a long time ago, as Lucy and her relatives and friends roamed the grass of East Africa some 3.2 million years ago.

Take romantic love. Even a happy lover shows all of the characteristics of an addict. Foremost, besotted men and women crave emotional and physical union with their beloved. This craving is a central component of all addictions. Lovers also feel a rush of exhilaration when thinking about him or her, a form of "intoxication." As their obsession builds, the lover seeks to interact with the beloved more and more, known in addiction literature as "intensification." They also think obsessively about their beloved, a form of intrusive thinking fundamental to drug dependence. Lovers also distort reality, change their priorities and daily habits to accommodate the beloved, and often do inappropriate, dangerous, or extreme things to remain in contact with or impress this special other. Even one's personality can change, known as "affect disturbance." Indeed, many smitten humans are willing to sacrifice for their sweetheart, even die for him or her. And like addicts who suffer when they can't get their drug, the lover suffers when apart from the beloved—"separation anxiety."

Trouble really starts, however, when a lover is rejected. Most abandoned men and women experience the common signs of *drug withdrawal*, including protest, crying spells, lethargy, anxiety, sleep disturbances (sleeping way too much or way too little), loss of appetite or binge eating, irritability, and chronic loneliness. Lovers also *relapse* the way addicts do. Long after the relationship is over, events, people, places, songs, or other external cues associated with the abandoning partner can trigger memories. This sparks a new round of craving, intrusive thinking, compulsive calling, writing, or showing up—all in hopes of rekindling the romance.

Because romantic love is regularly associated with a suite of traits linked with all addictions, several psychologists have come to believe that romantic love can potentially *become* an addiction.[24]

I think romantic love *is* an addiction—as I have mentioned, a *positive* addiction when one's love is reciprocated, nontoxic, and appropriate; and a disastrously *negative* addiction when one's feelings of romantic love are inappropriate, poisonous, unreciprocated, and/or formally rejected.[25]

## The Positive Addiction of Happy Love

"If an idea is not absurd, there is no hope for it," Einstein reportedly said. Few academics and laymen regard romantic love as an addiction—because they believe that all addictions are pathological and harmful.[26] Data do not support this notion, however.

When neuroscientists Andreas Bartels and Semir Zeki compared the brains of happily-in-love participants with the brains of euphoric addicts who had just injected cocaine or opioids, many of the same regions in the brain's reward system became active. Moreover, when my colleagues reanalyzed our data on seventeen men and women who were happily in love, we found activity in the nucleus accumbens (unpublished data), a brain region linked with all of the addictions—including the cravings for heroin, cocaine, nicotine, alcohol, amphetamines, opioids, even gambling, sex, and food.

Men and women who are intensely and happily in love are addicted to their partner. So my brain scanning partner, Dr. Lucy Brown, has proposed that romantic love is a *natural* addiction, "a normal altered state" experienced by almost all humans.[27]

And I have proposed that the brain circuitry for romantic love had evolved by Lucy's time—to motivate our ancestors to focus their mating energy on a specific partner, thereby conserving mating time and energy, initiating copulation and reproduction, and triggering feelings of attachment and subsequent mutual parenting to assure the future of their DNA.[28]

But romantic love can cause havoc in our lives—particularly when we've been dumped.

## The Negative Addiction of the Rejected Brain

To learn more about the neural systems associated with *rejection* in love, my colleagues and I used functional magnetic resonance imaging (fMRI) to study ten women and five men who had recently been dumped.[29] The average length of time since the initial rejection was sixty-three days. All participants scored high on the Passionate Love Scale,[30] a self-report questionnaire that measures the intensity of romantic feelings. All said that they spent more than 85% of their waking hours thinking of the person who rejected them. And all yearned for their abandoning partner to return.

The results were stunning.

Brain activations occurred in several regions of the reward system. Included were regions of the ventral tegmental area (VTA) associated with feelings of intense *romantic love*; the ventral pallidum, associated with feelings of deep *attachment*; the insular cortex and the anterior cingulate, associated with physical *pain*, *anxiety*, and the *distress* associated with physical pain; and the nucleus accumbens and orbitofrontal/prefrontal cortex, brain regions associated with *assessing one's gains and losses*—as well as *craving* and *addiction*.[31] Most relevant to our story, activity in several of these brain regions has been correlated with the craving for cocaine and other drugs.[32]

In short, as our brain scanning data show, these discarded lovers are still madly in love with and deeply attached to their rejecting partner. They are in physical and mental pain. Like a mouse on a treadmill, they are obsessively ruminating on what they've lost. And they are craving reunion with their rejecting beloved—addiction.

Few of us get out of love alive. In one American college community, 93% of both sexes reported that they had been spurned by someone they passionately loved, while 95% reported that they had rejected someone who was deeply in love with them.[33] And this can be just the first disappointment. Many may get dumped again in later life.

There is a pattern to this trajectory of abandonment and recovery. During the first stage, the *protest phase*, the deserted lover works obsessively to regain the abandoning partner's affection. As *resignation/despair* sets in, the lover gives up hope and slips into depression.[34] Both are linked with the dopamine system in the brain. And I suspect that both were deeply embedded in the hominin mind by the time Lucy was loving, perhaps even losing a beloved, long ago.

## The Protest Phase of Rejection

"The less my hope, the hotter my love." Over two thousand years ago, Terence, the Roman poet, perfectly captured this experience. When lovers encounter barriers to their romantic feelings, their passion intensifies— what I call *frustration-attraction*.[35] Adversity heightens feelings of romantic love. This phenomenon is rooted in the brain. When a reward is delayed in coming, neurons of the brain's dopamine system continue their activity[36]— sustaining one's feelings of intense romantic love. Addiction has set in.

Stress elevates this dopamine response. When mammals first experience severe stress, among their bodily reactions is an increase in the activity of central dopamine and norepinephrine and a suppression of central serotonin, known as the "stress response."[37]

Rejected lovers can also suffer from *frustration-aggression*, what psychologists call "abandonment rage."[38] Even when a rejecting partner departs with compassion and graciously honors his or her responsibilities as a friend or co-parent, many abandoned people oscillate between heartbreak and fury—another response with neural correlates. The primary rage system is closely connected to centers in the prefrontal cortex that anticipate rewards.[39] So as a person begins to realize that an expected reward is in jeopardy, even unattainable, these regions of the prefrontal cortex stimulate the amygdala and trigger rage, a trait that stresses the heart, raises blood pressure and suppresses the immune system.[40]

This rage response to unfulfilled expectations is well known in other mammals. When a cat is petted, for example, it purrs. When this pleasurable stimulation is withdrawn, it sometimes bites.

Indeed, romantic passion and abandonment rage have much in common. Both are associated with bodily and mental arousal; both produce obsessive thinking, focused attention, motivation, and goal-directed behaviors; and both cause intense yearning—either for union with or retaliation against the rejecting lover.[41]

Moreover, these feelings of romantic love and rage can act in tandem. In a study of 124 dating couples, Bruce Ellis and Neil Malamuth reported that romantic love and "anger/upset" react to different kinds of information. The lover's level of anger/upset oscillates in response to events that undermine the lover's goals, such as a mate's infidelity, lack of emotional commitment, and/or rejection. The lover's feelings of romantic love fluctuate in response to events that advance the lover's goals, such as a partner's visible social support during outings with relatives and friends, or a direct declaration of love and fidelity. Thus, romantic love and anger/upset can operate concurrently, adding intensity to one's rejection addiction.

We must have inherited this protest response, for it stems from a basic mammalian mechanism that gets triggered when *any* kind of social attachment is ruptured.[42] Take the puppy. When it is removed from mother and put into the kitchen by itself, it immediately begins to pace, frantically leaping at the door, barking and whining in protest. Isolated baby rats emit ceaseless ultrasonic cries; they hardly sleep because their brain arousal is so intense.[43] The purpose of this protest: to increase alertness and stimulate an abandoned creature to object, search, and call for help.

Protest, the stress response, frustration-attraction, abandonment rage, craving, withdrawal symptoms: all play a role in the worldwide incidence of crimes of passion.[44] Like all addictions, romantic love can lead to violence.

## Resignation / Despair

Eventually, however, the abandoned lover gives up. He or she stops the pursuit of the beloved, ushering in the second general phase of romantic rejection, resignation/despair.[45]

During this stage, the rejected one slips into feelings of lethargy, despondency, melancholy and depression,[46] known as the despair response.[47] In a study of 114 men and women who had been rejected by a partner within the past eight weeks, 40% experienced clinically measurable depression.[48] Some broken-hearted lovers even die from heart attacks or strokes caused by their depression.[49] Others commit suicide.

Surely most rejected lovers feel this sadness during the protest phase as well, but it's likely to escalate as all hope vanishes.

This despair has been associated with several brain networks. Yet, once again, dopamine circuits are most likely involved. As the rejected partner comes to believe that the reward will never come, dopamine-producing cells in the reward system of the brain *decrease* their activity,[50] producing lethargy, despondency, and depression.[51] Short-term stress escalates the production of dopamine and norepinephrine. Long-term stress suppresses the activity of these neurochemicals, producing depression instead.[52]

Hasn't nature overdone it?

Protest, stress, rage, resignation, and despair: this cataclysmic response to rejection seems highly unproductive. Rejected men and women have wasted precious courtship time and metabolic energy. They have lost essential economic and financial resources. Their social alliances have been jeopardized. Their daily rituals and habits have been altered. They may have lost property, even children. Their personal happiness and self-esteem have suffered.[53] And rejected lovers may have lost a vital reproductive opportunity, possibly even a parenting partner to help them rear their young—jeopardizing their genetic future. Romantic rejection has severe social, psychological, economic, and genetic consequences.

Why can't we just move on with life?

Because these feelings of protest and despair may be adaptive.

The protest response may have evolved to motivate the lover to entice a rejecting sweetheart to resume the partnership, while abandonment rage may have evolved to increase estrangement instead (no one likes angry people), obliging the disappointed lover to start looking for someone new. The despair response may have evolved to enable the rejected lover to send clear, honest signals to relatives and friends that they need help.[54] And the depression may have evolved to give rejected lovers time to rest and plan their future. Indeed, mildly depressed people make clearer assessments of themselves and others.[55]

We have inherited strong feelings and behaviors dedicated to helping us renew or depart from a failing partnership. Both strategies ultimately further our reproductive goals.[56] They were probably in place over three million years ago, along with our human drive to love and love again.

## Letting Go of Love

Sociologist Robert Weiss, a divorcé, began to study marital separation among members of two self-help groups, Parents without Partners and Seminars for the Separated. Then, from discussions with 150 people who attended these groups, he began to see more patterns to detachment,[57] data that adds the *psychological* component to this phenomenon: letting go of love.

First, he reported, the rejected man or woman is in *shock*, often the first stage after being dumped. Despite all of the bitter disappointments, failed promises, vicious battles, and rank humiliations, home continues to be where one's mate is; anywhere else is exile. If the relationship ends abruptly, the rejected person often responds with denial for several days, sometimes for as long as two weeks.

Eventually, however, reality sets in. "She" or "he" is gone.

Then, the *transition phase* begins. This psychological state seems to stretch across both of the biological phases, protest and resignation. Time hangs heavy. Many of life's daily rituals have evaporated; one hardly knows what to do with all the blanks. Protest, anger, panic, regret, self-doubt, and consuming sadness overcome the rejected individual. Some feel euphoria or a sense of freedom. But this joy can't last. Moods swing relentlessly; a decision made this morning vanishes this afternoon. Some turn to alcohol or drugs or sports or friends; others rely on psychiatrists, counselors, or self-help books. Some make ridiculous compromises or accept hideous battering for fear of losing "him" or "her." Like heroin addicts, they are chemically wedded to their mates.[58]

And they start to review the relationship—obsessively. Hour upon hour the rejected lover rewinds old memories, playing out the cozy evenings and touching moments, the arguments and silences, the jokes and snide remarks, listening endlessly for clues to why "he" or "she" departed. Then, with time, the tormented person develops an account of who did what to whom. Themes and key incidents dominate this mental narrative as the individual fixates on the worst humiliations. Eventually, however, they build a plot with a beginning, a middle and an end. This account is a bit like a description of an auto accident. Perceptions are garbled. But the process is important. Once in place, the story can be addressed, worked on, and, ultimately, discarded.

Sometimes this psychological transitional phase lasts a year. Any setback, such as an unsuccessful reconciliation or a rejection by a new lover, can hurl the sufferer back into shattered anguish. But as he or she develops a coherent lifestyle, the *recovery phase* begins. Gradually the abandoned individual acquires a new identity, some self-esteem, new friends, fresh interests, and some resiliency. The past begins to loosen its stranglehold. Now he or she can proceed with living.

But there was a provocative finding in Weiss's study. He noticed that the entire process of rejection and recovery regularly took *two to four* years, "with the average being closer to four than to two." The number four has come up again. Not only do we tend to form pair-bonds for about three to four years; we also tend to recover from them in a three to four-year period.

The human animal seems driven by a tide of feelings that ebb and flow to an internal beat, a rhythm that emerged when our ancestors first descended from the trees of Africa and developed a tempo to their relationships that was in synchrony with their natural breeding cycle—three to four years. Perhaps the brain's systems for dopamine, vasopressin, oxytocin, and other neurochemicals orchestrate this rhythm, escalating when you fall in love, changing as you begin to feel deep attachment and cosmic union, then eventually becoming desensitized or overloaded, leading to indifference or restlessness that slowly eats your love and leads to separation—a hardship that can trigger the mother of all addictions, addiction to a mate.

Each of us is unique, of course. People who were securely attached to their parents during childhood, those who can easily develop new friendships, those who are more self-confident, and those with other subtle psychological advantages may bounce back from a rejection faster. But we all suffer from addictive love—perhaps in different ways.

## Romance Junkies

As you know from chapter 2, I have proposed that humanity has evolved four broad, basic styles of thinking and behaving, each associated primarily with one of four basic brain systems: dopamine, serotonin, testosterone, and estrogen. I am speculating here, but I suspect that those men and women of each cognitive and behavioral style may be predisposed to handle the pain and craving of love addiction in a somewhat different way.

*Explorers*, those who express more of the traits linked with the dopamine system in the brain, may be more likely to become *romance junkies*. These men and women like novelty. They seek thrills and adventures—in the bedroom, in sports, travel, intellectual pursuits, alternate lifestyles, and/or drugs. Many are susceptible to boredom; and many tend to be impulsive, mentally flexible, curious, energetic, full of ideas, open to new experiences, and creative. So, despite their intense feelings of romantic passion, Explorers may have more difficulty committing to a long-term partner. And when they do, they may be more restless, more predisposed to infidelity, and more likely to abandon a mate to seek the dopamine rush of a new romance—romance junkies.

## Attachment Junkies

*Builders*, or those expressing more of the traits linked with the serotonin system, may be predisposed to becoming *attachment junkies* instead. These men and women observe social norms. They are inclined to follow rules, make plans, and adhere to schedules. They are cautious, conventional, and often religious. They like to go to familiar places and do familiar things. And they are willing to sacrifice their needs to obey the rules and fit in with their social group and society at large. Builders take their marital duties seriously. So I suspect these men and women may be disproportionately inclined to remain in a relationship long after it has become defunct—unwilling to break their vows, regardless of their pain and loneliness.

## Violence Junkies

Those more expressive of the testosterone system, what I call *Directors*, may be more likely to become violent when rejected. These men and women like action and take action. They also tend to be less empathetic, less able to express their frustrations verbally, and less socially skilled. So they may be more inclined to narcissistic stalking or impulsive physical violence—including impulsive suicide or homicide. Some data support my hypothesis: men are far more likely than women to stalk a rejecting partner, as well as batter or kill her.[59] And men are two to three times more likely to commit suicide after being rejected.[60]

## Despair Junkies

*Negotiators*, those who tend to express more traits linked with the estrogen and oxytocin systems, may be disproportionately susceptible to pathological rumination, clinical depression and attempted suicide—what I call *despair junkies*. I suggest this because these men and women (mostly women) tend to be agreeable, verbally skilled, intuitive, empathetic, trusting, nurturing, and driven to make social attachments. They are also emotionally expressive, introspective, and have a good memory. So Negotiators may tend to obsess about the partnership—continually raising the ghost and re-traumatizing themselves. This rumination may lead to a disproportionate susceptibility to clinical depression and attempted suicide.

Some data support my theory. Rejected women report more severe feelings of depression, as well as more chronic strain and rumination after being rejected.[61] Women are also more likely to talk endlessly about their trauma.[62]

## Animal Love

Are we alone in our drive to court and love and leave each other then love again? Or is the stallion that paws the ground, fills his nostrils with the scent of a receptive female, and mounts this mare feeling infatuation too? Does the dog fox feel attachment as he nudges an appetizing dead mouse toward his hungry vixen in their den? Are the robins that desert the nest in autumn glad to part? Do many animals seek a new partner with energetic zeal as the next mating season starts? Have billions of animals over millions of years felt the ecstasy of attraction, the peace of attachment, the agony of abandonment, and the return of passion when they begin a new mating dance with another?

Many scientists believe that the basic human emotions and motivations arise from distinct brain systems and that these brain networks derive from mammalian, even avian precursors.[63] For example, all birds and mammals have a hypothalamus deep in the brain. This little factory plays a major role in steering sexual behavior. It has changed very little in the last seventy million years and is very similar across mammalian species.[64] Animals feel lust.

The limbic system in the brain, which plays a central role in feelings of rage, fear, and pleasure, is rudimentary in reptiles. But it is well developed in birds and mammals. Higher animals are capable of fury, terror, and joy.[65]

The general pathways for the dopamine, vasopressin, and oxytocin systems—linked with feelings of attraction and attachment in humans—play similar roles among prairie voles and people. We even have similar genes in the vasopressin system,[66] suggesting that a related biological system plays a role in human attachment.

Most revealing: no free-ranging creature on this planet will have sex with just anyone who comes along. They are attracted to some and avoid others.[67] I call it animal magnetism or courtship attraction,[68] and I believe that animals feel this deep attraction to *specific* others (albeit often very briefly)—what we call romantic love.

Other creatures even express the same behaviors when they are "in love," including increased energy, focused attention, obsessive following, licking, patting, snuggling, and other affiliative gestures, possessive mate guarding, and intense motivation to win and keep a preferred mating partner at least long enough to ensure insemination or survival of the young.[69] Such, as you know, was Violet, the little pug dog who was fixated on another pug, Bingo; Throatpouch, the male orangutan in Borneo who was crazy about another orang, Priscilla; and the mallard duck who, as Darwin noted, "swam around the newcomer caressingly . . . with overtures of affection."

Other creatures also display feelings of attachment to a "spouse," building a mutual home in the trees, bushes, grass or dirt, feeding each other, grooming, patting, licking, kissing, maintaining close proximity, and sharing parental chores.

Perhaps all of the world's birds and mammals are servants of a few chemicals that surge through their various nervous systems, directing the ebb and flow of attraction, attachment, and detachment to fit their breeding cycles.

And if animals love, Lucy surely loved.

Lucy probably flirted with the boys she met when communities convened at the beginning of the dry season and then became infatuated with one who gave her meat. She might have lain beside him in the bushes and kissed and hugged, then stayed awake all night, euphoric. As she and her "special friend" wandered together across the plains in search of melons, nuts, or berries, she must have felt exhilaration. When they curled up together, she probably felt the cosmic warmth of attachment too.

But if Lucy's partner returned from scavenging with others and suspected her of philandering, he might have become enraged and attacked his rival with sticks and stones and fists. And if Lucy caught her mate with another female, she may have assaulted both with screams and bites, then tried to ostracize the female from the band. Perhaps she also became bored as they passed their days and nights together, and felt a thrill when she sneaked into the woodlands to kiss another. Probably she even mourned when she and her partner split up one morning to join separate groups. Then she fell in love again.

Like Lucy, those who felt the passion of infatuation formed more secure partnerships with "special friends." Those who sustained feelings of attachment long enough to raise their mutual child through infancy nurtured their own DNA. Those males who crept away occasionally with other lovers spread more of their genes, whereas those females who philandered reaped additional resources for their growing young. And those who left one partner for another had more varied babies. The children of these passionate individuals survived disproportionately, passing along to you and me the brain chemistry for romantic love, attachment, restlessness during long relationships, and the drive to love again.

What an incredible plot. The urge for sex, the intense passion of romantic love, the deep closeness of attachment, the seductive craving to philander, the torment and addiction of abandonment, the hope to mate anew—Lucy's children's children's children's children would pass these kernels of the human psyche through time and chance and circumstance along to you and me. And from this evolutionary history would arise an eternal struggle of the human spirit—the drive to pair, philander, divorce, and pair again.

Westerners adore love. We symbolize it, study it, worship it, idealize it, applaud it, fear it, envy it, live for it, and die for it. Love is many things to many people. But if love is common to all people everywhere and associated with tiny molecules that reside at nerve endings in pathways in the brain, then love is also primitive.

What consequences this brain chemistry would produce. The "husband," "father," "wife," the nuclear family, our myriad conventions of courtship, our human celebrations of marriage, our divorce procedures, our many punishments for adultery, our cultural mores for sexual comportment, and our patterns of family violence: countless customs and institutions would burgeon from our ancestors' simple drive to make and break pair-bonds millions of years ago.

Our restive, churning temperament would also create the evolution of our human sexual anatomy and some fantastical courtship tactics to lure prospective mates into the siren's web.

# 9

## Dressed to Impress

### Nature's Lures for Seduction

Why were we crucified into sex?
Why were we not left rounded off,
and finished in ourselves,
As we began,
As he certainly began,
so perfectly alone?

—D. H. LAWRENCE, "TORTOISE SHOUT"

Vermilion noses, crimson chests, puffy buttocks, stripes and spots and dapples, tufts, crowns, manes, horns, and hairless patches, such are nature's decorations; sexual beings are like ornamented Christmas trees, bearing an arsenal of accoutrements. We humans have a fantastic array ourselves. Among them are large penises, beards, fleshy breasts, puffy reddened lips, continual female sexual receptivity, and other beguiling gendered traits.

Darwin was annoyed by all these ornaments he saw in nature. What use was the peacock's bulky fan of tail feathers? He regarded all these traits as cumbersome, unnecessary handicaps that were detrimental to daily survival. Even worse, they undermined his theory that everything evolved for a purpose.[1] As he complained in a letter to his son, "The sight of a feather in a peacock's tail, whenever I gaze on it, makes me sick."[2]

## Sexual Selection

With time, however, Darwin came to believe that all these flashy embellishments evolved for an essential purpose: courtship—either to fight off wooing competitors, or to attract more and/or better mating partners.

If, for example, a bushy mane made a lion more threatening to other males, or more attractive to females, those males with bushy manes would breed more often and bear more young, passing along this otherwise unnecessary trait. Likewise, if large, strong male elephant seals fought off smaller, weaker ones and then lured a harem during the short breeding season, large males would breed more often—and pass along to their descendants these seemingly useless decorations.

Hence, through endless battles with competitors and magnificent courtship displays to catch the eye of potential partners, the stag evolved its antlers, the peacock its brilliant tail feathers, the elephant seal its lumbering size and excessive weight.

So in *The Descent of Man and Selection in Relation to Sex*, Darwin detailed a corollary to the concept of natural selection: sexual selection.[3]

Darwin was fully aware that sexual selection could not account for all of the differences between the sexes. But the eternal struggle of who will mate and breed with whom is the only explanation for the evolution of some of our more bizarre sexual accoutrements, including the human phallus.

Men have the largest penis in terms of thickness and length of any of our close primate relatives—and these separate assets may have evolved by different means of sexual selection.

Men's thick penises may have emerged in evolution simply because Lucy's female ancestors and their girlfriends *liked* thick penises. A fat phallus distends the muscles of the outer third of the vaginal canal and pulls on the hood of the clitoris, creating friction, making orgasm easier to achieve. And with orgasm, the female cervix may suck sperm into the womb, facilitating pregnancy. So males who had thick penises in Lucy's day may have had more "special friends" and more extra lovers. These males may have produced more children. And, thus, thick penises evolved.

As Darwin explained this female appetite: "The power to charm the female has sometimes been more important than the power to conquer other males in battle."

## Sperm Wars

Men also have long penises, extending, on average, about five inches. These are much longer than those of gorillas, a primate with three times a man's body bulk. Gorillas apparently have small phalluses because they do not compete with their genitals. These creatures live with stable harems. Males are twice the size of females, and they impress competitors with their bulk; long genitals are not part of their display. As a result, a gorilla's erect penis is, on average, about one and a quarter to two inches long.[4]

Male chimps, on the other hand, often solicit a female by spreading their legs, displaying an erect penis and flicking their phallus with a finger as they gaze at a potential partner. A prominent, distinctive penis (albeit on average only three inches long) helps broadcast a male's individuality and sexual vigor, which may lure female chimps. Perhaps our male forebears attempted to entice females with this display too.

The long human male penis may have evolved for a second reason as well—a form of sexual selection known as *sperm competition*. The theory of sperm competition was first developed to explain the mating tactics of insects.[5] Most female insects are highly promiscuous: they copulate with several partners, then they either eject the sperm of each or store it for days, months, or even years. So males compete inside the female's reproductive tract—with their sperm.

A male damselfly, for example, uses his penis to scoop out the sperm of previous suitors before he ejaculates. Male insects also try to dilute the sperm of competitors or push it out of place. Some insert a "mating plug" in the female's genital opening after copulation; others just guard the female until she has deposited her eggs.[6] The long human phallus may be the result of sperm competition too, designed to deposit these swimmers closer to the cervix, thus giving their sperm a head start.[7]

Interestingly, in a study comparing penis length to body size in a range of primate species, Alan Dixson has noted that penis size generally correlates with the living arrangements of the group. Thus male primates that live in a large community of several males and females tend to have larger penises, while males living in a one-male unit tend to have smaller penises for their body size. Humans are exceptional among our close ape relatives. But when compared with a far larger sample of primates, the size of the human phallus suggests that we evolved in groups of one-male units.[8]

Another artifact of early pair-bonding? Perhaps.

Further suggesting the early evolution of pair-bonding is the fact that men have average-sized testicles.

This feature may be best understood by studies of testicle size in chimps and gorillas. Male chimps have large testicles for their body size, and it is thought that they sport these factories because female chimps are promiscuous. Males must deposit a lot of sperm to outcompete other males. Quantity is important. Gorillas, on the other hand, have small testicles, most likely because they copulate infrequently and have little competition from other males.[9]

Men's average-sized testicles may be the result of our dual human reproductive strategy. With serial pairing—and clandestine adultery—our male forebears were subject to more sperm competition than gorillas, but far less than our closest chimp relatives.[10]

Another factor suggesting the early evolution of monogamy is the fact that men's testicles produce fewer sperm than those of chimps. Moreover, human sperm is of poorer quality; indeed, many are abnormal. And men have smaller reservoirs of sperm.[11] Chimps and males of other promiscuous or polygynous species cannot afford to run out of sperm. Nor can they afford to deliver poor-quality sperm that will lose in the battles constantly taking place with other males in the vaginal canal. But males of a monogamous species can afford to have fewer, poorer sperm, as well as less in reserve.

In fact, given our long evolutionary history of pair-bonding, why do men have as much sperm as they do? Perhaps ancestral females liked the shape and size of the male phallus and inadvertently also chose males with a dangling appendage packed with contents.[12]

～

Male–male competition; female choice. Scientists generally emphasize these two aspects of sexual selection because in nature males are more likely to fight among themselves for the privilege of breeding and females are more likely to be choosy about their lovers.[13]

This reasoning has genetic logic. For females of many species, the costs of reproduction are high. Females conceive the embryo, tote the fetus for days, weeks, or months, and often raise their infants largely by themselves. Females are also limited in the number of offspring they can produce. And it takes time to bear and raise each child, brood, or litter. So it is to a female's advantage to choose her partners carefully; she hasn't many opportunities to breed.

For males of most species the costs of reproduction are much lower. Males just donate sperm. Even more important, males can conceive off-spring much more regularly than females—as long as they can fight off other suitors, attract females, and withstand sexual exhaustion. So it is to a male's reproductive advantage to copulate relatively indiscriminately. Thus males of most species invest more time and metabolic energy in courtship, known as *mating effort*, while females of mammalian species invest far more time and metabolic energy in feeding, comforting and rearing infants, known as *parenting effort*.

Because of these differences in parental investment, it is generally males of the species that *compete* among themselves for females and generally females who *choose* between males.

But the alternative forms of sexual selection—males who choose between females and females who compete among themselves to breed—are also seen in nature. People are no exception. Just go to any bar or club or party and watch women compete with one another while men choose among them. As H. L. Mencken summed it up, "When women kiss it always reminds one of prize fighters shaking hands."

In fact, several important female traits may be the result of female–

female competition and males who chose between them in ancient times. Among the most conspicuous traits may be permanently enlarged female breasts.

## Why Did Big Breasts Evolve?

In the 1960s ethologist Desmond Morris proposed that when our ancestors became bipedal, the sexual signals that initially ornamented the rump evolved to decorate the chest and head instead.[14] Hence women evolved everted reddened lips to mimic the lips of the vagina and dangling fleshy breasts to mimic puffy buttocks. Ancestral males were attracted to females with these signs of sexual readiness. So females with bulging breasts bore more young—spreading this trait across the centuries.

Scientists have offered several alternative hypotheses, however. Perhaps breasts evolved to signal "ovulatory potential." Because women of prime reproductive age have more voluptuous breasts than do children or postmenopausal women, ancestral men may have seen these swellings as signs of likely fertility and chosen to mate disproportionately with big-breasted women.[15]

As another theory goes, among primates breasts swell only while a female nurses, so maybe these flags evolved to advertise a woman's ability to reproduce and feed her young[16]—the good-mother signal. Or they may even have evolved as a deceptive sign to trick males into thinking a female was a good reproductive bet.[17]

A last interesting proposition holds that breasts were primarily storehouses of fat, crucial reserves that could aid gestation and lactation, and be drawn upon if food was scarce.[18]

All these theories make genetic sense.

But what a bad design. These protuberances around the mammary glands seem poorly placed. They bobble painfully when a woman runs. They flop forward to block vision when she leans over to collect food. And they can suffocate a suckling child. Moreover, breasts (of any size) are sensitive to touch. A woman's nipples harden at the slightest touch. And for many, fondling the breasts stimulates sexual desire.

So I do not wish to entirely overlook Morris's original theory for the sexual purpose of the female breast: along with several other adaptive purposes for these pillowy appendages, ancestral males may have liked female breasts and bred more often with sexually responsive, busted women—selecting, in part, for this near-universal feminine decor.

⁓

As our early ancestors jockeyed for prized "spouses" and clandestine lovers, other fundamental aspects of human sexuality emerged.

Men have beards, while women have smooth complexions; men develop deep voices at puberty, while women retain mellifluous tones. How come?

Of facial hair, Darwin wrote, "Our male ape-like progenitors acquired their beards as an ornament to charm or excite the opposite sex . . ."[19] But beards could have evolved for several purposes. They enlarge the male face to look more dominant, more fierce. And they hide some of the nuances of facial expressions, making men appear less emotional, less vulnerable. These attributes could impress, even scare other males. Beards are built by testosterone, however, and this feature emerges as boys transform into men. So men's beards must have also appealed to ancestral women as signs of strength, maturity, and virility, while women's smooth complexions may have signaled youth, as well as displayed women's emotions and sexual interest more readily.

Men's low voices are also built by testosterone and signal sexual maturity, so men's gruff tones would have been another trait that menaced other males and attracted females. And maybe, the sweet feminine voice was childlike, unthreatening to men. Indeed, Darwin referred to the high female voice as a musical instrument, concluding, "We may infer that they first acquired musical powers in order to attract the opposite sex."[20]

For whatever reasons, in Lucy's day some males and females bore more young than others did, selecting for the peculiar body ornaments of these individuals—thick, long penises; permanently enlarged breasts; men's beards and low voices; and women's dulcet tones.

⁓

We are indeed naked apes, and the loss of body hair could have been, at least in part, another result of sexual selection. Actually we did not lose our body hair; we have the same number of hair follicles as do the apes. But our human body hair is less developed.

Explanations of this trait, our puny pelage, have cost a lot of ink and paper. The classic explanation is that it evolved as part of a revision in the body's heating and cooling system.

The sweaty jogger. Many believe that in order for our hunting-scavenging-collecting ancestors to lope long distances in search of game, insulating hair was replaced by body fat and sweat glands that poured a cooling liquid film across an exposed chest and limbs when they got too hot. Some argue instead that our ancestors lost their body hair to reduce the frequency of parasitic infestations. Still others think our hairlessness may have evolved in conjunction with our human trait of being born exceedingly immature.[21]

But these human hair patterns may have served as sex attractants too. With a diminutive pelage, the tender areas of the chest and around the groin became more visible, more exposed, more sensitive to touch. Not coincidentally, women evolved less hair around their lips and breasts—places where stimulation can easily lead to intercourse.

And where our ancestors retained hair seems just as much a stimulant to sex as where they lost it. Hair in the underarms and crotch holds the aromas of sweat and sex—odors that are sexually exciting to many people.

Like beards, deep voices, smooth chins, and high voices, some of these human hair patterns appear at puberty—the beginning of the sex season. So the simplest explanation is that all these traits evolved for *several* reasons—among them, to dazzle mates and paramours when our hominin ancestors first emerged from the shrinking forests of Africa to mate and raise their infants as a team.

## The Hourglass Figure

No one knows when ancestral women took on their shapely figure. But today men around the world gravitate to this form—as has been elegantly demonstrated.

Psychologist Devendra Singh displayed an array of line drawings of young women to a group of American men and asked them which body shapes they found particularly attractive.[22] Most chose women whose waist circumference was about 70% of their hips. This experiment was then redone in Britain, Germany, Australia, India, Uganda, and several other places. Responses varied; but many informants favored this same general waist-to-hip ratio.

Then, in a study of 330 artworks from Europe, Asia, the Americas, and Africa, some dating back 32,000 years, Singh found that most women were also depicted with a waist-to-hip ratio of this same general proportion.[23] Interestingly, *Playboy* centerfolds display these proportions too, as do today's supermodels. Even Twiggy, the gaunt supermodel of the 1960s, had a waist-to-hip ratio of exactly 70%.

A woman's waist-to-hip ratio is largely inherited; it is produced by genes. Moreover, although it varies from one woman to the next, this ratio adjusts during ovulation to come closer to 70%.

Why has nature gone to such extraordinary lengths to produce curvaceous women? And why do men around the world appreciate this particular waist-to-hip ratio in women?

Most likely for an evolutionary reason. Women with a waist-to-hip ratio of around 70% are more likely to bear babies, Singh reports. They possess the right amount of fat in the right places—due to high levels of bodily estrogen in relation to testosterone. Women who vary substantially from these proportions find it harder to get pregnant; they conceive later in life; and they have more miscarriages.[24] Egg-shaped, pear-shaped, stick-shaped: differently shaped women also suffer more from chronic diseases such as diabetes, hypertension, heart disease, certain cancers, and problems with circulation. They are prone to various personality disorders too.

So Singh theorizes that the male attraction to a specific female waist-to-hip ratio is a natural preference for healthy, fertile partners. In fact, because this preference is so deeply enmeshed in the male psyche, men of all ages express this taste, even when they have no interest in fathering young themselves.

And if men go for the hourglass feminine physique, women go for the wedge-shaped man. Known as the shoulder-to-hip ratio in men, women around the world find men more attractive if they have broad shoulders and narrow hips—signs of higher testosterone levels and physical strength. Indeed, the hourglass maidens and wedge-shaped young men have sex earlier in adolescence, as well as more sex partners.[25]

## Symmetry

Another sex lure we have inherited is body and facial symmetry. Both men and women seek well-proportioned mates. More than 2,500 years ago Aristotle maintained that there were some universal standards of physical beauty. One, he believed, was balanced bodily proportions—symmetry.

Symmetry is beautiful—to insects, birds, mammals, and people around the world.[26] Female scorpion flies seek mates with uniform wings. Barn swallows like partners with well-proportioned tails. Monkeys are partial to consorts with symmetrical teeth. And be you in New Guinea or New York, you (and just about anybody else) can pick out the beautiful people around you. Even two-month-old infants gaze longer at more symmetrical faces.[27] We all respond to symmetry.[28]

"Beauty is truth, truth beauty," Keats wrote in his "Ode on a Grecian Urn." Keats's words have puzzled many. But as it turns out, the beauty of symmetry does tell a basic truth. Creatures with balanced, well-proportioned ears, eyes, teeth, and jaws, with symmetrical elbows, knees, and breasts, have been able to repel bacteria, viruses, and other minute predators that can cause bodily irregularities. In fact, symmetrical men tend to have stronger immune systems. So, by displaying symmetry, animals and people advertise their superior genetic ability to combat diseases.[29]

So our human attraction to symmetrical suitors appears to be a primitive biological mechanism designed to guide us to select genetically sturdy mating partners.[30]

And nature has taken no chances: the brain naturally responds to a beautiful face. When scientists recorded the brain activity of heterosexual men aged 21–35 as they looked at women with attractive faces, the ventral tegmental area (VTA) lit up.[31] This is the brain region that produces "wanting." Not surprisingly, symmetrical women often have many suitors to choose from. As a result, exquisitely good-looking women tend to marry higher-status men.[32]

Highly symmetrical men also get reproductive perks. They begin to have sex some four years earlier than their lopsided peers; they also have more sex partners and more adulterous affairs.[33] Moreover, women orgasm more regularly with symmetrical men.[34]

And here's where their symmetry pays off: women prefer the smell of symmetrical men when ovulating,[35] and when an ovulating woman orgasms with a well-proportioned man, her contractions suck up more of his sperm,[36] favoring his DNA. Men with highly symmetrical faces tend to have better quality semen too,[37] good for baby-making.

Because symmetry expands one's choices in the mating game, women go to extraordinary lengths to achieve it. With powders they make the two sides of the face more similar. With mascara and eyeliner, they make their eyes appear more alike. With lipstick they enhance one lip to match the other. And with plastic surgery, exercise, belts, bras, and tight jeans and shirts, they mold their forms to create the symmetrical proportions men prefer.

Nature helps. Scientists have found that women's hands and ears are more symmetrical during monthly ovulation.[38] Women's breasts become more symmetrical during ovulation too.[39] Moreover, young men and young women are often quite symmetrical; we take on more lopsided proportions as we move beyond our reproductive years.

## The "Special Effects" of Kissing

Academics often hold that kissing is another of nature's ploys to assess a mate, charm him or her with erotic fireworks and win the mating game.

But in only 40% of eighty-eight cultures recently studied do men and women kiss erotically—touching their lips together long enough to exchange saliva.[40] And most of these cultures are complex agrarian and industrial societies. In fact, until Western contact, kissing was reportedly unknown among the Somali, the Lepcha of Sikkim, and the Siriono of South America; whereas the Tsonga of South Africa and other traditional peoples found kissing disgusting.[41] Erotic kissing is not a universal human trait; hence many think it did not evolve as a mechanism for seduction or pair-bonding.

But there are other sides to this issue. Kissing can bolster a partnership. Men and women in Western societies say that kissing brings them emotionally closer to their partner.

They've got this right. Kissing a long-term partner elevates the activity of oxytocin, the brain chemical associated with feelings of trust, attachment, and emotional union. Kissing also reduces the stress hormone cortisol—contributing to these feelings of attachment. Kissing even boosts your pulse and blood pressure, dilates your pupils, and deepens breathing—aspects of the sexual response that may propel you on to coitus with your beloved. And as you know, with orgasm comes a spike of oxytocin—and more feelings of attachment.

It has been said that the best thing you can do for your children is to love your partner. Perhaps as kissing enhances one's feelings of attachment to a mate, it subtly contributes to one's reproductive and parenting capacity too.

But kissing may also be a direct tool for seduction. Saliva has testosterone in it—the hormone of sexual desire.[42] Men tend to like sloppier kisses than women do.[43] So they may be unconsciously trying to inject this sexy chemical to woo a potential lover into bed. A woman's breath and saliva change across the menstrual cycle. So with his sloppy kiss, a man may also pick up this signal of her fertility.[44] In these ways, kissing may have evolved as an adaptive means of sexual enticement, as well as aiding pair-bonding and reproduction.

A good first kiss may even trigger feelings of romantic love. Any kind of novelty triggers the dopamine system in the brain. And, as you know, dopamine is associated with feelings of romance. So if a first kiss is exciting, it might push you over the threshold into falling in love—the beginning of the mating process.

So I suspect that kissing *is* a biological mechanism, that it evolved to help initiate and sustain a pair-bond. But this inherited mechanism became altered in some societies as our forebears began to create rules of sexual decorum.

⤳

Kissing is dangerous, however. With this little act, you learn a huge amount about your would-be lover. You can see them clearly, as well as smell, taste, hear, and feel them. Instantly these messages from your senses are picked up by five of your twelve cranial nerves and escorted directly to the brain. Here they detonate, giving you firsthand information about this individual's health, their eating, drinking, and smoking habits, and their state of mind. A kiss is not just a kiss.

In fact, the first kiss can be disastrous. In a recent study of 58 men and 122 women, 59% of men and 66% of women said they had ended a romance after the first kiss.[45] It was the kiss of death.

Not everybody kisses, of course. But in cultures where men and women find kissing revolting, they regularly pat, suck, lick, or caress the face of a beloved—as do males and females of other species. Dogs lick one another's lips and face. Moles rub noses. Elephants put their trunk in one another's mouths. Albatrosses tap their bills together. Bonobos, our closest chimp relatives, smooch with deep tongue action, the "French" kiss.

Our erotic human lip-lock may be part of a much larger repertoire of courtship practices that are expressed in different species in different ways and serve several different purposes—among them, to get to know, perhaps even to impress, a potential mating partner.

⤳

Of all our human sexual decorations and habits, the most striking and pleasurable to both men and women are three bizarre traits: women's ability to copulate face to face; women's intense but fickle pattern of orgasm; and women's remarkable ability to copulate around the clock. About these feminine lures men have rhapsodized for centuries, if not millennia.

Did Lucy copulate face to face?

I think she did. All modern women have a downward-tilted vagina rather than the backward-oriented vagina of all other primates. Because this is tipped, face-to-face coitus is comfortable for women. In fact, in this position the man's pelvic bone rubs against her clitoris, making intercourse extremely stimulating.

Not surprisingly, face-to-face coitus in the missionary position is the preferred copulatory posture in most cultures, although variations abound.[46] The Kuikuru of Amazonia sleep in single-person hammocks strung around a family hearth, so lovers have little privacy. Moreover, one false move and both are pitched into the night fire. Because of these inconveniences, spouses and paramours make love in the forest, where the ground is uneven and often wet. Here a woman cannot lie on her back to copulate. Instead, she squats, leans back, and holds her buttocks and back above the ground with flexed arms and legs. Still, she makes love while looking at her partner.

People have invented dozens of other positions for intercourse. But face-to-face copulation is depicted in artworks around the world; it is probably a badge of the human animal.

If Lucy had a tipped vagina and encouraged face-to-face coitus, her partners could see her face, whisper to her, gaze at her, and pick up the nuances of her expressions. Face-to-face copulation fosters intimacy, communication, and understanding. So I suspect that the downward-tilting human vaginal canal evolved via sexual selection.[47] Like those ancestral females with pendulous, sensitive breasts, those with tipped vaginas and those who made love face to face forged stronger bonds with their "special friends" and bore disproportionately more young—passing these traits to modern women.

## Female Orgasm

Another dazzling trait of most women is their ability to orgasm.

Some scientists don't believe that female orgasm is an adaptive trait, one that evolved for reproductive purposes. They reason that orgasm is critical to men because these pulsations push sperm into the vagina. But a woman's egg pops naturally from her ovary once a month, regardless of her sexual response. Moreover, women vary widely in when, where, and with whom they "come," whereas men are highly consistent in their sexual response, also suggesting that female orgasm isn't necessary for reproduction.[48] Most important, women who orgasm regularly have no more children than those who don't.[49] Nor do orgasmic women have more sex partners across their life or any other known reproductive payoffs.[50]

So, many hold that female orgasm was never selected in the past.

Some even compare female orgasm to the nipples on men—a useless characteristic in females dragged through evolution because it was of such vital reproductive importance to ancestral men. Female orgasm, they conclude, is not an adaptation at all.[51]

Wait a minute. The clitoris is not a relatively inert patch of tissue like the male nipple; it's a remarkably sensitive clump of nerves that serves a primary role in inducing orgasm. And for a woman orgasm is a journey, an altered state of consciousness, another reality that escalates to chaos, then elicits feelings of calm, tenderness, and attachment. Surely, feelings of attachment to her partner strengthen the pair-bond, and thus enhance the survival of their young.

Female orgasm signals something too: satisfaction. Men like women to climax because it reassures them that their partner is gratified and perhaps less inclined to seek sex elsewhere. So female orgasm may serve to produce feelings of attachment in her partner too.[52] Moreover, a mind-bending orgasm is likely to stimulate a woman to seek more coitus with this partner, further enhancing feelings of attachment in both of them.

In fact, women tend to climax with men who are sexually attentive, and with longtime, committed partners. Women achieve orgasm more regularly with husbands, for example, than with secret lovers or during casual hookups or one-night stands. And streetwalkers who copulate with strangers climax less frequently than do call girls with better-paying, more considerate, and return customers. Perhaps female orgasm also evolved to prefer a caring, patient Mr. Right to a cavalier, restive Mr. Wrong.

Female orgasm could facilitate conception with Mr. Right as well. Orgasm triggers the uterus to rhythmically contract which may suck sperm into the womb through the cervix.[53] Orgasm also relaxes a woman, thus motivating her to remain lying down—keeping sperm in the vaginal canal. In fact, after sex, women retain more of the sperm of men who give them orgasms.[54]

So I'll stick with the unpopular view that female orgasm evolved for genuine purposes: to encourage females to seek sex with Mr. Right instead of Mr. Wrong; and to initiate and sustain a pair-bond with a healthy, caring reproductive partner.[55] In short, female orgasm may not have evolved to produce *more* offspring, but instead, to guide females to choose partners who were better equipped, both mentally and physically, to help them raise their offspring in a stable partnership—thus enabling their children to disproportionately survive.

In fact, female orgasm probably evolved long before our ancestors descended from the trees. All female primates and higher mammals have a clitoris. A chimp's clitoris is larger than that of a woman, both relatively and absolutely. And once a female becomes sexually excited, she begins to copulate at a fevered pitch—suggesting that female chimps climax several times. Females of many mammalian species also experience changes while having sex, including alterations in blood pressure, respiration, heart rate, muscular tension, and hormone levels; they also make distinctive vocal tones. All these traits resemble the human female sexual response during orgasm.[56] So orgasm most likely occurs in many other creatures.[57]

Lucy probably inherited the ability to orgasm from Ardi and her other ancestors living largely in the trees and passed this blissful phenomenon along to us.

## Will She or Won't She?

Of all the sexual ploys women have acquired to seduce, none is so captivating to scientists—and so enjoyable to men and women—as the female's remarkable ability to copulate when she wants to. As you recall, to males and females of almost all other species, sex is not constantly available. Why? Because females of sexually reproducing genera have a period of heat, or estrus, and when they are not in heat they generally refuse to accept a male.

There are exceptions, of course.[58] But women fall at the far end of a long continuum of behavior: we regularly can and do copulate throughout our entire monthly menstrual cycle; we can engage in intercourse throughout most of pregnancy; and we can and often do resume coitus as soon as we have recovered from childbirth—months or years before a child is weaned.

Critics say that continual female sexual readiness exists only in the fears of old men and the hopes of young boys. This is not the point. If a woman *wants* to, she *can* copulate anytime she pleases.

American married women copulate, on average, one to three times a week, depending on their age.[59] In many cultures women reportedly make love either every day or every night, except when rituals of war, religion, or other local customs intercede.[60] Sex does not end with menopause or aging, either.[61] This is not to say that a woman always has a high libido. But the human female has lost her period of heat, enabling her to have sex any time, anywhere, under any circumstances.

Several theories have been offered for the loss of "estrus periodicity."[62] The classic explanation holds that ancestral females lost estrus in order to cement a pair-bond with a male. With the ability to copulate at any time, a female could keep her "special friend" in perpetual attendance.

But many birds and some mammals are monogamous, and none except women display continual sexual availability. There must be a richer explanation for this remarkable human female trait.

Perhaps adultery selected for the loss of estrus. If clandestine copulations provided Lucy and her female companions with extra protection and support, then it would have been to their advantage to copulate with clandestine lovers whenever the opportunity arose. And to philander, you must seize the moment. If your "special friend" is away scouting and scavenging and his brother joins you to collect nuts, you can't wait until your period of estrus returns: you must make love then.

Continual sexual receptivity enabled females to pursue *both* of their fundamental reproductive strategies: sustaining a pair-bond with one mate and attaining ancillary copulations with other lovers.

~)

So if Lucy had a slightly longer monthly period of sexual receptivity, last-ing, let's say, twenty days as opposed to ten, she would have maintained a longer sexual relationship with her "special friend" *and* clandestine lov-ers, garnering more of their protection, more of their scavenged meat. She would have lived. Her young would have lived. And the propensity for longer and longer periods of sexual receptivity evolved.[63]

Moreover, those females who copulated throughout more of their pregnancy and sooner after delivering a child most likely also received extra gratuities and survived disproportionately, contributing to modern women the trait of continual sexual availability.

## Silent Ovulation

So magnificent is this bizarre trait, continual sexual availability, that it must have been the culmination of several environmental and reproduc-tive forces. But did women lose estrus or acquire perpetual estrus?

They lost estrus. Women exhibit almost no signs of mid-cycle ovu-lation. Shortly before the egg pops from the ovary, the tacky mucus on the cervix becomes slippery, smooth, and stretchable. Some women feel cramping. A few bleed slightly at this time. Others have unusually oily hair, their breasts become sensitive, or they have more energy than usual. A woman's body temperature rises almost a full degree at ovulation and remains normal or above until the next menstruation. And as her body voltage goes up, a woman becomes more electrically charged as well.[64] With these exceptions, ovulation is silent.

Women do not become sex-crazed at mid-cycle either—unlike other female primates who sport puffy, conspicuous genitals at estrus and flaunt ovulation with alluring aromatic scents and persistent courting ges-tures.[65] Instead, most women do not even know when they are fertile. In fact, a woman must copulate regularly in order to get pregnant and take precautions if she does not want to bear a child. For women ovulation is concealed.

What a dangerous inconvenience "silent ovulation" is. It has led to millions, perhaps billions, of unwanted pregnancies. But it is easy to speculate on the advantages of silent ovulation in Lucy's day.

If Lucy's partner did not know when she was fertile, he was obliged to copulate with her regularly in order to bear a child. Silent ovulation kept a "special friend" in constant close proximity, providing protection and meat the female prized. Paramours did not know whether Lucy was ovulating either. So she could count on their attentions too. And because primate males that consort with a female are often solicitous toward her young, these ancillary lovers may have doted on her children.

Silent ovulation got the female more of what she needed—males.

Males got more sex. With the loss of estrus, a female mate was continually sexually available. Extra female lovers were consistently sexually ready too. With silent ovulation a "husband" did not have to fight off other suitors either, because his "wife" never signaled fertility. Silent ovulation kept the peace.[66]

Of all the payoffs of this magnificent human female trait, however, the most staggering was choice. Unchained from the ovulatory cycle of all other animals—and a continual sex drive—Lucy could finally begin to *choose* her lovers more carefully.

Though female chimps definitely have favored sex partners and sometimes avoid intercourse with those they dislike by moving at key moments or refusing to get into a mating pose, female chimps cannot conceal their receptivity, feign tiredness or a headache, or drive off suitors with nonchalance or insults. They are compelled by chemistry to copulate while in estrus. Hence the word *estrus* is derived from the Greek word meaning "gadfly."

Freed from this monthly hormonal flood, however, ancestral women gained more *cortical* control of their sexual desire. They could copulate for myriad new reasons—including power, revenge, companionship, resources, and love. "Will she or won't she?" came into vogue.

Large penises; men's beards and deep voices; women's smooth complexions, mellifluous tones, and dangling breasts; face-to-face copulation; female orgasm; continual sexual receptivity: the evolution of serial pair-bonding and clandestine adultery would start to change our bodies. With time, we would become dressed to impress.

As ancestral men and women paired and worked as a team, selection would also build the brain. Now the human psyche would take flight.

## The Mating Mind

Psychologist Geoffrey Miller was troubled by all of our exceptional human skills. So in a highly original book, *The Mating Mind*, Miller added to Darwin's theory of sexual selection, proposing that humans evolved a host of extravagant human *mental* talents largely to impress potential mating partners.

Our human intelligence, linguistic skills and musical abilities, our drive to create visual arts, stories, myths, comedies, and dramas, our agility at all kinds of sports, our intense curiosity, our ability to solve complex math problems, our moral virtue, our religious fervor, our impulse for charitable giving, our political convictions, sense of humor, even our courage, pugnacity, perseverance, and kindness, Miller argued, are far too ornate and metabolically expensive to have evolved solely to survive another day.[67] These exceptional human traits must have emerged, at least in part, to help us win the mating game.

We are "courtship machines," Miller writes.[68] His reasoning: Those ancestors who could speak poetically, draw deftly, dance nimbly, craft better tools, build better huts, or deliver more fiery moral speeches were regarded as more attractive by the opposite sex. Thus, these talented men and women had more lovers and produced more babies. And gradually our myriad stunning human capacities became inscribed in our genetic code. Moreover, to distinguish themselves, our forebears specialized—creating the tremendous variety in human skills we see today.

Miller acknowledges that in their simple forms, many of these traits were also useful to survive on the grasslands of ancient Africa; these talents had *many* purposes. But if our forebears had earnestly needed these advanced aptitudes to survive, chimpanzees would have developed these abilities as well. They didn't. So our myriad mental aptitudes most likely became more and more complex *because the opposite sex liked them* and chose to mate with verbal, musical, artistic, or otherwise talented men and women.

Miller concludes: "The mind evolved by moonlight."[69]

⌒

But how did ancestral men and women come to prefer these extraordinary traits in particular suitors? Some brain mechanism must have simultaneously evolved in the "display chooser" to become attracted to the fancy rhymes, lyric tunes, pleasing drawings in the dirt, and other flashy traits that "display producers" paraded for their pleasure.

My brain scanning partners and I may have stumbled on an answer. When participants in our studies looked at photos of particularly good-looking men and women (not a beloved) while in the brain scanner, they showed activity in the *left* ventral tegmental area (rather than the right VTA, associated with romantic love). We concluded that this response in the left VTA is associated with an aesthetically pleasing experience, rather than feelings of romantic love.

Perhaps this brain circuitry plays a role in *all* aesthetically pleasing experiences. So as Lucy's suitors courted her with an array of tuneful songs, exciting drawings, a dead-eye shot, or some other exceptional talent, she found some suitors particularly pleasing and seduced only them. Then, as other girls and boys seduced those with different talents and bore their young, our ancestors gradually developed our myriad and magnificent human faculties and capacities.

## Courtship Deception

And I'm not surprised that both sexes exaggerate their talents to impress. Courtship is not about honesty; it's about winning. Don't get me wrong: honesty pays off. But no courting moose tries to make his antlers look smaller; he shows them off. So it is with humans. Thus, "courtship deception" may be yet another skill our forebears developed, at least in part, to win the mating game.

Take men's height. Around the world women are more attracted to tall men—perhaps because tall men tend to get better jobs and make more money, resources that women naturally seek for their forthcoming young. So men lie about their height, particularly on contemporary Internet dating sites where women must decide to meet a man before seeing him. Men hope their fib will be overlooked as they proceed to captivate the woman with their more appealing qualities.

Women fib about their weight—another unconscious mating strategy. As you know, women whose waist circumference is about 70% of their hip measurement have the right balance of estrogen, testosterone, and other hormones to produce healthy babies. So it's adaptive for men to be attracted to a woman with a supple, balanced figure.

But why lie about height and weight—such obvious deceptions?

Because, as Mae West said, "It's better to be looked over than overlooked." Throughout the animal world, males and females hope to get past a false first impression to seduce with more winning traits.

And many have succeeded. Intelligence, playfulness, curiosity, creativity, sense of humor, a person's values, their interests, their compassion, their ability at math or music and many other exceptional human qualities must have evolved because Lucy, her companions, and numberless others in our long ancestry sought different talents in their "special friends" and lovers. Hence those deficient in some abilities won a beloved by parading other skills.

Nature has excluded almost no one from the mating dance.

# 10

## Men and Women Are Like Two Feet: They Need Each Other to Get Ahead

### Gender Differences in Mind

Breathes there a man with hide so tough
Who says two sexes aren't enough?

—SAMUEL HOFFENSTEIN

"**M**an is more courageous, pugnacious and energetic than woman, and has a more inventive genius. . . . Woman seems to differ from man . . . chiefly in her greater tenderness and less selfishness." Darwin wrote these words in 1871. Man the aggressor, woman the nurturer: he believed these gender qualities were the "birthright" of humankind, acquired from our distant past.

Darwin also thought men were naturally smarter. This superior male intelligence, he proposed, arose because young men had to fight to win mates. Because ancestral males had to defend their families, hunt for their joint subsistence, attack enemies, and make weapons, males needed higher mental faculties, "namely, observation, reason, invention or imagination." So, through ancestral competition among males and the survival of the fittest, intelligence evolved—in men.

An aggressive, intelligent Adam; a gentle, simple Eve: proof of the gender inequality Darwin saw everywhere around him. The poets, merchants, politicians, scientists, artists, and philosophers of Victorian

England were overwhelmingly men. Moreover, Paul Broca, the eminent nineteenth-century French neurologist and authority on race, had confirmed the belief in feminine intellectual inferiority. After calculating the brain weights of over a hundred men and women whose bodies were autopsied in Paris hospitals, Broca wrote in 1861, "Women are, on the average, a little less intelligent than men, a difference which we should not exaggerate but which is, nonetheless, real."[1]

Broca had not corrected his calculations for the smaller body size of women. He had used an impeccable "correction formula" to prove that the French were just as capable as the Germans. But he did not make the necessary mathematical adjustments on his female skulls. Everyone knew that women were intellectually inferior anyway; such was the climate of the times.

⁓

This sexist credo saw a bitter reaction after World War I. Anthropologist Margaret Mead was among the intellectual leaders of the 1920s who emphasized the predominance of nurture over nature. The environment, she said, molded personality. As she wrote in 1935, "We may say that many if not all the personality traits which we have called masculine and feminine are as lightly linked to sex as are the clothing, the manners and the form of headdress that a society at a given period assigns to either sex."[2]

Mead's message spelled hope for women—as well as for ethnic minorities, immigrants, and the poor—and helped spread the belief that people are essentially all similar.[3] Strip men and women of a few cultural ornaments, and you have basically the same animal. Society and upbringing make women behave like women and men act like men. The 1930s and following decades saw a flood of scientific treatises proclaiming that men and women were inherently alike. Biology be gone.

But new data have emerged. And today almost all broadly educated scientists and laymen have come to realize that the sexes have, *on average*, some differences. Moreover, some of these gender differences are either built into brain architecture by fetal hormones as the brain develops in the womb, or by floods of hormones across one's life.

When egg meets sperm and conception occurs, the embryo has neither male nor female genitals. But around the sixth week of fetal life a genetic switch flips and the SRY gene on the Y chromosome begins to direct the precursors of the gonads to develop into testes if the child is to be a boy. The die is cast. The differentiating testes begin to produce fetal testosterone. And as this powerful male hormone surges through embryonic tissues during the third month of fetal life, it builds the male genitals—and aspects of the male brain. If the embryo is to be a girl, however, it develops without the stimulus of male hormones; and many believe that the DAX-1 gene on the X chromosome also kicks into action to direct the development of the female genitals, along with aspects of the female brain.[4]

So hormones "sex" the fetal brain. And this brain architecture plays a role in creating some of the gender differences that appear in later life.

Some of these gender variations, I suspect, come across the eons, selected in a time long gone—when ancestral men and women began to pair and raise their children as a team.

## The Gift of Gab

In tests of verbal abilities in America, it is becoming clear that, *on average*, little girls speak sooner than little boys. They speak more fluently, with greater grammatical accuracy, and with more words per utterance. By age ten, girls regularly excel at verbal reasoning, written prose, verbal memory, pronunciation, and spelling. They are better at foreign languages. They stutter less. They exhibit dyslexia four times less often than boys. And far fewer girls are remedial readers.[5]

Several cultural explanations have been marshaled to prove that verbal skills are culturally instilled more regularly in girls than in boys.[6] Some academics have suggested, for example, that women's superior linguistic skills occur because infant girls are born more mature than boys. Thus girls enter life with a slight edge in language ability that parents and schools then cultivate as they age.[7]

But scientists now cite a host of data that, *on average*, this gender difference has a biological foundation. For example, women are more verbally fluent not only in the United States but in places as diverse as England, the Czech Republic, and Nepal.[8] Moreover, the International Association for the Evaluation of Educational Achievement has reported that in some 43,000 writing samples of students in fourteen countries on five continents, girls express their thoughts more clearly on paper.

Moreover, women's verbal superiority is now linked with estrogen.[9] In a study of two hundred women of reproductive age, psychologists have shown that during the middle of the monthly menstrual cycle, when estrogen levels peak, women are at their best verbally.[10] When asked, for example, to repeat the tongue twister "A box of mixed biscuits in a biscuit mixer" five times as fast as possible, they performed particularly well at mid-cycle. Directly after menses, when estrogen levels are much lower, these women's speed declined. However, even at their worst, most of these women outstripped men on all verbal tasks. And prenatal estrogen priming has now been associated with women's superior linguistic abilities; while prenatal testosterone priming has been linked with men's lesser ability at several verbal aptitudes.[11]

This is not to say that boys are inarticulate; or that *all* boys have weaker verbal skills than *all* girls. Men vary; women vary. In fact, there is more variation within each gender than there is between them.[12] And culture always plays a role. Proof lies in our Western heritage. For the past several thousand years, Western society has suppressed women's opportunities to be orators, writers, poets, and playwrights, and cultivated male geniuses. Not surprisingly, the vast majority of our public speakers and literary giants have been men.

## The Math Gap

Men excel, *on average*, at higher mathematical problems (not at arithmetic). And they are generally better at reading maps, solving mazes, and completing several other visual-spatial-quantitative tasks.[13] These aptitudes also appear to have a biological foundation.

Foremost, these skills appear in early childhood, long before culture trains the mind. Infant boys are better at tracking a blinking light across a TV screen. Little boys take more toys apart, explore more of the space around them, and see abstract patterns and relationships more accurately. By age ten, more boys can rotate three-dimensional objects in their mind's eye, more precisely perceive three-dimensional spaces on flat paper, and begin to score higher on some other mechanical and spatial tasks.

Then at puberty boys begin to outstrip girls in algebra, geometry, and other subjects involving visual–spatial–quantitative skills.[14] In one test of nearly 50,000 American seventh-graders who took the standard Scholastic Aptitude Test, for example, 260 boys and 20 girls scored over 700 (out of 800) on mathematical problems—a ratio of 13 to 1.[15] And these gender differences in spatial acuity and interest in mathematics are seen in several other cultures.[16]

Like verbal skills in girls and women, these abilities observed in boys and men clearly have a large cultural component. But there is also a direct link between the predominant male hormone, testosterone, and enhanced visual-spatial perception and mathematical skills.[17] Girls who experience abnormally high doses of male hormones in the womb exhibit tomboyish behavior in childhood—and do better on math exams in teenage. Conversely, pubescent boys with low levels of testosterone do poorly on spatial tasks; men with an extra Y chromosome (XYY) score higher on visual-spatial tests; and those with an extra female X chromosome (XXY, or Klinefelter's syndrome) have a poorer spatial aptitude.[18]

Most interesting to me, when my brain scanning colleagues and I put men and women into the scanner (using fMRI), we found that those men and women who scored high on the traits linked with testosterone (in my personality questionnaire, the Fisher Temperament Inventory) also showed more activity in brain regions linked with visual/spatial acuity— brain factories built by fetal testosterone. And those individuals who scored high on my scale measuring estrogen-related traits showed more activity in brain regions built by estrogen.[19]

I am not suggesting that women have developed *no* superior spatial skills. On the contrary, scientists Irwin Silverman and Marion Beals uncovered an intriguing feminine spatial aptitude. In a room, Silverman and Beals displayed several dissimilar objects as well as objects drawn on a sheet of paper; then they instructed men and women to memorize these items. Later they asked the participants to recall what they had memorized. The results: women were able to remember many more of these stationary objects, as well as their locations.[20]

Each gender has specific spatial skills.

≈

Does society train girls to fail at math and boys to fail at English?

Several cultural explanations have been proposed to explain these gender differences. Teachers' assumptions and their treatment of students; parents' attitudes toward their children and how they raise boys and girls; society's perception that math is masculine; the different games and sports that boys and girls play; each gender's self-perception and ambitions; the many social pressures on adolescents; even the way that tests are designed and how scientists interpret the results: all undoubtedly affect test scores.[21] Scholastic Aptitude Test scores, for example, vary as much with social class and ethnic background as with gender. And the gap between male and female performance on standardized math tests has declined since the 1970s.

Is biology destiny? Not at all. Culture plays an enormous role in molding human aptitudes and actions.

But the body of data on gender differences in infants; the persistence of male/female differences on tests other than the SATs; the fact that adolescent girls do not fall behind on *other* skills because of social pressure; the corroborative data from other countries; the literature linking testosterone with spatial skills and estrogen with verbal aptitudes; our brain scanning experiments: all support the view that the sexes exhibit gender differences in some spatial and verbal abilities—and that these gender differences stem, at least in part, from male/female variations in biology.[22]

Moreover, these gender differences make evolutionary sense. As ancestral males began to scout, track, and surround animals more than two million of years ago, those males who were good at maps and mazes would have disproportionately survived. Ancestral females needed to locate vegetable foods within an elaborate grassy landscape. So those who could remember where these resources were located would have also lived another day—passing on this female spatial skill. Moreover, superior verbal aptitudes must have been critical tools to ancestral women as they soothed, scolded, educated, and played with their growing young.

Hence it is likely that as pair-bonding emerged and the human hunting-gathering-scavenging tradition took shape, selection favored these gender differences in aptitude.

Other variations between the sexes have a biological foundation and most likely evolved during our long nomadic past.

## Women's Intuition

"It is generally admitted," Darwin wrote, "that with woman the powers of intuition . . . are more strongly marked than in man."[23]

Science is proving Darwin right. Tests show that, on average, women read emotions, postures, gestures, tone of voice, context, and other non-verbal information more effectively than men.[24] A slight twist of the head, lips pulled taut, shoulders hunched, a shift of body weight, a change in vocal timbre—any of these subtle signals can lead a woman to feel that someone is uncomfortable, fearful, angry, or disappointed. Could the aptitude for reading people, what scientists now call *theory of mind*, stem from brain anatomy?

I think so.

Women have, on average, more nerve fibers that connect the two hemispheres of the brain.[25] They may have more long-distance connections within each hemisphere as well.[26] Men, on the other hand, have more short nerve connections between nearby brain regions within each hemisphere. So the female brain is, *on average*, better connected; while the male brain is more compartmentalized.[27]

This gender difference is particularly apparent in hospitals. From several hundred examples of stroke victims and patients with brain tumors and injuries, women more easily recover—by employing a wider range of brain factories to relearn their skills.

So, with these data and many experiments on healthy men and women, scientists now believe that this female brain architecture develops in the womb, is built by fetal estrogen,[28] and is then sustained across the life course by more estrogen and the activities of a closely related neurochemical, oxytocin.[29] Moreover, this female brain architecture may contribute to women's intuition—enabling them to collect data from a wider range of visual, aural, tactile, and olfactory senses, as well as centers for memory and cognition. Hence women connect disparate bits of information quickly, giving them that ready insight that Darwin extolled.

## Web Thinking

I have proposed that women's intuition is part of a broader feminine aptitude, what I have termed *web thinking*[30]—the tendency to take a broad, contextual, holistic, and long-term view of just about any issue.[31]

We all collect reams of data when we think, put these bits of information into patterns, and weigh these variables as we make decisions. As Plato said, "When the mind is thinking; it is talking to itself." A committee meeting is in progress in your head.

But psychologists report that when women think, they collect more data, put these factoids into more complex patterns, and think of more ways to proceed.[32] Women generalize; they synthesize; they take a more global perspective of anything they ponder. They think in webs of factors, not straight lines—web thinking. In contrast, men tend to focus on the goal; they discard what they regard as extraneous information and proceed toward their decision in a more linear, causal manner— what I call *step thinking*.

Both are fine ways to cogitate. And I suspect that the brain architecture for web thinking and step thinking evolved long ago for practical reasons: ancestral men had to focus on the hunt. The goal: to hit that buffalo in the head with a rock. This narrow, deep focus could have selected for men's more compartmentalized mind. Women, on the other hand, had to coddle the baby, stoke the fire, build the hut, cook the supper, and do myriad other chores all at once. So women's work selected for women's more widely connected mind.

"Get to the point!" he said. "Which point?" she said. This misunderstanding between the sexes may come from our distant past.

Web thinking has given women other natural perks. It enables women to better tolerate ambiguity. It most likely also contributes to women's mental flexibility, their propensity for long-term thinking, and their vivid imagination.[33]

⁓

Male excellence at math and spatial tasks, female verbal skills, intuition, and web thinking: these are not the only intellectual differences between the sexes that appear to have biological foundations and have developed during our long prehistory.

Women of all ages have better fine motor coordination, manipulating tiny objects with ease. (Just ask a man to undo your necklace or even thread a needle—then wait.) And this feminine dexterity increases during the middle of the menstrual cycle, when estrogen levels peak—suggesting a physiological element to this fine manual prowess.[34]

In contrast, boys and men are, on average, more dexterous at gross motor skills requiring speed and force, from running and jumping to throwing sticks and stones and balls.[35]

Once again, these gender differences make evolutionary sense. As ancestral women gathered more tiny seeds and berries and more regularly picked the grass, dirt, and twigs off of their young, those with superior fine motor coordination may have disproportionately survived—selecting for this trait in modern women. On the other hand, it seems likely that as men hurled more weapons at predators and prey, the male aptitude for gross motor coordination emerged.

## Boys Will Be Boys

A last trait distinguishes most men and women: just as Darwin said, men are, on average, more aggressive, while women are, on average, more empathetic and nurturing.

In a classic study of aggressiveness in villages in Japan, the Philippines, Mexico, Kenya, and India, as well as in "Orchard Town," an anonymous New England city, anthropologists Beatrice and John Whiting found that boys were more aggressive in each culture.[36]

Psychologists confirm this for Americans. Boy toddlers grab and scratch. Nursery school boys chase and wrestle. Teenage boys like contact sports. Rough-and-tumble play is almost exclusively a male preoccupation throughout childhood, as it is in other primates. More men are drawn to the violent acts of war. And the vast majority of homicides around the world are committed by men, often by young men with high levels of testosterone.[37]

This aggressive spirit certainly would have served our male ancestors well as they strode forth to confront their predators and enemies on the grasslands of Africa millions of years ago.

I am not suggesting that women are unaggressive. We all know that women can be exceedingly tough-minded, sometimes backstabbing, sometimes physically violent—particularly when they protect their young. Just threaten a baby to see a mother's rage. But scientists think that, in women, the environment plays a larger role in women's aggressive interactions, whereas men's aggression is more governed by hormones, particularly testosterone.[38]

Nurturing is often considered to be the female counterpart to male aggressiveness. Women of every ethnic group and culture around the world (and every other primate species) show more interest in infants and more tolerance of their needs. Moreover, in every society on record, women do the majority of daily infant-rearing tasks.[39]

Some would like to attribute this feminine nurturance to learned behavior. But data indicate that this too has a biological foundation.[40] Nurturing behavior has been linked with the activity of fetal estrogen as it washes over the developing brain.[41] And the effect can be seen in girls long before culture begins to sculpt their minds and actions.

Infant girls chatter, smile, and coo to people's faces, seeking to connect, while boys are just as likely to babble at objects and blinking lights. Little girls have longer attention spans, they are more patient, and they devote more time to fewer projects, while boys are more distractible, more active, and more exploratory. Girls are more drawn to novel people, while boys are more drawn to novel toys. And girls are better at discerning your emotional state from your tone of voice. Moreover, girls born with only one X chromosome, or Turner's syndrome, are "extremely feminine"; they show less interest in sports and childhood fighting and are more interested in personal adornment than are normal girls. They also score extremely low on tests of mathematical and spatial tasks. But these girls are very interested in marriage and are strongly drawn to children.[42]

## Women Are "Pro-Social"

In her classic book *In a Different Voice*, psychologist Carol Gilligan proposed that women have an outstanding sensitivity for interpersonal relationships. In interviews with over a hundred men and women, boys and girls, she and her colleagues found that women cast themselves as actors in a web of attachments, affiliations, obligations, and responsibilities to others. Then they cultivate these ties. Indeed, during stressful situations, women express their anxiety with a social strategy known as "tend and befriend"; they reach out to those around them for comfort and connection. Men, on the other hand, tend to become aggressive when they are stressed.[43]

This feminine drive to make social attachments is also associated with the estrogen system in the brain. Women are what scientists call "pro-social"; they more naturally express empathy,[44] a trait now associated with estrogen priming in the womb. Oxytocin, the largely female hormone, is also associated with several pro-social traits, including trust, reading emotions in others, and intuition.[45] In fact, when I and my brain scanning partners put two groups of people into the scanner (using fMRI), we found that those who scored high on my personality scale measuring traits linked with the estrogen system in the brain also showed more activity in brain regions linked with empathy, brain areas built by estrogen.[46]

Most likely women's gift for gab, their intuition and web thinking, their natural interest in people's faces, their patience, mental flexibility, and long-term view, their sensitivity to interpersonal relationships and their need for social affiliations, are all tools of the feminine psyche that evolved as ancestral females nurtured their young long ago.

"If it's true we are descended from the ape, it must have been from two different species. There's no likeness between us, is there?" says a man to a woman in August Strindberg's 1887 play *The Father*. The misogynistic Swede was exaggerating. But men and women are, on average, endowed with several different skills that evolved during our human hunting-gathering-scavenging tradition—when men and women began to pool their energy, food, and abilities to rear their young as mated pairs.

Nevertheless, neither sex is more intelligent.

Here Darwin was wrong—a product of his times. Intelligence is a collage of thousands of separate abilities, not a single trait. Some people excel at reading maps or recognizing faces. Others can mentally rotate objects, fix a car, or write a poem. Some people reason well when faced with a thorny scientific problem, while others reason well in difficult social situations. Some people learn music rapidly; others can learn a foreign language in weeks. Some remember economic theories; others recall philosophical ideas. Some people just remember more of everything but can't express what they know or apply it meaningfully; others know far less but express themselves creatively and have a greater capacity to generalize or use their knowledge or ideas. Some women are brilliant mathematicians, composers, or chess players; some men are the world's finest orators, playwrights, interpreters, and diplomats. There is a magnificent variety in human sagacity, wit, and personality.

But the sexes are not identical. A good deal of data now indicate that, on average, each gender has an undercurrent, a melody, a theme.

And selection for men's spatial aptitudes and women's verbal skills, for women's intuition and web thinking, for men's gross and women's fine motor coordination, for men's aggressiveness and women's nurturing behavior, may have begun even before our female and male forebears emerged in the woodlands of the ancient world to start scavenging, hunting, and collecting for a living.

⌒

"Darwinian Man, though well-behaved, / At best is only a monkey shaved." So goes the ditty written by the English librettist W. S. Gilbert.

Scientists are not the first to think there is continuity between man and beast. Confirming it, however, is anthropologist William McGrew, who has found rudiments of these gender differences among chimpanzees.[47]

As you recall, male chimps living along Lake Tanganyika in East Africa hunt. They stalk, chase, and kill animals. These are spatial, quiet, aggressive tasks. Males also scout along the border of their range and guard the community territory—occupations that are also spatial, silent, and aggressive. And male chimps throw more foliage and rocks—gross motor tasks.

Female chimps gather. They engage in termite fishing and ant dipping three times more often than males do. These tasks require fine manual dexterity; one must maneuver a slim stick down the mud corridors of these insects' homes. Female common chimps also engage in more social grooming, using fine motor coordination to pick tiny specks from one another and their young for hours at a time. And while they forage and groom their companions, female chimps interact with their children too, touching and vocalizing. This has honed their verbal skills. Like their counterparts among other higher primate species, male chimps tend to bark, growl, and roar, making more strident aggressive sounds while females make more "clear calls," appeals for affiliation.[48]

These data suggest that some of the modern differences between the genders *preceded* our descent onto the ground of ancient Africa. Then, as our forebears began to collect small game, to scavenge, and to forage for seeds and berries in the woodlands and out on the open plains, these gender roles became critical to survival—selecting for today's male/female differences in spatial and verbal skills, as well as in intuition, web thinking, hand-eye coordination, and aggressiveness.

## "The Gorge"

We have, of course, no physical evidence of male scavenging and hunting or female gathering among Lucy and her relatives who strolled through the trees and grass of Africa between 3.6 and 3.2 million years ago. We have only footprints and old bones.

But the fossil record becomes more abundant by two million years ago. And some peculiar archaeological remains suggest that human gender roles—and gender differences in the brain—had started to emerge.

The most abundant data come from Olduvai Gorge, Tanzania, a barren, desiccated canyonland where, over the last 200,000 years, a river has cut a deep seam between the rocks, exposing a layer cake of ancient geological strata. In the 1930s Mary and Louis Leakey began to dig in this crevasse, looking for evidence of early humankind. And in 1959 Mary discovered a site at the bottom of the gorge, Bed I, that exposed life as it was between 1.7 and 1.9 million years ago.

The area was then a shallow, brackish, emerald-colored lake surrounded by marsh, bush, and trees. Pelicans, storks, herons, and hippos waded through the tranquil pools. Crocodiles floated in the brine. And ducks and geese nested in the papyrus reeds at the water's edge. Sloping off the lake, the brush merged into high open countryside, dotted here and there with acacia trees. At the horizon were forests of mahoganies and evergreens that stretched up mountain slopes toward volcanic peaks.

On the eastern edge of the extinct lake, where salty marshes were once fed by freshwater streams, Mary Leakey unearthed over 2,500 ancient tools and fragments of worked stone.[49] Someone with a good eye had made these tools. Some were big chunks of lava, quartzite, or other stones that had a few edges whacked off to make a single sharpened edge. Others were fragmentary flakes that had been chipped from larger rocks. Débitage, small slivers of sharp stone, and manuports, hunks of unworked stone carried from far away, were strewn along the shore.

Some of these tools were of local stone; others came from outcroppings, stream channels, and lava flows kilometers away. Some had been made elsewhere and then left whole beside the lake. Others had been chipped or worked at the marsh and carried off, leaving only their detritus behind. Here, then, was a tool factory and depository.

Known as Oldowan tools, these primitive choppers and scrapers are not the oldest ever found. Two and a half million years ago someone left tools in Gona, Ethiopia and someone may have made tools even earlier. But these utensils at Olduvai, Bed I, were special.

Near them lay some 60,000 bits of animal bones. Elephants, hippos, rhinos, pigs, buffalo, horses, giraffes, oryx, elands, wildebeests, kongoni, topis, waterbucks, bushbucks, reedbucks, Grant's gazelles, Thompson's gazelles, and impalas made up the larger species. The remains of turtles, elephant shrews, hares, and ducks, and the bones of hundreds of other smaller animals and birds lay here as well. In the 1960s and 1970s the Leakeys uncovered five more sites along this ancient lake. At one, an elephant had been butchered.

Like palimpsests, these assemblages at Olduvai are blackboards half erased. But the field of taphonomy has begun to establish what happened beside this lake so long ago.

## Bone Puzzles

Taphonomy is the ingenious science that studies fossilized bones by working backward.[50] By looking at how modern people butcher meat, how other carnivores such as lions and hyenas chew on bones, and how water and wind spread bones across the landscape, taphonomists establish how ancient bones arrive in the positions and conditions they are in.

For example, taphonomists have watched hunters cut up carcasses, and they report that when hunters remove the flesh, they leave cut marks in the center of the long bones. To harvest skin and tendons they etch distinctive cut marks at the ends of bones instead. Hyenas, on the other hand, chew the feet and ends of bones, leaving quite different marks on bone refuse.

Using these and many other taphonomic clues, anthropologists have tried to piece together what happened at Olduvai some two million years ago. Convincing is the work of Henry Bunn and Ellen Kroll.[51]

After studying all of these ancient bones, these anthropologists proposed that our ancestors caught the turtles, shrews, herons, and other little creatures with cord traps or with their hands. Because lions would have dragged off the entire carcass of middle-sized animals, such as gazelles, our forebears most likely hunted and killed those whose bones remained here. The larger animal bones without carnivore teeth marks on them probably were those of animals our ancestors collected at the end of the dry season, when animals collapsed from thirst. And the bones with carnivore teeth marks on them our forebears undoubtedly scavenged.

Maybe they drove their carnivore competitors from a meal just long enough to steal joints, the "bully sneak" strategy. Perhaps they picked over the remains after their rivals had wandered off to snooze. They could also have stolen the carcasses that leopards dragged into trees.[52]

Our ancient forebears not only collected, scavenged, and hunted animals, but they must have also butchered these beasts. Some of the tools have microscopic scratches that come from cutting meat off bone. Many of the bones have parallel cut marks in the middle of the shaft where someone must have sliced off chunks of flesh. And other fossil bones have tool cut marks at the joints where someone disarticulated limbs and carried these long bones to the shore. Last, the disproportionately large number of meaty limb bones from middle-sized animals like wildebeests suggests that our ancestors had enough meat for "cooperative group sharing."

"People" had begun to butcher, carry, and share meat almost two million years ago.

But why are the bones and stones in discrete heaps? After lengthy analysis of the bones, the tools, and the sites, as well as computer simulations combining all these data with factors like energy expenditure, time of travel, and other variables, anthropologist Richard Potts has theorized that these piles of bones and stones at Olduvai were "stone caches," places where our ancestors stashed their tools and stone raw materials.[53] Here they made tools, left tools, and brought animal parts to be processed quickly. Then, after chopping off meat, extracting marrow, and harvesting skin or tendons, they abandoned the butchery station before the hyenas arrived. When they were in the area again with meat in hand, they revisited one of these stone caches.

Year upon decade upon century the bones and tools and raw materials accumulated. Then Mary Leakey found these garbage heaps.

These refuse dumps say something important about women, men, and the evolution of gender skills. If our ancestors two million years ago had stone caches dotted across the landscape, complete with tools and raw materials to butcher meat, then clearly these early peoples coordinated their activities, engaged in the dangerous pursuit of getting meat from middle- to large-sized animals, delayed eating it, carried joints to specific shared locations beside the lake, butchered meat, and had enough food to share it with relatives and friends. And it is highly unlikely that many ancestral females, often carrying small children, engaged in the dangerous activities of hunting or scavenging even medium-sized animals.

## Woman the Gatherer—and Provider

For decades after Darwin initiated the "man the hunter" concept, academics ignored the roles of ancestral females. But in the early 1980s revisionist anthropologists began to set the record straight.[54] And today most think ancestral women engaged chiefly in the far more productive, dependable activity of collecting nuts, berries, vegetables, and delicacies such as eggs and fruit.

Unfortunately the principal tools of gathering—the digging stick and the pouch—do not normally fossilize. But scientists have recently found broken long bones of antelopes in the cave at Swartkrans, in southern Africa, with polished ends. Microscopic wear patterns near the tips indicate that someone used these implements for digging vegetables. Teeth from this era suggest that our ancestors also ate a lot of fruit.[55] In fact, Potts suggests that meat composed less than 20% of the diet.

So if men did more of the hunting and scavenging, whereas women did the bulk of collecting fruit and vegetables, women had essential jobs two million years ago.

With time, these emerging gender roles (which may have begun to develop among earlier primate relatives) would select for men's knack for maps, mazes, and other spatial skills, their aggressiveness, and their gross motor coordination. And as days turned into centuries, women's spatial memory for stationary objects, their verbal acuity, their facility for nurturing, their fine motor abilities, and their uncanny intuition and web thinking would also become firmly established.

## The Nature of Intimacy

These gender traits may explain some misunderstandings between the sexes.

We struggle, you and I, with intimacy. In poll after book after article women express their disappointment that their mates do not talk out their problems, do not express their emotions, do not listen, do not share—verbally. Women derive intimacy from talking.

Sociologist Harry Brod reports that men often seek intimacy differently. "Numerous studies," he writes, "have established that men are more likely to define emotional closeness as working or playing side by side, while women often view it as talking face to face."[56] Men, for example, derive intimacy from playing and watching sports. I'm not surprised. What is a football game but a map, a maze, a puzzle, spatial action, and aggressive competition—all engage skills that appeal to the male brain. In fact, watching a football game on television is not very different from sitting behind a bush on the African plains, trying to judge which route the zebras will take.

No wonder most women don't understand why men get such pleasure from watching sports; these pastimes don't ring a chord in their evolutionary psyches. Indeed, perhaps women should adopt at least one nonverbal, side-by-side leisure activity that their lovers enjoy, whereas men could improve their home lives if they took time out to sit face to face with their mates and engage in conversation with "active listening."

Another possible gender variation in intimacy may stem from our ancestry. Psychologists maintain that women more regularly seek to feel included, connected, and attached, while men more often enjoy space, privacy, and autonomy.[57] As a result, women say they feel *evaded* by a partner, while men report that they feel *invaded* by a mate.

Could a woman's drive to be included come from a time when women's roles as nurturers selected for those who sought the social comfort of a group? Perhaps men's need to seek autonomy harks back to those days too, when men made their living as solitary, stealthy scouts and trackers.

Men puzzle over the age-old question "What do women want?" Women, on the other hand, regularly say, "Men just don't understand." I suspect our ancestors had begun to mystify one another by two million years ago, when males and females began to split up to hunt and forage around the emerald lake at Olduvai and our fundamental human gender skills started to emerge.

Who were these "people" at Olduvai?

The bones of two separate species of early hominins have been recovered from Bed I, the bottom sedimentary layer of the gorge. But anthropologists trace our ancestry to only one of them, "Handy Man" or *Homo habilis.*

These people had gracile skulls and small molar teeth. The original four fossil specimens found were nicknamed Twiggy (a crushed cranium and seven teeth), George (teeth and skull fragments), Cindy (a lower jaw, bits of an upper jaw, some teeth, and a piece of skull), and Johnny's Child (more bits of jaw and cranial fragments). All died near streams where fresh drinking water tumbled into salty marsh on the eastern margin of the lake some two million years ago.[58]

Twiggy and these other specimens of Handy Man were special. They may have stood only three feet tall. But they had a cranial volume of 600 to 700 cubic centimeters, well above that of Lucy and other australopithecines, who had an average cranial capacity of about 450 cubic centimeters, and about half that of you and me.

Our gang was getting smarter.

Anthropologist Ralph Holloway has exposed the contours of their brains by making latex casts of the insides of these fossil skulls. He reports that the frontal and parietal areas of the cortex—the portions of the brain used to discriminate, categorize, reflect, and reason—had begun to assume a modern shape. Twiggy and her relatives had probably developed the ability to plan ahead.

They may have discussed their plans too. Holloway's endocasts show a slight bulge in Broca's area, named after the nineteenth-century neurologist I mentioned at the beginning of this chapter. Broca's area is a portion of the cortex above the left ear that directs the mouth, tongue, throat, and vocal cords to produce speech sounds. In the brain of Handy Man, this language section had begun to swell.[59]

Language is a hallmark of humanity. Yet no one really knows how or when our ancestors first began to arbitrarily assign words to objects (like *dog* for the tail-wagging, four-legged creature we play with in the yard), to break down these words into separate sounds (like d–o–g), or to recombine these tiny noises to make novel words with novel meanings (like g–o–d). But with all our meaningless little squeaks, clicks, and hisses, strung together to make words, with all our words linked to one another according to grammatical rules to make sentences, humankind would eventually dominate the earth.

Did Twiggy call hello to her lover as she returned from collecting nuts? Did she verbally describe the animal tracks she had seen on the plains or whisper that she loved her mate as she curled up to sleep? Did George and Cindy reprimand their infants, tell jokes, weave tales, lie, give compliments, discuss tomorrow and yesterday—with words? Certainly not the way you and I do. Postures, gestures, facial expressions, and intonations were probably critical to the message. Scientists now believe that human language could not have evolved earlier than some 500,000 years ago. But since Broca's area was expanding in the brain, Twiggy may have conversed with primitive, *prehuman* language.

Man the scout, tracker, explorer, scavenger, hunter, and protector. Woman the gatherer, nurturer, mediator, and educator. We may never know which early peoples first began to do separate, gendered tasks and share their spoils. But someone carted bones into the reeds and stripped them of their meat two million years ago.[60] And I do not think that females with small children were the hunters or the butchers. I suspect that our human sexual division of labor had begun.

There is no reason to think that either sex had rigid, formal roles, however. Probably females without children joined, even led, scavenging and hunting parties. Certainly males often gathered plants, nuts, and berries.

Probably some couples beat the grass together to catch small animals. But our ancestors had begun to collect, butcher, and share meat. The sexes had started to make their living as a team.

Times had changed. Now men and women were like two feet; they needed each other to get ahead. This hunting-gathering-scavenging life-style would produce an intricate balance of women, men, and power.

# Women, Men, and Power

## The Nature of Sexual Politics

> History always enunciates new truths.
>
> —FRIEDRICH WILHELM NIETZSCHE

Tens of thousands of women, their faces smeared with ashes, wearing loincloths and wreaths of ferns, poured from villages across southeastern Nigeria one morning in 1929 and marched to their local "native administration" centers. There the district's British colonial officers resided. The women congregated outside these administrators' doors and shook traditional war sticks, danced, ridiculed them with scurrilous songs, and demanded the insignia of the local Igbo men who had collaborated with this enemy. At a few administration centers women broke into jails to free prisoners; at others they burned or tore apart native-court buildings. But they hurt no one.

The British retaliated, opening fire on protesters in two centers, slaughtering sixty women. So ended the insurrection. The British "won."

History often records the words of victors, and this Women's War, as the Igbo called it, soon acquired its British name, the Aba Riots.[1] But the British never comprehended what this war was all about—that it was orchestrated entirely by women, for women. The notion of a violation of women's rights was beyond their grasp. Instead, most of the British officers were convinced that Igbo men had organized this demonstration, then directed their spouses to revolt. Igbo wives had rioted, colonial officials reasoned, because they thought the British would not fire on the weaker sex.[2]

A colossal cultural chasm stretched between the British and the Igbo—a gulf that gave rise to the Igbo Women's War and symbolized a profound European misunderstanding about women, men, and power in cultures around the world.

For centuries these Igbo women, like women in many other West African societies, had been autonomous and powerful—economically and politically. They lived in patrilineal villages where power was informal. Anyone could participate in Igbo village assemblies. Men engaged in more of the discussions and normally offered the final settlement on disputes. Men had more resources. So they could pay the fees and hold the feasts that brought them more titles and prestige. And men controlled the land. But at marriage a husband was obliged to give his wife some property to farm.

This soil was a woman's bank account. Women grew a variety of crops and took their produce to local markets run entirely by women.[3] And women came home with luxury goods and money that they kept. So Igbo women had independent wealth—financial freedom, economic power. Thus, if a man let his cows graze in a woman's fields, mistreated his wife, violated the market code, or committed some other serious crime, women did what they would do to the British administrators. They assembled at the offender's home, chanted insults, sometimes even destroyed his house. Igbo men respected women, women's work, women's rights, and women's laws.

Enter the British. In 1900 England declared southern Nigeria a protectorate and set up a system of native-court areas. Each district was governed by a British colonial officer from a district seat, the native court. This was unpopular enough. Then the British appointed one representative from each village, a warrant chief, to membership in each district's native court. Often this was a young Igbo who had curried favor with the conquerors rather than a respected village elder; always it was a man. Steeped in the Victorian belief that wives were appendages of their husbands, the British could not conceive of women in positions of power. So they excluded women, one and all.

Igbo women lost their voice.

Then, in 1929, the British decided to take inventories of women's goods. Fearing impending taxation, Igbo women met in their market squares to discuss this crippling economic action. They were ready to rebel. And after a series of flare-ups between women and census-takers in November, they dressed in traditional battle garments and went to war, an uprising that erupted over six thousand square miles and involved tens of thousands of women.

After the British quashed the revolution, Igbo women requested that they too serve as village representatives in the native courts. To no avail. As far as the British were concerned, a woman's place was in the home.

## "It's a Man's World"

The Western conviction that men universally dominate women has passed like a deleterious gene from one generation to the next.[4] Is this true? Did men universally dominate women in Twiggy's day, some two million years ago? To explore the deep evolutionary roots of women, men, and power, let me first unravel what we know of gender relations in societies around the world today.

Before the women's movement of the 1970s, American and European anthropologists simply assumed that men were always more powerful than women, and their research reflected their convictions. Accounts of the Australian aborigines provide a striking example.

Several academics—mostly men—wrote that these people's marriage system, in which infant girls were married to men thirty years their senior and men had several wives, was the crowning example of male rule. From their perspective, aboriginal women were pawns, commodities, currency in the marriage manipulations of men.[5] They explained the aborigines' separate men's and women's religious ceremonies as evidence of women's subordination too. And as for women's work, Ashley Montagu summed it up in 1937, calling the women no more than "domesticated cows."[6]

Today we know that this picture of aboriginal life is distorted. Women ethnographers have gone into the Australian Outback and talked to women. From conversations during gathering expeditions, at swimming parties, across the firelight, these scholars have established that Australian aboriginal women politick avidly in the betrothal poker game and begin to choose their own new husbands by middle age. Women regularly engage lovers. Some tribes have a *jilimi*, or single women's camp, where widows, estranged wives, and visiting women live or visit, free of men. Far from being a battered wife, a woman sometimes hits a lazy husband with her "fighting stick." Women hold some rituals that are closed to men. And women's economic contributions are vital to daily life.

Although women's and men's activities are often segregated, Australian aboriginal women appear to be every bit as powerful as men.[7] Neither sex dominates—a concept that was apparently foreign to Western scholars. A Western obsession with hierarchy, in concert with deeply ingrained beliefs about gender, has traditionally colored scientific analyses of other peoples.

This perspective changed during the women's movement, culminating in the late 1970s and early 1980s when feminist anthropologists began to challenge the dogma of universal female subordination. They argued that because men had done most of the fieldwork, spoken mostly to male informants, and primarily observed men's activities, many anthropological reports were biased. The voices of women had not been heard.

Some charged, moreover, that male anthropologists had misconstrued what they saw, denigrating women's work as "housework," women's conversations as superficial "gossip," women's artistry as "crafts," and women's participation in ceremonies as "non-sacred," while aggrandizing hunting, men's arts, men's religious rituals, men's oratory, and many other male pursuits.[8] Because of this selective blindness, androcentrism, or sexist bias—call it what you wish—women's work and women's lives had been ignored, distorting anthropological reports.

These accusations are not entirely true. In a classic study, sociologist Martin Whyte compared studies of gender roles in ninety-three traditional societies and noted that in some of these reports, data on women's roles were neglected or minimized; in others, aspects of men's power were disregarded. However, these omissions were random, rather than systematically biased against women. Moreover, the oversights were not linked specifically to male or female authors. Androcentrism may not be as pervasive as some reported.[9]

Nevertheless, even a casual reader of the literature can point to some classic ethnographies in which women look like faceless drones. And the ubiquitous articles of earlier times about "man the hunter" have now become balanced by literature on "woman the gatherer." So the feminist era turned the tide, adding a necessary lens to scholarly investigations of other peoples, women as well as men.

This newer focus on women's lives uncovered a reality of extreme importance. Like the Igbo women of Nigeria, women in a great many traditional cultures were relatively powerful—*before the coming of the Europeans*.[10] Some survived Western influence with their power intact. Many others, like the Igbo, fell victim to European mores.

Anthropologist Eleanor Leacock arrived at this conclusion while studying the Montagnais–Naskapi Indians of eastern Canada. Most instructive to her were the journals of the Jesuit Paul Le Jeune. Le Jeune took up his post as superior of the French mission at Quebec in 1632. Here he wintered with the Montagnais–Naskapi. To his horror, he saw indulgent parents, independent women, divorced partners, men with two wives, no formal leaders, a peripatetic, relaxed, egalitarian culture in which women enjoyed high economic and social status.

This state of affairs Le Jeune resolved to change. He was convinced that discipline for children, marital fidelity, lifelong monogamy, and, above all, male authority and female fealty were essential to salvation. As he told the Indians, "In France women do not rule their husbands."[11] Within months Le Jeune had converted a handful of these "heathens." Ten years later, some had started to beat women.

How many women have colonialism tethered?

It's impossible to say. But the Igbo Women's War was no fluke of history. As one scientist summed up the situation, "The penetration of Western colonialism, and with it Western practices and attitudes regarding women, has so widely influenced women's roles in aboriginal societies as to depress women's status almost everywhere in the world."[12]

## Power Plays

Knowing, then, that women have indeed been powerful in many traditional societies around the world, what can we infer about life in Africa during our long nomadic prehistoric past—millennia before European guns and gospels skewed power relations between men and women?

We have two ways of gaining insight: by examining daily life in modern traditional societies and by dissecting power relations among our close relatives, the apes. Let's begin with the power plays of people.[13]

Anthropologists generally agree that power (the ability to influence or persuade, as opposed to authority, formal institutionalized command) regularly resides with those who control valued goods or services and have the right to distribute this wealth outside the home.

## The Gift

If you own the land, rent the land, give away the land, or distribute resources on the land, like water holes or fishing rights, you have power. If you have a special service, like doctoring, or a connection with the spirit world that others need, you have power. If you kill a giraffe and give away the meat, or make baskets, beads, blankets, or other products for trade, you can make friends—alliances that bring economic ties, prestige, and power. So who collects what, who owns what, and who gives, rents, sells, or trades what to whom matters in the power dance between the sexes.[14]

The traditional north Alaskan Inuit (or Eskimos) offer a good example of this direct relationship between economic resources and social control.

In the barren north, where only moss and grasses appear above the permafrost for much of the year, there were no plants to gather. As a result, women traditionally did not leave home for work as gatherers or bring back valuable goods to trade. Men did all the hunting. Men left the house to chase seals or whales throughout the winter months and fished or hunted caribou during the long Arctic summer days. Men brought home the blubber for the candle oil, the skins for parkas, trousers, shirts, and shoes, sinew for cord, bone for ornaments and tools, and every scrap of food. Women depended on these supplies. Eskimo men depended on their wives to tan the hides, smoke the meat, and make all the heavy clothing. So the sexes needed each other to survive.

But men had access to the fundamental resources. And Eskimo girls realized early in life that the way to succeed was to "marry well."[15] Young women had no other formal access to power.

⋧

Traditional !Kung women of the Kalahari Desert, on the other hand, were far more economically powerful. And they did not marry as a career. As you know, when anthropologists first recorded their lifeways in the 1960s, women commuted to work and came home with much of the evening meal. !Kung women had economic power. They also had a voice.

But !Kung wives, unlike their husbands, did not distribute their food within the larger social group.

This distinction is important. When men returned from a successful hunting trip, they divided the precious meat according to rules as well as fanfare. The owner of the arrow that killed the animal got the prestigious task of distributing the catch. The man who first saw the beast got certain choice sections, those who tracked it got others, and so forth. Then each hunter gave steaks and ribs and organ meats to his family and other kin. These were "investments," however, not offerings. !Kung hunters expected to be reimbursed. For when the hunter gave his neighbors these hunks of meat, he garnered honor and obligations—power. And although women "had a formidable degree of autonomy," both !Kung men and women thought that men were slightly more influential than their wives.[16]

It's better to give than to receive, the adage goes. The !Kung and many other peoples would agree. Those who hold the purse strings have substantial social power—an economic formula that suggests that ancestral women, as well as men, had a good deal of social pull.

⋧

Power, of course, is not always a matter of economics. Can anyone be sure, for example, that economically powerful women or men are powerful in the bedroom too? It's not necessarily so.

Inuit women may marry well to get ahead, but there's no knowing whether these wives feel subordinate to their husbands. Although !Kung men distribute a prized resource, meat, !Kung women provide most of the daily meal. And who's to know whether the farmer who presides at the dinner table also dominates private conversations with his wife.

In fact, in peasant societies today—where men monopolize all the positions of rank and authority and women tend to act deferentially toward men in public—women have a great deal of *informal* influence. Despite men's strutting and public posturing in these cultures, anthropologist Susan Rogers has reported that neither sex actually thinks men rule women. She concludes that the sexes sustain a rough balance of power, that male dominance is a myth.[17]

So although economics undoubtedly played an important role in the power relations of men and women millennia ago, the sexes were most likely engaged in a much more complicated duel.

In an effort to unravel this subtle power dynamic between women and men, Martin Whyte mined the Human Relations Area File, a modern data bank that records information on over eight hundred societies.[18] From this file and from other ethnographic reports, he compiled data on ninety-three preindustrial peoples: one-third were nomadic hunter-gatherers; one-third were peasant farmers; one-third were peoples who herded and/or gardened for a living. Societies ranged from the Babylonians living around 1750 B.C. to present-day traditional cultures. Most had been studied by anthropologists since 1800 A.D.

Whyte then culled from these data the answers to a number of questions about each culture: What were the sexes of the gods? Which sex received more elaborate burial ceremonies? Who were the local political leaders? Who contributed what to the dinner table? Who had the final authority to discipline the children? Who arranged the marriages? Who inherited valuable property? Which gender did individuals think had the higher sex drive? Did people believe women were inferior to men? He cross-correlated these and many other variables in order to establish the status of women in societies around the world.

Whyte's findings confirm some widely held beliefs.[19]

There was *no* society in which women dominated men in most spheres of social life. Myths of Amazon women, tales of matriarchs who ruled with a velvet fist, were just that: fiction. In 67% of all cultures (mainly agricultural peoples), men appeared to control women in *most* circles of activity. In a fair number of societies (30%) men and women appeared to be roughly equal—particularly among gardeners and hunting-gathering peoples. And in 50% of the cultures, women had much more *informal* influence than societal rules accorded them.

Whyte uncovered an even more important fact: there was no single constellation of cross-cultural factors that together added up to *the* status of women or of men. Instead, each society revealed a series of pluses and minuses. In some cultures women made an enormous economic contribution but had less power over their marital and sex lives. In others, they could divorce easily, but had little say in religious matters or held no formal political offices. Even where women owned valuable property and had considerable economic power, they did not necessarily have extensive political rights or religious sway.

*Power in one sector of society did not necessarily translate into power in another.*

This fact is nowhere more obvious than in the United States. In 1920 women won the right to vote; their political influence increased. But they remained second-class citizens in the office. Today women's power in the workforce is rising; many are highly educated as well. At home, though, married working women still do more of the cooking, washing, and cleaning up. Because Americans assume that status is a single phenomenon, we cannot understand why working women still do more of the housework. But one's status in one sector of society does not necessarily affect one's position in another.

Instead, the power game between the sexes is like a crystal ball: turn the sphere a little and it casts a whole new light. Hence Twiggy and her pals may have been economically powerful and wielded a great deal of informal influence some two million years ago, yet were not necessarily leaders of the group.

What else can a study of traditional peoples say about women, men, and power in the past? Well, class, race, age, sex appeal, accomplishments, and kinship ties also contribute to the mosaic we call power.

Under certain circumstances the most insipid member of a higher class or dominant ethnic group can reign over a smarter, more dynamic person of a lower station. And although Westerners traditionally made sweeping judgments about the miserable status of women in Asia, an elderly Chinese or Japanese woman is often just as dictatorial as any man. In many societies age counts. So do sex appeal, wit, and charm. A barmaid can rule a businessman with sex; a cartoonist can puncture a politician with a drawing; a student may beguile her vastly better-educated teacher with a gaze.

Kinship also plays a part in who runs whom. In traditional patrilineal societies, where men regularly owned the land and children marked their descent from father, women tended to have little formal power in most sectors of society. On the other hand, women in matrilineal societies owned more property and this gave them much more influence in the community as a whole.

Last, the genders derive power from their society's symbolic world. As a culture evolves, it develops a "sexual template" or social script for how the genders are supposed to behave, as well as beliefs about the powers of each sex.[20] These scripts people carry in their minds. Mbuti pygmies of Zaire, for example, think women are powerful because only women give birth. The Mehinaku of Amazonia and many other people bestow power on menstrual blood: touch it and you get sick. Westerners have immortalized women's power to seduce men in their fable of Adam, Eve, the serpent, and the apple. Ultimately what a society designates as symbolically powerful becomes just that.

Power, then, is a composite of many forces that work together to make one man or woman more influential than the next.

What, then, of Twiggy, George, and the other hominins discussed in the last chapter who left their bones beside a blue-green lake at Olduvai two million years ago? Were those men and women social equals?

Undoubtedly these early "people" did not have class or ethnic distinctions. It is also unlikely that they had a cultural life rich with symbolic associations of power. But we can say a few things with some degree of certainty about Twiggy and her companions. They did not live like the Inuit, whose men collected all of the food while women stayed at home. There was no permanent home. And women worked. The double-income family was the rule. But Twiggy and her friends ate meat. And hunting and scavenging are not logical pastimes for pregnant women or mothers with small children. So Twiggy probably let her "special friend" collect the meat, the sinew, and the marrow from dangerous beasts, while she gathered fruit, vegetables, seeds, and small game with her female friends.

With her shopping expeditions, however, Twiggy made an enormous contribution to the evening meal—and she was, most likely, economically and sexually powerful as well.

But how did Twiggy live? Who actually bossed whom?

Not only do traditional cultures give us a clue; so do other species. In fact, we can glean a great deal of insight into Twiggy's daily power plays by examining a fascinating colony of chimpanzees in the Arnhem Zoo (officially known as Burgers' Zoo) in Holland.[21] To these chimps, maneuvering for rank and power is the spice of life.

## Chimpanzee Politics

Since 1971 a colony of chimps have resided in this zoo. At night they sleep in separate indoor cages; then after breakfast the chimps are free to enter a two-acre outdoor yard. It is surrounded by a moat and a high wall in the rear. About fifty oak and beech trees, each cloaked in electric fencing, loom inaccessibly above them. Rocks, tree trunks, and a few dead oaks for climbing are spread across the pen. Here the chimps engage in all of their political power plays—after the great escape.

On one morning, soon after the chimps arrived in this new home, they inspected their outdoor acreage inch by inch. Then that afternoon, after the last of the anthropologists, zookeepers, and trainers had departed, they staged their getaway. Some of them wedged a five-meter tree limb against the back wall. Then several chimps quietly scaled the fortress. Reportedly a few even helped the less surefooted with their climbing. Then they all descended nearby trees and availed themselves of the park's facilities. Big Mama, the oldest female of the group, made a beeline for the zoo cafeteria. Here she helped herself to a bottle of chocolate milk and settled among the other customers.

Bedlam reigned. With time the chimps were enticed back into their cages. But they have engaged in perpetual power struggles among themselves ever since—maneuvers that shed light on Twiggy's life in ancient times, as well as on the nature of modern human power plays.

The male chimps negotiate regularly for rank. A male begins his "intimidation display" by puffing up his hair, hooting, and swaying from side to side or stamping, often holding a rock or stick in his hand. Then he dashes past his rival, pounds the ground, and crows. This ritual is normally enough to persuade his adversary to defer. The retreat is accompanied by a distinctive gesture; the subordinate emits a short sequence of panting grunts as he bows deeply to his superior or crouches with his hair flat against his body to look small.

Aggressors enlist allies too. At the beginning of the intimidation display, the attacker often tries to get a companion to back him up, holding out a hand, palm up, toward a potential friend—inviting him to side with him. If he succeeds in recruiting a supporter, he may charge his opponent, pelting him with stones, screaming, pummeling him with fists, and biting him on the hands, feet, or head. But he also keeps an eye on his ally. If his deputy seems to waver in his allegiance, the aggressor renews his begging gestures to him.

"There is no such thing as a free lunch," they say, and it's just as true of chimpanzee politicians as of human ones. When one chimp backs up another, he expects his favor to be returned. In fact, chimps seem to feel obliged, rousing themselves from a perfectly peaceful doze to stand near an argument or join the fray. Alliances count.

On one occasion at Arnhem, the male who was second in command groomed one female after the next, patting each and playing with her children. These rounds completed, he immediately threatened the alpha male. Had he bribed these females to support his cause? Probably. Like politicians who kiss babies and speak out on women's issues, male chimps cultivate female friends.

Some male coalitions last for years; many more last only minutes. Status-hungry male chimps make fickle friends. But when an individual gets into a scrape, he "pulls strings," hollering until allies come to root or join the brawl. Sometimes four or five males participate in the melee, a huge knot of yelling, tumbling, gouging apes.

Perhaps when Twiggy and her hominin comrades rested at midday, a male flaunted his high status, huffing, hooting, and swaying threateningly until a subordinate bowed to him. Occasionally fights must have broken out. And males probably cultivated Twiggy for her support and that of her female pals.

## Networking

Curiously, male and female chimps at Arnhem arrange themselves in quite different power structures. Each is much like that of contemporary humans and may also hark back to Twiggy's times.

Male chimps are connected in a web of hierarchical intrigues with friends and enemies that add up to a flexible dominance ladder with one male at the top. These ranks are clearly demarcated at any one moment. But as a male wins more allies and more skirmishes, the dominance ladder slowly changes. Finally a series of confrontations or a single vicious fight swings the balance and a new individual emerges as king of the male hierarchy.

This ruler has an important job—sheriff. He steps into a brawl and pulls the adversaries from one another. And he is expected to be a nonpartisan referee. When the alpha male keeps fights to a minimum, his chimp underlings respect him, support him, even pay him homage. They bow to him, plunging their heads and upper bodies rapidly and repeatedly. They kiss his hands, feet, neck, and chest. They lower themselves to make sure they are beneath him. And they follow him in an entourage. But if the leader fails to maintain harmony, his inferiors shift their allegiance, and the hierarchy slowly changes until peace is reached. Subordinates create the chief.

Female chimps do not establish this kind of status ladder. They form cliques instead—laterally connected subgroups of individuals who care for one another's infants and protect and nurture one another in times of social chaos. Females are less aggressive, less dominance oriented, and this network can remain stable—and relatively egalitarian—for years. Moreover, the dominant female generally acquires this position by sheer personality, charisma, and age, rather than by intimidation.

Female chimps quarrel, though, and, like males, they use their allies to settle scores. On one occasion a threatened female called on a male friend for help. Amid high-pitched "indignant" barks, she pointed with her whole hand (rather than a finger) toward the assailant, at the same time kissing and patting her male ally. When her pleas became more insistent, her male friend counterattacked the antagonist while the female stood by and watched approvingly.

Do men naturally tend to form hierarchal ranks and then jockey for better positions, whereas women form more egalitarian, stable cliques? Yes. A host of data suggest they do.[22] Moreover, men's sensitivity to rank is linked with the activity of testosterone,[23] while women's drive for cooperation and group harmony is linked with the activities of estrogen.[24] There is biology to this gender difference.

So two million years ago *Homo habilis* males, such as George, may have spent a good deal of time jockeying for rank, while Twiggy probably had a network of more stable relationships with her female friends.

Twiggy's most powerful role may have been as group arbiter, however. At Arnhem, Big Mama played this part. She broke up arguments between juveniles just by standing near them, barking and waving her arms. It was always Big Mama who coaxed the vanquished from the dead tree in the center of the enclosure. And after any battle, the loser always fled whimpering to her side.

Other females at Arnhem acted as mediators too. Once during a male's "bluff display," a female strolled up to him, peeled his fingers from around his rock and walked away with it. When the male found a new rock, she took it away too. This confiscation process occurred six times in a row. Other mediators behaved differently. Some simply jabbed the victor's side with a hand, driving him until he sat down beside his enemy and began the grooming ceremony.

This grooming ritual has a pattern, and it suggests perhaps the single most important thing about power relations in our past: peacemaking was a staple of daily life.[25] Within minutes after a brawl, or hours or even days later, chimp enemies walk up to each other, grunt softly, shake hands, hug, kiss each other on the lips, and gaze deeply into each other's eyes. Then they sit, lick each other's wounds, and groom each other. Chimp rivals also spend inordinate amounts of energy suppressing their animosity, indeed, grooming each other particularly furiously when they are very tense.

Chimps and all other primates work hard to mollify their companions. Violence is the exception; placating is the rule—as it probably was among our ancestors in Twiggy's day.

From the perpetual power struggles at the Arnhem Zoo, primatologist Frans de Waal established several things about power among these apes, principles that most likely applied to our ancestors on the grasslands of Africa two million years ago and that have been carried across time to modern humankind.

First of all, power shifts. Ranks are formalized; but animals are part of a pliable network of relationships. Moreover, the ability to rule does not always depend on strength, size, speed, agility, or aggressiveness; it often depends on wits, on whom you know, and how you pay your social debts. Last, power can be either formal or informal. As supporters and arbiters, females are major players in the power game. And under the right set of circumstances, a female can even reign.

In fact, when visitors asked de Waal which were more powerful, male or female chimps, he shrugged and explained it thus. If you look at who greets whom, males dominate females 100% of the time. If you count who wins aggressive interactions, males win 80% of the time. But if you measure who takes food away from whom or who sits in the best spots, females win 80% of the time. And to emphasize the complexity of power, de Waal liked to add, "Nikkie [male] is the highest-ranking ape but he is completely dependent on Yeroen [male]. Luit [male] is individually the most powerful. But when it comes to who can push others aside then Mama [female] is the boss."[26]

De Waal confirmed the two things that anthropologists have observed in human cultures: status is not a single, monolithic quality measured in a single way; and male dominance, if it implies power over females in every sphere of life, is a myth.

## The Old Girls Network

A final factor may have contributed to Twiggy's power—her family status. In several primate species, such as baboons, groups of related females usually stick together, while the males often switch from troop to troop. Within each troop, one matriline tends to dominate the next, and so forth—a relatively stable hierarchy of dynasties, an "old girls" network.[27] Hence a juvenile of a high-ranking female clan can often dominate a mature female from a less prestigious family.

Moreover, children often assume their mother's rank. Among wild chimps at Gombe, where females are not organized into matrilines but form cliques instead, the children of the sovereign female, Flo, grew up to become influential in the community, whereas the offspring of a submissive peer became subservient adults as well.

## Gender Relations at Ancient Olduvai

Power relations in traditional human cultures and politics among chimpanzees suggest how our ancestors could have lived and jockeyed among themselves for status at Olduvai Gorge some two million years ago.

Twiggy's first memory may have been that of looking across the waving grass as she rode on her mother's hip. By the time she was three or four, she knew where the cashews grew and how to dig for roots. She probably played at water holes as her mother collected crabs and lolled below the fig trees when grownups gathered blossoms or sweet fruit. If her mother was powerful, like Big Mama, Twiggy probably rested in the shady spots. If mother's "special friend" was a good scavenger, she dined on tongue and other delicacies of wildebeest. And maybe when all lined up to slurp water trickling from a rock, Twiggy went first.

Whether these ancestors traveled in groups of related males or related females, we will never know. But every morning some ten to fifty members of Twiggy's band must have awakened, chattered, drank, relieved themselves, and abandoned their night nests to wander along the lake or out into the grass. Regularly males split off to scout or scavenge and returned later in the day, while groups of females went gathering together. Then all settled in early evening to share their food with their partner (and others if they had enough) and sleep in a clump of fig trees, on a grassy cliff, or in a dried-up streambed on the ground. The next morning they began again.

As the days passed, Twiggy probably became used to seeing males and females bow to her mother as they marched along. When she grew older, she probably tagged along beside her older sister, formed a clique with other girls, and spent her time grooming them, playing tag and tickle, and chasing boys. Undoubtedly Twiggy knew her place in the social network and grinned, bowed, and kissed the hands and feet of her superiors. When Twiggy got into battles with other children, her mother (or father) defended her and she won. And by wits and charm, Twiggy made friends with boys, then coaxed them into sharing bits of meat.

After Twiggy reached puberty, she must have formed a pair-bond with a "special friend." Maybe he was someone from a different group she met when her band made its annual pilgrimage in the dry season to camp beside the blue-green lake. Together Twiggy and her lover walked through the open plains; together they shared their food; together they bore a child. If the partnership became acrimonious, she probably waited until her infant had stopped suckling, then picked up her digging stick and pouch and joined a neighboring band or orchestrated his departure from the group. Economic autonomy enabled Twiggy to "divorce" her mate as soon as her infant could join a multi-age playgroup and be cared for by additional members of the band.

Twiggy may have been powerful in other aspects of daily life as well. If she consistently remembered where to find honey and prized vegetables, she was admired. Perhaps she was an arbiter too, taking rocks and sticks from her "husband's" hand as he swayed and shouted at a rival. Undoubtedly she had one or two girlfriends who always defended her in a quarrel. And if Twiggy was charismatic, bright, respected, and clever at keeping friends, she could well have become a leader in the group. Among primates the law of the jungle is not just strength but also brains.

These brains soon harnessed fire and invented new tools and weapons. Then, like a rocket, our ancestors shot into "almost human" social life.

# 12

## Almost Human

### Genesis of Kinship and the Teenager

It is indeed a desirable thing to be well descended, but
the glory belongs to our ancestors.

—PLUTARCH, *MORALS*

Fire.

Ever since our ancestors descended from the trees, they must have fled to lakes and streams when volcanoes disgorged rivers of molten rock or lightning licked the prairie and flame spread across the grass. While the plains still smoldered, they probably picked their way back through the embers to collect hares, lizards, fallen bees' nests, seeds, even large mammals, then gorged on the roasted food.

At the mouths of caves, where the dung of owls, bats, saber-toothed cats, and other cave dwellers collected in rich deposits, the embers may have flickered on for days or even weeks, and gradually ancients learned to sleep beside these coals, even feed the thirsty flame with dried branches until passing game, the promise of distant flowering fruit trees, or lack of water pushed a tiny band to abandon the warm, protective glow.

Fire was humankind's companion—an enemy when it raged, a friend when it subsided. But when our ancestors first learned to control flame, to carry embers in a baboon skull or wrapped in fleshy leaves, fire became their greatest asset.

With fire they could harden wood to make more deadly spears. With burning moss they could smoke out rodents from their burrows or drive rabbits toward their snares. With hearths they could ward off stealthy nighttime predators from carcasses they had half consumed. With smoke they could signal friends. And with burning branches they could drive hyenas from their lairs, then usurp these cave homes and sleep within the halo of the flame. Now injured band members, older men and women, pregnant females, and small children could stay in camp. There was a camp. No longer servants of the sun, our ancestors could stoke the embers and lounge about in morning, mend their tools at dusk, and reenact the day's events late into the night.

Darwin wrote that the art of making fire was "probably the greatest [discovery], excepting language, ever made by man."[1] For when our forebears began to harness fire they could also cook their meat and their vegetables, roots, and tubers. Cooking dramatically increased the caloric value of most foods, providing significantly more nutrition. It also gave our forebears far more metabolic energy. It produced healthier children. And it brought longer life.[2]

Most important: *cooking with flame enabled the evolution of the human brain.*[3]

Brains need glucose for energy. Our modern brains gobble about 20% of our bodily energy budget; we need this energy or we will die. In humans, a diet rich in calories can provide this energy—but only in conjunction with a reduced gut, necessary for digestive efficiency. So anthropologist Richard Wrangham and others have proposed that cooked food—in association with changes in the teeth, jaws, stomach and gut—enabled our ancestors to build bigger brains and leap toward modernity.[4]

This brain growth would produce vast new changes in human sexuality, love, and family life.

◈

We may never know exactly when humankind first began to control fire. Anthropologists do not agree. But someone living around Lake Turkana in northern Kenya may have built a campfire some 1.5 million years ago.[5]

I had a profound experience with this particular hearth, an event that occurred in 2010.

I had joined a team of scientists digging in the Lake Turkana area at a site known as Koobi Fora. One morning, drained by the 110-degree heat, I found a small rock cairn where I plopped down to rest—until our leader, anthropologist Jack Harris, informed me that I was sitting atop this ancient fireplace, marked with these rocks for further excavation. I leapt up. But I still wonder who sat there last. He or she may have been eating cooked meat, for a gene responsible for building our weak human jaw (now associated with cooked food) seems to have proliferated among our ancestors about 2.5 million years ago.[6]

Clearer evidence of campfires comes from the Swartkrans cave, in South Africa, where anthropologists collected 270 charred bits of ancient animal bones.[7] These fossil bones had been burned at between 200 and 800 degrees Centigrade. This is within the temperature range created today by a campfire of stinkwood branches.

Someone may have collected dead limbs from the many white stinkwood trees that have covered this area for eons and enjoyed fire here at least 1.5 million years ago. And once our ancestors began to make campfires, they built them over and over again. More than twenty separate levels of fire-burned debris have been found at Swartkrans. Still more evidence of man-made hearths has been found in Ethiopia and other parts of Kenya.

What "people" warmed their hands, burned these bones and sat around these hearths' protective glow some 1.5 million years ago? Most anthropologists are convinced that someone new had emerged, that these more advanced *Homo erectus* peoples fed these ancient flames. Why? Because *Homo erectus* peoples were far more intelligent than any of their forebears: their brains had burgeoned; they were well on their way toward humanity.

These "people" appear in the fossil record at Olduvai Gorge, Tanzania, at Koobi Fora, Kenya, and in the Omo River valley in southern Ethiopia by 1.9 to 1.8 million years ago. But a telling early *Homo erectus* site is Nariokotome III.[8]

# Nariokotome Boy

Here, in arid sediments near the western shore of Lake Turkana, Kenya, a youth died in a marsh some 1.6 million years ago. The robustness of the face and shape of the hips indicate that this individual was most likely a boy. Nariokotome Boy, as he is called, was about twelve years old and somewhat less than five feet three inches tall the day he passed away. His hands, arms, hips, and legs were very much like ours. His chest was more rounded than the chest of modern men, and he had one more lumbar vertebra. But if this young man had walked fully clothed down your street on Halloween wearing a mask, you would not have noticed him at all.

Had he removed the disguise, you would have fled. Although he was far more human-looking than Twiggy and her *Homo habilis* pals, his rugged, protruding jaw and big teeth, the heavy brow ridges above his eyes, his sloping, flattened forehead, his thick skull, and his bulging neck muscles would have stunned even the corner cop.

Nevertheless, the boy was reasonably smart. He had a brain volume of almost 900 cubic centimeters, much larger than that of Lucy and her *Australopithecus afarensis* pals, who had a brain volume of some 450 cubic centimeters, and of Twiggy and her *Homo habilis* contemporaries, who had an average brain volume of some 612 cubic centimeters, and just below that of modern men and women, whose average cranial capacity is about 1,350 cubic centimeters. Later *Homo erectus* skulls would show even larger cranial capacities, reaching over 1,200 cubic centimeters.

Interestingly, chimpanzees understand fire.[9] Chimps living in captivity like to smoke cigarettes, and they are adroit at lighting a match and blowing out the flame.[10] More remarkable, wild chimps in Senegal deftly watch a wildfire that is coming their way, size up the behavior of the flame, and move away from it calmly as they monitor its direction.[11] So it is likely that *Homo erectus* men and women, with a much bigger brain than those of chimps, understood the behavior of fire, could start it, fuel it, and ignite and extinguish it in campfires in South Africa, Ethiopia and Kenya by 1.5 million years ago.

With their advanced "thinking caps," these creative individuals would start to build our modern human social and sexual world.

Foremost, *Homo erectus* developed sophisticated tools.

While Twiggy and her relatives had made simple Oldowan tools—no more than water-worn rocks with a few edges whacked off to make a sharpened edge—ingenious *Homo erectus* peoples had begun to chip delicate flakes from larger stones. They probably used these small flakes to cut, slice, scrape, and dig. More impressive were their bifacial tools, including cleavers and large six- to seven-inch stone hand axes, called Acheulean hand axes because they were first discovered in Saint-Acheul, France. With a rounded butt end and careful flaking along both edges to make a tapered point, these tools look like large almonds, pears, or tear-drops of stone.

Like golf balls in a water trap, these hand axes have been found strewn along ancient streams and rivers, on channel bars, at lake margins, in swamps and bogs and marshes across southern and eastern Africa, as well as along watercourses in Europe, India, and Indonesia. So although some must have been used to dig for vegetables that grew along the banks, it has long been thought that early *Homo erectus* peoples used these massive streamlined tools mainly to skin and disarticulate carcasses at the shore, then chop meat from bone, cut sinew, and crack bones for marrow.

This may have been the fate of a baby hippo whose remains were found at Lake Turkana, in what was a shallow, muddy lake some 1.5 million years ago. Acheulean hand axes lay nearby. And seven footprints of a *Homo erectus* individual were imprinted nearby in the mud.[12] Perhaps the individual, who stood about five and a half feet tall and weighed some 120 pounds, had waded silently into the water and slain the wallowing beast.

Fire. Fancy tools. Hunting large animals. The bodies of *Homo erectus* had also become well adapted for endurance running; indeed their limb proportions, buttock muscles, and tendons had taken on our modern form.[13] Moreover, these peoples had begun to establish home bases, campsites that they returned to for days or weeks.[14] *Homo erectus* men and women had started to perfect the basic elements of the hunting-gathering way of life.

Our expanding brain created a complication, however, that would speed the journey toward you and me.

## Born Too Young

Since the early 1960s, anthropologists have reasoned that at some point in hominin evolution the brain became so large in proportion to the mother's pelvic birth canal that women began to have difficulty bearing their large-brained young. With its growing head, the infant couldn't get out.

This tight squeeze is known as the *obstetrical dilemma*.[15] Nature's solution: to bear young at an earlier (smaller) stage of development and extend fetal brain growth into postnatal life. As Ashley Montagu summed up the infant's problem: "If he weren't born when he is, he wouldn't be born at all."[16]

Indeed, we are born too soon; the human newborn is really just a fetus. All of the primates bear immature (altricial) young, and the degree of altriciality (immaturity) increases from monkeys to apes to humans. Human babies are born even more immature than those of our closest relatives, a characteristic known as secondary altriciality.[17] Not until six to nine months of age does the human infant acquire the chemical responses of the liver, kidneys, immune system, and digestive tract, or the motor reactions and the brain development displayed by other primates shortly after birth.

Scientists estimate that our ancestors began to bear exceedingly immature, helpless babies when the brain reached an adult cranial capacity of 700 cubic centimeters—most likely among *Homo erectus* peoples more than a million years ago.[18]

⁓

What an impact this single adaptation had on human patterns of marriage, sex, and love. Foremost, these helpless young must have dramatically increased the "reproductive burden" of *Homo erectus* females, further stimulating selection for the brain circuits of romantic love, attachment, and pair-bonding. Now a "special friend"—indeed, a long-term steady partner—was even more critical to the survival of the help-less child.[19]

Anthropologist Wenda Trevathan thinks that the complications of this tight squeeze at birth also stimulated women's first specialized occupation—midwifery.

In her book *Human Birth: An Evolutionary Perspective*, Trevathan looked at human parturition from the viewpoint of an animal behavior-ist. She proposed, for example, that when a human mother strokes her newborn, this gesture stems not just from a psychological need to bond, but also from the mammalian practice of licking one's young to stimu-late breathing and other bodily functions. Because human newborns are covered with a creamy fluid known as the vernix caseosa, new mothers probably evolved their patting habit to rub in this fatty gel—lubricating the skin, protecting the infant from viruses and bacteria. Trevathan also noted that, regardless of their handedness, new mothers hold their infants in the left arm, directly over the heart, probably because the heartbeat soothes the child.

More important to our story, Trevathan proposed that by *Homo erectus* times birthing had become so complicated that women needed a helper to "catch" the infant. Thus the human tradition of midwifery emerged. Perhaps these helpers became bonded to the newborn too, widening the circle of adults who felt responsible for the child.[20]

Grandmothers may have become necessary helpers too—contributing to the evolution of a universal human female trait: menopause. Known as the *grandmother hypothesis*, this theory proposes that with the evolution of menopause, middle-aged women could forgo the burden of bearing more of their own young in order to help rear their children's children.[21] Quality over quantity. By "stopping early" women could conserve their strength, avoid reproductive competition with their own daughters, and focus their energy on helping their living offspring survive.

"There is no greater power in the world than the zest of a post-menopausal woman," Margaret Mead reportedly said. Post-menopausal women brought new vigor to the eternal struggle to pass one's DNA into tomorrow.

More changes were to come.

# Origin of Teenage

Our *Homo erectus* ancestors most likely acquired another burden—the teenager. From characteristics of ancient teeth and bones, it appears that at some point (perhaps some 900,000 to 800,000 years ago) the human maturation process slowed down.[22] Not only did women now bear exceedingly helpless babies, but childhood had also become prolonged.

Hail the origin of teenage, another hallmark of the human animal, another distinct divergence from our relatives the apes. A chimpanzee reaches puberty at about age ten. Girls in hunting-gathering societies, however, often did not reach menarche until age sixteen or seventeen (although today in Westernized societies female menarche is far earlier). Boys went through a prolonged adolescence too. In fact, today humans do not stop growing physically until about age twenty.

Even more remarkable, human parents continue to provide food and shelter for their teenagers. After chimp mothers have weaned their infants, these youngsters feed themselves and build their own nests every night. The juvenile chimp still stays near mother much of the time. But mother no longer feeds or shelters her offspring.

Not so humankind. At age five the human child can barely dig a root. Even the most sophisticated youngster in a hunting-gathering society cannot forage and survive until they are years older. So human parents continue to rear their offspring for many years after their children have been weaned.[23] With the evolution of our slow human maturation process, our childhood and adolescence would eventually become almost twice as long as that of chimps and other primates.

Why did the human maturation process become so extended?

To gain time: time in childhood to learn about an increasingly complex world. Boys needed to learn where to quarry flint and other stones, how to hit these rocks at the precise angle to remove a flake, and how to fashion their weapons for perfect throwing. Boys had to watch the animals, learn which creatures led the herd, understand how the winds and seasons changed, as well as which prey to track, how to track, where to surround, how to fell their quarry, how to cut the game and divide the spoils, and how to carry flame.

Girls had even more to learn: where the berry bushes grew, what bogs to avoid, where to find birds' eggs, what the life cycles of hundreds of different plants were, where small animals burrowed or reptiles sunned, and which herbs were best for colds, sore throats, and fevers.

All this learning took time, trial and error, and intelligence. Perhaps the young also had to commit to memory long tales, stories like morality plays that taught them about the weather and the habits of the plants and animals around them.

Equally important, they had to learn the nuances of the mating game. With the evolution of teenage came all of those extra years to experiment at courting, sex, and love—crucial parts of life in a social world where men and women needed to pair up to share their food and raise their children as a team.

## Brotherly Love

As the brain expanded and women began to bear helpless young with a long teenage, pressures on parents must have mounted—stimulating the evolution of another human hallmark: our formal human kinship systems.

Many animals, including all of the higher primates, tend to hang around with mother, are highly familiar with their siblings, and have specific relationships with all the other members of the group. The informal roots of human kinship lie deep in our mammalian past. But when our ancestors began to develop *categories* of relatives, each with prescribed ties and duties, they had begun to build the social glue of traditional human social life.

The evolution of our human kinship systems is among the oldest arguments in anthropology. Basic to the debate has been the question, which came first: matriliny (tracing your lineage through your mother's line) or patriliny (tracing your lineage through your father's line)? Today many tribal peoples, as well as many contemporary postindustrial peoples, trace their descent through both their mothers' and fathers' lines, a bilateral kinship system. But this kin structure is not generally found in nature. So, our *Homo erectus* forebears most likely grew up with either their mother's or their father's blood relatives and others who joined the community.

Primitive matriliny or patriliny? The lives of our close relatives give conflicting clues.

Among savanna baboons, groups of related females travel as a unit, whereas males depart for other troops as they mature—the kernel of matriliny, the kinship system based on female genetic ties.

Among common chimpanzees the reverse is true. Related males tend to remain together to defend their community, whereas females typically leave the group at puberty to seek mates in neighboring groups. Here are the seeds of patriliny, the kinship system based on male blood ties. Interestingly, an ingenious study of fossils (dating from more than two million years ago) suggests that females dispersed farther than males,[24] perhaps to join novel partners in a different group, a sign suggesting primordial patriliny.

But in most of today's hunting-gathering societies, both young men and young women are free to leave or remain in their natal group; moreover, when they marry, a couple may live with either the husband's or the wife's kin. Indeed, they often live with both kin groups, switching their residence when they choose.[25] Yet some hunter-gatherers trace their descent through mother; some hark to their father's line; and some regard themselves of members of both kin groups simultaneously—a bilateral kinship system.[26]

Because kinship structure varies among primates, including humans, it is impossible to make an informed guess about the kin networks of these early *Homo erectus* bands. With a few exceptions: almost certainly all members knew one another and could recognize "mother." With the evolution of pair-bonding, they must have also included in their inner circle mother's "special friend."

Then at some point, they began to expand this network to include mother's or father's genetic relatives and their relatives' special friends— affinal relatives related only by "marriage." Hence they began to convert these *biologically unrelated* men and women into family members. And as these formalized social networks took shape, the concepts of "clan" and "tribe" most likely arose.

I suspect that Nariokotome Boy and his *Homo erectus* relatives grew up in formalized kin networks. They had to. Mother and her "special friend" needed extra relatives to help them raise their tiny, helpless infants through a long childhood and teenage.

What an ingenious twist: a web of consanguineal and affinal relatives locked in a formal network of ties and obligations—an eternal, unbreakable kinship system dedicated to nurturing their mutual DNA.

As a child, a *Homo erectus* girl probably expected her mother's "special friend" to share his meat, protect her, and hold her when she cried. With him she had a specific tie that became "daughter–father." She probably became obliged to help care for her male sibling, an obligation that would evolve into the duties of "sister–brother." And some of her mother's or father's sisters and brothers and their "special friends" she came to know as aunts and uncles.

With the escalation of big-game hunting, the intensified division of labor between the sexes and the vicissitudes of raising helpless babies through a long teenage, our *Homo erectus* forebears began to classify relatives into specific social niches—each with distinct obligations, responsibilities and social roles. Moreover, as these formalized kinship systems emerged, our forebears would begin to develop their first prescribed rules and taboos regarding sex, romance, attachment, and who could "marry" whom—the foundation stones of human reproductive life.

## Out of Africa

Our *Homo erectus* ancestors also began to spread across the globe. They had reached western Asia by 1.7 million years ago, Indonesia by at least 1.6 million, and China by 1.15 million years ago.[27]

Why our ancestors left Africa, we do not know. Perhaps because they could.

By 1.8 million years ago the earth's temperature had taken another dramatic plunge. To the north, in Europe and Asia, snow piled in the high country during the longer, colder winters, and less snow melted during the chilly summer days and nights. Century upon century, ice sheets grew into mile-high glacial crusts. Then gravity pulled these ice fortresses from the mountain peaks, carving valleys, moving rocks, felling trees, extending the bitter weather to the south. Each cold spasm lasted several thousand years.

With each bout of freezing weather, more and more of the ocean's water became locked in ice. So, with time, the sea level dropped some four hundred feet, exposing wide land bridges—highways to the north.

Not only could our ancestors now walk north; maybe they had to.

As they grew more efficient at hunting game, they probably needed to look farther afield for prey. Moreover, with fiery torches with which to hunt and protect themselves, as well as efficient tools with which to butcher game, they could probably collect more meat—enabling more children to survive.[28] So when a tiny band appeared at the Swartkrans cave, another group had already moved in, or the fig groves and crabbing pools were picked clean when a band arrived. Last, skirmishes with neighbors or quarrels among themselves might have driven splinter groups or whole communities out of their native lands.

Whatever the reasons for the migration, our ancestors gradually explored new river valleys and new trails that led them out of Africa. Some followed reindeer, musk ox, bison, giant elk, and other massive beasts through what is now the republic of Georgia in western Asia; others spread into northern China; others trickled south to Java, where they left their remains along the steamy Solo River; still more left their bones in today's Israel. Moving no more than ten miles every generation, they would have reached Beijing in less than 20,000 years.

They did just that.

The biggest cache of evidence is at Dragon Bone Hill, a rich complex of caves along this hill about thirty miles from Beijing, well known to anthropologists as Zhoukoudian.[29] Here Chinese fossil hunters had been collecting ancient bones for centuries, treasures they sold to local chemists who ground the fragments into a sour-tasting powder that they peddled as medicinal elixirs. After hearing of these expeditions, Canadian anatomist Davidson Black launched his own pilgrimage in 1927.

Since then, over a dozen parts of skull caps and facial fragments, some

147 teeth, and many postcranial bones of *Homo erectus* individuals have been unearthed at Dragon Bone Hill—along with the bones of wild pigs, elephants, rhinos, horses and thousands of stone tools.[30] *Homo erectus* men and women camped here many times, some 500,000 years ago. Perhaps they came mostly in the autumn when the mammoths and mastodons, rhinos, deer, and ancient horses lumbered past their front doors heading south to warmer, wetter weather.

## Love Among *Homo Erectus* Peoples

What, then, of sex, love, and life among the *Homo erectus* men and women who stalked hippos in Lake Turkana, warmed their hands around hearths in South Africa, and left their bones in the jungles of Java and on the slopes of Dragon Bone Hill in China?

These men probably valued women for their work as gatherers and mothers. Their wives and lovers must have known every stand of yarrow, every honey tree, the tiniest berry shrub, every site where water dribbled from a rock, and every hillock, cave, and trail for over a hundred miles around them—even in plains as seemingly uniform as the Pacific Ocean. On most mornings women must have left camp carrying their infants in skin pouches on their backs. Every afternoon they returned with nuts, berries, firewood, and often information concerning the whereabouts of herds, water, enemies, and relatives. Men counted on their women to survive.

Women must have appreciated men for their bravery in the hunt, for their gifts of steaks and roasts and chops, and for their protection against enemies. Women needed the skins of these slaughtered animals for shawls and blankets, the skulls for containers, the bones for tools, and the sinews for string and cord.

Surely men and women smiled and joked when they returned at night to feed the embers and recount the day's events. Undoubtedly they flirted as they sucked on bones and berries across the smoky haze. And most likely they slipped in next to one another as the campfire faded and sometimes kissed and held each other long into the night. But what these people dreamed, who they loved, or what they thought as they drifted off to sleep is gone with the firelight.

These were not ancient replicas of modern people. They painted no pictures of bears or bison on cave walls. No small bone needles suggest they made tailored coats. No amulets indicate they worshiped the sun, the stars, or a god. They left no graves. But they were *almost* human beings. They had big brains. They nurtured flame. They bore very helpless babies, as we do today. Immature teenagers trailed along with parents and other members of the band. Old and young were all intertwined in an elaborate network of socially related kin. And the fireside had become synonymous with "home."

Some from among these ancestors would emerge into archaic forms of modern men and women. Now our world of sex and love would take its completely human form.

# 13

## The First Affluent Society

### "That Short but Imperious Word, 'Ought'"

> Two things fill the mind with ever-increasing wonder
> and awe, the more often and the more intensely the
> mind of thought is drawn to them: the starry heavens
> above me and the moral law within me.
>
> —IMMANUEL KANT, *CRITIQUE OF PURE REASON*

Beneath the quiet towns of southwestern France, the Pyrenees, and northern Spain, restless ancient torrents carved out a labyrinth of caves. Here, in the windless chasms deep below the ground, stalagmites and stalactites attend like ghostly ivory soldiers. Bullets of dripping water make a metallic ping in the utter quiet. The sounds of bats dance off craggy pits and hollows. And the roar of still-living rivers rushes up through chutes, funnels, and "cat holes," then vanishes into stillness at some hairpin turn.

What nature built, our ancestors came to decorate perhaps as early as 40,000 years ago, leaving behind thousands of cave paintings and engravings, evidence that modern humanity had burst onto earth.

In the giant underground rotundas in the cave at Lascaux, near Les Eyzies, France, someone painted dozens of stampeding herd animals. In a recess of the cave of Les Trois Frères, in the Pyrenees, another artist incised a magical beast—with the head of a man, the antlers of a stag, and the body and tail of a horse. In the La Juyo cave, in Spain, our forebears carved a monstrous stone head, half man, half cat. In over thirty caves giant bison, reindeer, mammoths, ibex, bears, and other beasts are outlined in red or black, their fur and muscles filled in with carefully placed strokes that use the natural fissures and protrusions of the rock.

And where real figures give way to magical ones, headless horses, duckbilled people, wolf-headed bears, disembodied hands with missing fingers, floating arms and legs, snake patterns, and dots and dashes dance along the walls and ceilings. Some of these paintings appear in large galleries; others are painted in cul-de-sacs so remote that professional cavers have fainted from claustrophobia trying to gain access to these crypts.

In these sunless tunnels, amid heightened sounds and cool, stagnant air, something of significance was going on. No one lived here. Our ancestors came to paint and gather for communal purposes instead. Perhaps they held ceremonies to ensure a good hunting season, to celebrate the birth of a son or daughter, to cure the sick, or for a host of other purposes.[1] John Pfeiffer, in his classic book *The Creative Explosion*, proposed that they may have held complex initiation rituals as well.

Pfeiffer believed it possible that young initiates were left in isolated tombs in the bowels of the earth until fear, isolation, and monotony stripped them of their normal senses and put them in a trancelike state of receptivity. Then their elders, using trickery and illusion, led these spellbound youngsters through convoluted alleys while they told them important clan traditions, clan history, and clan legends, the accumulated wisdom of the tribe.

To emphasize an incident in an elaborate tale, these sorcerers may have held a lamp beneath a painting. The flickering torch lit a hand or bird or fish, then suddenly a dancing, snorting elk or a swimming stag, to animate a specific point in the storyline. Then after each meandering trek, these priests assembled their disoriented students in large subterranean theaters where the brainwashed youths underwent more ordeals and repetitions that permanently etched these "textbooks" in their minds.

What were the elders saying? Why this first flowering of human art? What does the outpouring of artistic expression say about human romance and sexuality during this creative burst?

Pfeiffer proposed that these people were experiencing an "information explosion," produced by vast changes in technology and expanding social networks. And because the footprints of children are prevalent in many of these caves, he theorizes that the young were taken into these surreal mazes to participate in initiation rituals designed to teach them all these new facts.

Even today this strategy is common. Human beings around the world store concepts and data in art form. One look at the German swastika can elicit a panoply of remembered information about Hitler and the Nazis, while a cross encapsulates a tremendous number of facts and ideas for Christians. Another vivid example is the Australian aborigines, who use their myths and arts as mnemonics (as well as for many other purposes). It was the inventiveness of these people that led Pfeiffer to his theory about the European cave art.

The traditional Australian aborigines lived in the world's most barren desert. If they were to find water regularly, they were obliged to remember every rise, every dip, every tree, rock, and hole in an area of several hundred miles. So every physical feature of the landscape was woven into elaborate tales of mythical ancestral beings. The dots, squiggles, and figures they painted on their tools, on walls, and on themselves often symbolically depicted the water holes and rock formations where these apparitions visited. Thus their myths, songs, and art were actually maps of the Australian Outback. As one memorized the escapades of the gods, the smallest details of the desert became committed to memory too.

To teach their children all this lore, Australian aborigines put their young through excruciating ordeals. Traditionally, the Arunta of central Australia took their male initiates into the desert far from home and family, denied them food and clothing, and sang, danced, and acted out these survival tales.[2] On the final night of the ritual the youngsters were concealed under blankets beside a roaring fire. And after the chanting, darkness, isolation, and fear engulfed the youths, their penises were slit from tip to base. A horrible experience. But these boys never forgot the script they had learned; it would forever guide them from one water hole to the next.

The cave paintings of these early European peoples, Pfeiffer proposed, were just the same, cue cards for epic tales—part of a "survival course" in an era of dangerous social change.

~

Pfeiffer had it right.

These people were experiencing population pressure. Continually inclement weather—due to the most recent glacial age—was raging in the north. The land where London is today lay under a mile-high rind of ice. But along what is now the Mediterranean stretched vast grasslands much like today's Serengeti. Here woolly mammoths, woolly rhinos, reindeer, ibex, bison, ancient horses, and many other hooved animals grazed in droves. Pushed by glaciers to the north and deserts to the south, our ancestors congregated on these savannas too, in what is today France and Spain.

And as people became hemmed in by one another, they were most likely forced to forge new social networks and create all sorts of new traditions to survive.

No wonder these people led their children through the belly of the earth and scared them half to death to train them for adulthood. Life had become vastly more complex.

## Abstract, Symbolic Thinking

We will never know exactly what occurred in the bowels of the earth so long ago. But one thing is clear: humankind had become richly endowed with abstract, *symbolic* culture.

Anthropologists use the term *symbolic thinking* to mean the ability to arbitrarily bestow an abstract concept upon the concrete world. The classic example is holy water. To a chimpanzee, the water sitting in a marble basin in a cathedral is just that, water; to a Catholic it is an entirely different thing, holy water. Likewise, the color black is black to any chimp, while to you it might connote death, or even the newest fashion.

With this capacity for symbolic thought, humankind could fully develop such essential concepts as morality, conscience, and our vast store of culturally coded beliefs, rituals, taboos, and rules about sex, romance, and attachment. The modern human mind had emerged.

## The Mysterious Neanderthals

It has long been debated whether the closest relatives of these cave painters, the Neanderthals, engaged in symbolic thinking or whether symbolic thinking sprang into life among these modern human cavern artisans.[3] To be expected, the fossil record offers a mixed bag of clues.

Many believe the Neanderthals split off from our own ancestors some time between 500,000 and 270,000 years ago, although even this is controversial. Others regard them as a racial variety of our species. But all agree that by 100,000 years ago, these men and women were living in Europe, as well as in the Near East and Central Asia.

The Neanderthals were a curious combination of physical traits. They had heavy brow ridges above their eyes, rugged teeth and jaws, and muscular, thick-boned, stocky, barrel-chested bodies. If you saw one on a street in America today you would definitely think him brutish. But these people with beetle brows had skulls *larger* than ours—as well as larger brains.

Moreover, their brains were organized just like yours and mine. We know this from studying the contours of their ancient skulls, which is done quite easily by means of endocasts.

These are ingenious inventions. You take some latex, pour it into a Neanderthal cranium, let it set, and remove the lumpy blob. On the surface of this endocast are all the tiny impressions of the skull that the brain engraved when it once squeezed against its bony helmet. So the design of seams, grooves, and fissures on the surface of the rubber shows how the brain's lobes were organized. These endocasts illustrate that the Neanderthal brain was constructed like our own.[4]

These people thought.

They also spoke. Indeed, compelling evidence suggests that the ancestors of the Neanderthals *and* modern humans may have been using human language by some 500,000 years ago.[5] But most anthropologists would agree that Neanderthal men and women were regaling one another with stories about the hunt and whispering about their love affairs with human language by 100,000 years ago. Why?

Because the remarkable discovery of a Neanderthal hyoid bone,[6] the tiny U-shaped bone that lies suspended in the throat and aids in speech, as well as two hyoid bones from ancestral relatives of the Neanderthals,[7] indicate that the Neanderthals had a vocal tract sufficient for speaking as we do today. The construction of their inner ear also suggests that some sort of language system had evolved,[8] as do aspects of Neanderthal handedness.[9] Moreover, the Neanderthals share with modern humans the FOXP2 gene, a gene linked with language ability.

Scientists argue about what language actually is, when and how it evolved, and the data that support their various opinions.[10] But all believe that by the time the Neanderthals were roasting mammoth steaks and lying with one another in the caves of ancient France, Spain, Russia, Siberia, and Croatia they spoke with some form of human language.[11] Indeed, they may have developed exceedingly complex languages—because peoples living in small, isolated groups tend to speak in intricate tongues.[12]

⌒

But did the Neanderthals "believe" in anything? Had they created the concept of the soul or an afterlife? Did they live in a *symbolic* world?

In several caves across Europe archaeologists have found what look like shallow graves where Neanderthals may have interred their dead, tucked in sleeping positions.[13] Kin may have left grave offerings as well, for some of the skeletons were surrounded by stone tools, or carefully placed stones, bones, and horns of animals.

In a cave high in the hills of northern Iraq, friends and lovers may have laid bouquets of flowers on a deceased Neanderthal relative some 60,000 years ago. Around the bones were scattered the fossilized pollens of holly-hocks, grape hyacinths, bachelor's buttons, yellow-flowering groundsel, and other wildflowers of the area.[14]

Red ocher found at several Neanderthal sites suggests that they also decorated themselves, their tools, and weapons—for people around the world use red ocher to color their faces, hands, figures, and regalia before a ceremony. Someone marked some bear teeth with shallow grooves. Another punctured a fox tooth. Another perforated a reindeer bone. And a series of cross-hatched lines etched into the rock wall of a cave in Gibraltar suggests that the Neanderthals held rituals.

If the Neanderthals believed in an afterlife, if they decorated themselves and their surroundings, if they engraved symbols into the rocks of caves as part of ceremonies: they could symbolize. And if they created art, they must have appreciated the arts as well.

## What Is Art For?

Ethologist Ellen Dissanayake has an interesting proposal for the evolution of this human drive to create and value the arts.

In her book *What Is Art For?* she traces all of the arts back to an apparent human need to shape, to embellish, to beautify, to make things and activities "special." Those who made an event or tool "special" with decorations or ritualistic fanfare remembered the occasion. And remembering these rituals was important to survival. So those who produced art and appreciated the arts lived on—selecting for the aesthetic sense, the biological predisposition to appreciate the arts.

Actually, there is some evidence that this aesthetic appreciation may have evolved long before the Neanderthals strode the earth, because some 250,000 years ago, two individuals in England each chipped a flint hand axe with a fossil shell prominently displayed at its center. These people must have found these fossils embedded in a rock, then fashioned their tools around the shells—making their tools "special." Perhaps these individuals even designed their hand axes for use in special ceremonies.

At about the same time someone also left globs of red, yellow, brown, and purple ocher in a sea cliff cave in France. Maybe these people had begun to make themselves and their belongings "special" too.

Why art? Geoffrey Miller would add that good artists also attracted more lovers and had more babies—selecting for our genetic disposition to make art and appreciate the arts.[15]

The Neanderthals did not leave an impressive inventory of aesthetic expression. Nevertheless, they had begun.[16] So Dissanayake (and now many others) is convinced that the Neanderthals were indeed ritualistically burying their dead, embellishing these gravesites, using ocher for decorative and symbolic purposes, and wearing bear and fox teeth for emblematic as well as ornamental purposes. Were they the original "old masters"? Not likely. But an artistic predisposition was gradually becoming part of human nature, encoded in our DNA.

These people engaged in abstract, symbolic thought.

These people also loved, not only their own, but also their neighbors. Groundbreaking new genetic data collected by paleogeneticist Svante Paabo and his colleagues indicate that at least some of these men and women had sex with some fully modern Europeans and Asians about 50,000 years ago[17]—*because today many modern Europeans and Asians carry some Neanderthal DNA.*[18]

First Paabo extracted DNA from the bones of three female Neanderthals who had lived in Vindija cave in Croatia over 38,000 years ago. Then they compared this Neanderthal DNA with the DNA of five modern humans: a member of the San people of southern Africa, a member of the Yoruba tribe in West Africa, a Papua New Guinean, a Han Chinese, and a Frenchman.[19] To the amazement of the scientific world, the modern European, Asian, and New Guinean shared 1–4% of their DNA with the Neanderthals. The Africans shared none.

So Neanderthal men and women must have interbred with modern people *after* these moderns left Africa and before our tribe spread into Europe, Asia, Australia, and New Guinea.

## Neanderthal Romance

Perhaps these Neanderthals and early modern folk lay together in Europe between 50,000 and 30,000 years ago—when the Neanderthals coexisted with modern folk in these northern climes.

In the Middle East, however, they may have started to have sex together even earlier. By some 100,000 years ago modern men and women were living in caves in what is Israel today. Pushed south by severe cold, the Neanderthals began to live here by 80,000 years ago as well. These different peoples could easily have met one another, traded with one another, and slipped into the bushes for an afternoon of sex. And many bore young—for, as Paabo says, "In a sense, the Neanderthals are then not altogether extinct; they live on in some of us."[20]

More of the Neanderthals, we do not know—except that they lived in small, nomadic bands, made sophisticated stone tools, did some long-distance trading across Europe, hunted big game, and ate a great deal of meat. Several thousand bones of mammoths, woolly rhinos, reindeer, and bison have been excavated below sheer rock walls where these hunters drove the beasts from plateaus above. This "cliff fall" hunting marked another innovation: these hunts were organized, systematic, planned.[21]

Then the hapless Neanderthals vanished about 30,000 years ago, absorbed and/or replaced in Western Europe by fully modern men and women—called Cro-Magnon peoples after the place in France where their bones were first discovered. These men and women looked just like you and me.[22]

## The First Affluent Society

And with the appearance of modern men and women, human art and cultural life exploded.

Indeed, cave art was only one of their innovations. About a dozen people must have worked a week stacking the jawbones of ninety-five mammoths, one atop the next in a herringbone design, to build the sides of an oval hut found in the Ukraine, dating to some 15,000 years ago.[23] Others in this area also arranged the long bones of mammoths to make oval-shaped huts. Then these early architects threw skins over the bones or chinked the structure with mud and grass to keep out the winter wind.

Cro-Magnon people also built houses of skin and wood at the fords of rivers where the great herds came to drink, atop hillsides with a vista, and on sunny floodplains that straddled migration trails. Usually these homes faced south to take advantage of solar heat. And near their houses they dug storage pits, indicating that our relatives had begun to settle down, at least seasonally.

Cro-Magnon people invented new tools and weapons. Although the Neanderthals had a complex stone tool technology (and must have sewn skin clothes and shoes), these men and women began to make utensils of ivory, bone, and antler, as well as lightweight barbed harpoons, fishhooks, spear-throwers and miniature projectile points—perhaps used in the first bows and arrows.

Impressions of plaited strands found on a bit of clay in the Lascaux cave, France, indicate that they also made cordage—probably rope, twine, netting, and fishing line. And because amber mined in the Baltic has turned up in Cro-Magnon homes on the Russian plains and because seashells from the Atlantic are found over a hundred miles away in Les Eyzies, France, these people must have established networks of exchange and engaged regularly in long-distance trade for precious stones and lithic raw materials.[24]

Life took on new gaiety too. Cro-Magnon people invented the flute, the whistle, and the drum. They wore necklaces of bear and lion teeth, bone bracelets and pendants, and hundreds upon hundreds of ivory, shell, and stone beads.[25] Bone needles as small and sharp as any found in a modern sewing kit were used to sew hooded parkas and make shirts with collars and cuffs, tunics, leggings, boots and other tailored clothing. Palm-sized figurines of big-busted, fat-buttocked women (known as Venus figurines), as well as sculptured animals of ivory, bone, and ceramics, have been found in places ranging from the Pyrenees to the Urals. Perhaps these were fertility symbols, aids to divination, good-luck charms, or gifts to a relative, friend, or sweetheart.[26]

Theirs was the first affluent society. They enjoyed music, dance, and song. They buried their dead with grave goods. They wore fox skin coats, braided their hair, donned jewelry and styled their clothes. They used stone lamps with burning oil to paint in caves and light the night. They sat around well-built hearths, roasted large chunks of meat, and talked with entirely human language. And most likely they had created myths, magic, rituals, and gods.

They may have also developed social strata. When two children were buried near Moscow, our Cro-Magnon ancestors bedecked the bodies with rings, anklets, spears, darts, daggers, and some 10,000 beads. These youngsters could not have earned fame as mighty hunters or leaders of any sort. Were they of an upper class?

Perhaps most important, these people lived cheek by jowl in the world's first *seasonal* villages. These needed to be organized. They must have developed moral codes about sex, marriage, adultery, and divorce.

What were these codes for love?

## Forbidden Fruit

All human societies have some sort of incest taboo.[27] At times in history the Egyptians, Iranians, Romans, and others sanctioned brother–sister incest for their royalty. But with these few exceptions, mother–son, father–daughter, and brother–sister mating has been forbidden. Because the incest taboo is universal to humankind, it was probably in place by Cro-Magnon times—largely because it was practical.

Foremost, if a Cro-Magnon girl mated with her brother or her father and produced a baby, the group then had a helpless new member and no new adult to help support the infant. It was far more economical to breed with an outsider and enlist this foreigner as manpower to help rear the child.

Incestuous mating would have caused endless family conflict too. We humans are jealous, possessive. So if a Cro-Magnon girl mated with her father or a Cro-Magnon boy mated with his mother, this would have caused serious domestic rivalry—undermining the relationship between wife and husband and disturbing domestic life.[28]

With incest, our forebears also lost the opportunity to make political gains. As the old axiom goes, "It is better to marry out then to be killed out."[29] So if your daughter leaves the group to mate with a man in the next valley, relations with these people will improve; they become *affinal* kin—relatives by marriage instead of blood. If she stays home and mates within her nuclear family instead, she and her relatives have forged no new trading, warring, or social ties.

Last, "breeding out" was important to avoid the possibly dangerous physical effects of inbreeding.[30]

Cro-Magnon people could not afford all these economic, social, political, and genetic liabilities. So it seems likely that by the time our earliest real relatives were donning bead necklaces and fur coats, they also had rules prescribing that parents and siblings were not fair game for sex or love. In fact, they may have even inherited a *biological* distaste for incestuous relationships—a predisposition to mate and breed outside the nuclear family.

## Biology of Incest Avoidance

Could there be a genetic tendency to avoid sex with mother, father, or siblings?

This is not a new idea. In 1891 Edward Westermarck first proposed this, saying that children develop a natural physical repulsion toward those they grew up with.[31] Since then, this aversion has been confirmed by studies of sexuality in Israel.

Investigations began when Melford Spiro watched infants as they grew up together in a kibbutz, a common living, sleeping, and bathing quarter where a group of age-mates lived throughout their juvenile years.[32] Here boys and girls played at sex, lying under bedcovers together, examining one another in a game they called "clinic"—which consisted of kissing, hugging, and touching one another's genitals. By age twelve, however, these children became shy and tense in one another's company; by age fifteen they developed strong brother–sister bonds.

Although these unrelated youngsters were free to copulate and marry, to Spiro's knowledge not a single one wed or even engaged in intercourse with another member of the same kibbutz group.

Pursuing this investigation in the early 1970s, sociologist Joseph Shepher obtained records on all known kibbutzim marriages. Of 2,769 weddings, only thirteen occurred between individuals of the same peer group. And none of these spouses had entered their common childhood living arrangement until after the age of six. Shepher thinks there is a critical time in childhood between ages three and six when people develop a natural sexual aversion to those they see regularly.[33]

## Animal Incest

This physical aversion to sex with nuclear family members may have evolved long before our ancestors were playing flutes, using bows and arrows, and decorating the walls of caves in France and Spain—because incest avoidance has extensive correlations in the animal community.

Among mammals, birds, and even insects, opposite-sexed creatures reared together also prefer to mate with strangers. In fact, other species have developed so many ways to avoid inbreeding that biologists think the human incest taboo derives from animal anticedents.[34]

Higher primates, for instance, recognize kin, and adolescents rarely breed, or even mate, with close relatives, particularly mother. This was nicely illustrated by young male rhesus monkeys on Cayo Santiago Island, east of Puerto Rico. Here males grew up under the tutelage of mother and her close female kin. As these juveniles matured, they rarely approached their mother sexually. Instead, they saw mother as an authority figure and a wailing wall. Rather than court her, they became infantile—climbing into her arms, cooing, and nuzzling instead; some even tried to suckle.[35] Men and women occasionally regress too, becoming quite childlike in the presence of their parents.

Brother–sister and father–daughter matings are rare in nature for a different reason. In many species, either the pubescent male or female leaves the social group. Chimpanzee siblings sometimes end up in the same community, however; and at the Gombe Stream Reserve, Tanzania, Jane Goodall saw a few incestuous copulations. During these sexual events, either the sister appeared extraordinarily bored or the brother and sister had a vicious fight. Fifi, for example, hung screaming from a branch as her brother, Figan, forced her into coitus.

Probably earlier than four million years ago, Ardi, Lucy, and then Twiggy and the rest of our early hominin ancestors regarded those they grew up with as sexually unattractive. They sought their mother or her "special friend" for succor, not for copulation; and boys *or* girls switched communities at puberty. Incest was rare. Then, when humankind evolved a mind capable of recognizing a broad array of formal kin, as well as the brainpower to make, remember, and follow sexual rules, people readily sensed the economic, social, and political disadvantages of incest. And what had been a natural tendency among their forebears became a cultural dictum too.[36]

Surely by the time Cro-Magnon women and men were learning the legends of their ancestors in eerie caverns beneath the Pyrenees, they knew whom they could court and marry and who was "forbidden fruit."

Incest had become taboo.

꩜

Undoubtedly these people had other sexual prohibitions.

Postpartum taboos have traditionally been the most universal of these mores, existing in some 94% of all traditional cultures on record.[37] Generally couples were supposed to abstain from sex for about six months after a child was born. These rules probably evolved so that mother—and father—could attend to the helpless infant. Cro-Magnon people may have lived with this stricture too.

Most likely Cro-Magnon couples also had sex in the dark or out of view. Nowhere in the world do people regularly copulate in public.

Men may have avoided making love before setting out to hunt as well. Indeed, some American football coaches are still convinced that their players do better if they avoid sex prior to a game.

Cro-Magnon peoples may have also bestowed power on menstrual blood, as do people in the vast majority of traditional societies. Indeed, our European ancestors were steeped in superstition about menstruation. "In various parts of Europe," wrote Sir James Frazer, the great explorer of worldwide folklore, "it is still believed that if a woman in her courses enters a brewery the beer will turn sour; if she touches beer, wine, vinegar or milk, it will go bad; if she makes jam, it will not keep; if she mounts a mare, it will miscarry; if she touches buds, they will wither; if she climbs a cherry tree, it will die."[38] Until the 1950s American women still called menstruation "the curse," and many avoided sex when it occurred.

Cro-Magnon peoples must have also observed codes for sexual modesty.

Even in the steaming jungles of Amazonia women and men wear clothing, although you might not recognize it as such. Traditionally, Yanomamo women wore no more than a thin cord around their waists. But if you asked a woman to remove her string belt, she showed just as much anguish as does an American woman if you ask her to take off her clothes. A Yanomamo man wore a string about his abdomen, and he carefully tucked the foreskin of his penis into it so that his genitals lay snugly against his stomach. When a man's penis slipped from its mooring, however, he responded with the same embarrassment that a tennis player does if his penis flops from his shorts.

Be it a string belt in Amazonia or a full-length dress in Victorian England, men and women give symbolic power to apparel. Without this drapery they feel vulnerable and ashamed. Since our Cro-Magnon ancestors were wearing leather tunics and necklaces of lion's teeth, they undoubtedly had clothing codes for their genitals as well. And most were fastidious about their sexual decorum.

Perhaps most important, our immediate forebears must have had precepts about adultery and divorce. Hunting-gathering and gardening peoples are generally less upset about infidelity than those in many Western industrial societies. So maybe the punishment for philandering in a Cro-Magnon community was no more than an afternoon of public ridicule, a mild beating, or a few fierce arguments. But surely these ancestors had developed strictures about fidelity—and both men and women knew these rules.

Even the most hotheaded must have also honored basic customs for divorce. In small groups, where gossip is a perennial pastime and ostracism is tantamount to death, no one wishes to risk too much alienation. So long before a Cro-Magnon man or woman stomped off to join another band, he or she must have spent time staring across the meadows or into the firelight, ruminating on how to break the news, deciding when it was most appropriate to go, and how to depart according to etiquette.

## Origins of "Ought"

Rules, rules, rules. How did Cro-Magnon people curb their sexual desires and abide by all these strictures? Had they feelings of morality? A sense of right and wrong? A conscience?

Probably.

"Of all the differences between man and the lower animals," Darwin wrote, "the moral sense or conscience is by far the most important." He defined conscience, saying, "It is summed up in that short but imperious word, 'ought.' "[39] How did this extraordinary ability, our human conscience, evolve?

Anthropologist Robin Fox has reasoned that as human social life became more and more complex, young men had to follow stringent new rules concerning whom to court and whom to avoid, intensifying their need to restrain their natural sexual and aggressive drives. "The upshot of this selection process," Fox writes, "was to produce a creature who was capable of becoming extremely guilty about his sexuality.[40]

And Fox is convinced that our conscience is "soft-wired" in the brain. He describes this predisposition as "a syndrome of genetically determined behaviors which make humans susceptible to guilt."[41]

Indeed, we now know some of this brain wiring. From studies of brain-damaged men and women, it has been established that the ability to feel guilt and weigh ethical dilemmas lies in parts of the brain right behind and above the bridge of your nose, in regions where we make decisions.[42] These people know right from wrong; they reason; but they don't feel guilt or the need to follow moral codes.

# Stages of Morality

Scientists now believe that the potential for moral reasoning is present when a neonate emerges from the womb.[43] For example, an infant will begin to cry when it hears another sob. Known as "global empathy," this generalized sympathy, this "foundation-stone" of morality, as Darwin called it, is the first twinkle of what will blossom into the child's moral code.

Then between the ages of one and two, children achieve a sense of "self" and "other" and begin to express specific care about those around them. Toddlers feel shame, and slightly later, guilt. They understand rules of right and wrong. And they try to adhere to convention, honoring secrecy, stealth, and social propriety. From these beginnings, they absorb their culture's moral rules and build their personal styles of adhering and cheating.[44]

Definitions of morality vary with age, status, and from one individual and one culture to the next, of course.[45] What is virtuous behavior in New Guinea is not necessarily virtuous in the United States. But scientists now believe that the human animal is built to understand the concepts of right and wrong; then we absorb our culture's mores as we grow up; then, with our conscience, we wrestle with our inner disposition and cultural needs to follow or bend the rules. Hence, no one has to teach you to feel guilty. Your culture just teaches you *what* to feel guilty about.

Philosophers, psychologists, and laymen of many stripes have offered ingenious theories regarding what morality actually is, when it evolved, and how moral thought and action develops across the life course.[46] But I'd like to offer a strictly Darwinian addendum. I have come to believe that morality develops in four broad stages across one's life, each with a specific adaptive purpose.

Foremost is children's moral code. Regardless of their global empathy, children are regularly focused on themselves. And from a Darwinian perspective they *should* be self-centered. A child's primary goal is to survive childhood—a time when they are particularly vulnerable to accidents and disease.

Second comes teenage morality—focused on their peers. Teenagers will, for example, steal from parents to please or provide for a friend. From the Darwinian perspective, this behavior is adaptive too. In our hunting-gathering past, teenagers needed to establish essential alliances with their comrades—individuals with whom they would travel, hunt, and gather throughout their lives.

Third is the moral code of parents. This is focused on their children. Parents are likely to steal from friends to feed their young, another adaptive mechanism—this time to guarantee the future of their DNA.

Last is the morality of older men and women. These people tend to focus on the future of the community. Many become philanthropic, spending their time, energy, and resources on building a better neighborhood, a stronger tribe or nation, saving the planet, or engaging in some other "cause." Post-reproductive people tend to concentrate (unconsciously) on building a world in which their DNA can flourish decades, even centuries, down the road.

## The Unfolding Conscience

When our human predisposition for moral judgment and behavior evolved is another matter. Darwin noted that many animals exhibit "social instincts," such as defending their young, comforting others, and sharing their food.

Primatologist Frans de Waal takes this argument much further, showing that many creatures, from whales to elephants, to dogs, to monkeys and chimps, have social rules, a sense of fairness, sympathy, cooperation, and the concept of mutual aid—the building blocks of our human conscience.[47]

As de Waal writes, "Aiding others at a cost and risk to oneself is widespread in the animal world."[48] Dolphins support injured companions. Birds make warning calls to help their peers escape while drawing attention to themselves. Vampire bats call on buddies to regurgitate and share blood when they are hungry after a luckless night of hunting. Monkeys expend their metabolic energy protecting blind juveniles. Elephants bury their dead, piling leaves and branches over the body. Chimps hug a friend who has just been beaten up by another. And chimps remember their social debts and reciprocate with support and kindness days, even weeks, after they have been helped. These creatures aren't human—but many are humane.

"The capacity to care for others," de Waal notes, "is the bedrock of our moral systems."[49] Indeed, de Waal speaks of the "moral ability" in many animals as similar to the "language ability" in people. Moral codes, he believes, are at the core of mammalian social life.

Because morality has analogues in nonhuman creatures, Darwin proposed that our ancestors also had these social instincts; that these drives "served him at a very early period as a rude rule of right and wrong. But as Man gradually advanced in intellectual power . . . so would the standard of his morality rise higher and higher."[50]

It is not difficult to imagine that the evolution of serial monogamy and clandestine adultery triggered the escalation of this moral wiring perhaps four million years ago. What conflict this dual reproductive strategy must have produced! To form a pair-bond *and also be adulterous* required our forebears to weigh a range of consequences to their actions.

The roots of human morality may have been set by the time Ardi walked among the trees of ancient Ethiopia some 4.4 million years ago. This predisposition for moral responses then gradually expanded as Lucy, then Twiggy, then Nariokotome Boy walked the earth. Psychologist Jonathan Haidt proposes that by the time our ancestors were clearly engaging in cooperative big game hunting more than 700,000 years ago, they had crossed the Rubicon, having evolved a "rudimentary moral matrix that helped them work together."[51]

But all would agree that by the time the Neanderthals (with modern brains) were warming their hands around fires in southern France some 50,000 years ago, they had concrete codes for right and wrong, a host of moral rules, and a sense of duty to abide by these group credos.

Indeed, at several Neanderthal sites are the remains of crippled individuals and those with chronic diseases.[52] Someone had taken care of these people, despite their inability to contribute to the group.

Then, as Cro-Magnon men and women became enmeshed in larger and larger social networks, more stringent moral rules probably evolved to reduce social chaos, along with our human feelings of embarrassment, guilt, shame, remorse, indignation, and a full-blown moral streak or conscience—particularly a conscience about sex and love.

What a remarkable addition to the human biological repertoire. Modern men and women no longer needed to be admonished, attacked, or ostracized by others for their misdeeds. With the flowering of conscience, they could reprimand *themselves* instead. "A society works best when people want to do what they have to do," said psychoanalyst Erich Fromm. He knew the power of the conscience as social glue.

⌒

What, then, of Cro-Magnon men and women? Carefree savages, free to wander, copulate, and desert their partners? Certainly not.

"The heart of man is made so as to reconcile contradictions," the eighteenth-century Scottish philosopher David Hume once said. I suspect that more than one Cro-Magnon man and woman lay awake in their warm skin hut, tossing, listening to the sighing of the embers and the breathing of their mate as they debated whether to meet a clandestine lover in a secluded glade the following afternoon.

Such men and women would not be the last to struggle with the fickle passions of humanity.

# Fickle Passion

## Romance in Yesteryears

I am the family face;
Flesh perishes, I live on,
Projecting trait and trace
Through time to times anon,
And leaping from place to place
Over oblivion.

The years-heired feature that can
In curve and voice and eye
Despise the human span
Of durance—that is I;
The eternal thing in man,
That heeds no call to die.

—THOMAS HARDY, "HEREDITY"

"Up the stream, past the overhanging rock, you'll see some small white pebbles on the trail that lead into the bush. Follow these. Not far along the animal path you'll come across water dripping from an overhanging rock. Above the rock is a piney overlook. Wait there. I'll come." He sat and listened, thinking of her laugh, her good directions, this secret spot. As he mused, he whittled a fist-sized ivory horse. He'd give her the gift today, he thought.

How many million men and women have loved each other in all the seasons that preceded you and me? How many of their dreams have been fulfilled? How many of their passions spent? How many nights did our ancestors beseech the stars for a change in fortune or thank the gods for their tranquility as they nestled in each other's arms? Sometimes I walk through the halls at the American Museum of Natural History and wonder about the great love stories that still live in the little ivory horses, the shell beads, the amber pendants, and the old tools and bones and stones that now rest in the museum cases.

How did our ancestors love?

We have one final clue to the nature of sex and love in yesteryear—the lives of traditional peoples around the world today. So I have picked two to write about, the !Kung of the Kalahari Desert of southern Africa and the Mehinaku of Amazonia, largely because anthropologists Marjorie Shostak and Thomas Gregor have so vividly described the traditional sexual attitudes and behaviors of these peoples.[1]

Neither culture represents life as it was when our Cro-Magnon ancestors had begun to moralize and worry, to worship and obey, to carve big-busted women and draw on the walls of dank caverns deep beneath the soil. But these traditional societies do have patterns of sexuality in common. These themes, these similarities, these basic patterns of romance are also seen in other societies across the continents. So they must have evolved with the dawn of modern humankind—if not long before.

## Sex on the Kalahari

Nisa's first sexual memories were of lying beside her parents in their tiny hut of brush and sticks, just large enough to lie in. If Nisa feigned sleep, she could watch her parents "do their work." Daddy would wet his hand with saliva, put this liquid on Mommy's genitals and move up and down on top of her. Sometimes during a trip into the bush to collect vegetables, her mother would set Nisa down beneath a tree and go off to copulate with another man. Once Nisa got so impatient that she screamed through the bush, "I'll tell Daddy he had sex with you!"

Nisa knew in infancy that sex was yet another thing that grownups did and that it had rules that were often broken.

After Nisa was weaned, she no longer accompanied her mother on her gathering expeditions. The !Kung say children walk too slowly; they are nothing but a nuisance. Instead, Nisa stayed in camp and played with friends. Regularly the gang of children left the circle of five or six huts, however, to build a "pretend village" some distance into the bush. Here they played at hunting, gathering, singing, "trancing," cooking, sharing—and "marrying."

"Marrying" consisted of pairing up, sharing their "pretend catch" of food with a "make-believe spouse," and playing with this partner—sexually. The boys would remove the leather aprons the girls were wearing, lie down on top of them, wet their genitals with saliva and poke around with a semi-erection as if they were having intercourse. At first Nisa was not an avid player, she told the anthropologist, but she liked to watch.

Boys and girls also sneaked into the bush to meet and play at sex with forbidden lovers. The boys normally initiated this pastime, saying, "We'll be your lovers because we already have wives in the other huts over there. We'll come and do what lovers do, then go back to them." "Being unfaithful" was another variation of the game. Once again the boys began, saying to the girls, "People tell us that you like other men." The girls would deny it. But the boys would insist the girls had philandered, threatening to hit them so that they wouldn't take extra lovers any more. This way, as Nisa says, "they played and played."

!Kung parents did not approve of these sexual games, but they did nothing more than scold their children and tell them to "play nicely." With teenagers they just looked the other way.

Nisa's first teenage crush was on Tikay. She and her boyfriend built a little hut, and every day they played at sex, "doing everything but screw." But Nisa noted, "I still didn't understand about sexual pleasure—I just liked what Tikay did and I liked playing that play." Nisa did not want to share her lover either. She became fiercely jealous when Tikay decided to "take a second wife," playing one day with Nisa and the next day with the other girl.

Did our Cro-Magnon ancestors begin in childhood to play at marrying and being unfaithful, then start in teenage to have infatuations?

Probably. American children play doctor, invent all sorts of other softly sexual pastimes, and begin a series of puppy loves. These childhood games and crushes are quite common around the world; they probably emerged long ago.

Nisa's sex life as an adult—her several marriages and numerous love affairs—strikes another familiar chord.

Around the age of sixteen or seventeen !Kung girls "begin the moon" or start to menstruate. Often they enter a marriage arranged by parents at this time, although many marry somewhat before puberty begins. Parents have definite opinions about a suitable match. They generally select a man several years older than their daughter. Because boys must go through secret initiation ordeals and also kill a large animal before they become eligible to wed, grooms are often as much as ten years older than their brides. Parents also seek good hunters and responsible men who are unmarried, rather than a married man looking for a second wife.

Girls seem not to express opinions about whom they want to wed. Young men, however, say they want young, industrious, attractive, pleasant, fertile women. And when Shostak asked a man whether he would marry a woman who was smarter than himself, the man replied, "Of course. If I married her, she would teach me to be smart too."

Nisa married before puberty. Her parents picked an older boy—but responsible he was not. As was customary, after the bargaining and the preliminary exchange of gifts, her wedding ceremony took place. At sunset friends led the couple to their new marriage hut built some distance from the camp. They carried Nisa over the threshold and laid her down inside while her new husband sat outside the door. Then Nisa's family and the relatives of the groom brought coals from their hearths to start a new fire in front of the marriage hut, and everyone sang and danced and joked until well after dark. The following morning both wife and husband were ceremonially rubbed with oil by their partner's mother—a normal celebration.

But Nisa had a bizarre wedding night—and a marriage that lasted only a few angry days. Nisa had not begun to menstruate, and as is normal among the !Kung, an older woman bedded with Nisa and the groom in their marriage hut to reassure the pubescent bride. But Nisa's chaperone had other ideas. She took the new husband as her own lover, bumping Nisa with her ardent copulating. Nisa couldn't sleep. When her parents heard of the goings-on two days later, they became incensed. After announcing that the marriage was finished, they stormed out of camp, taking Nisa with them.

~

Nisa's second marriage had other problems. Virginity is not a prerequisite for betrothal among the !Kung; in fact, Shostak could find no word for virginity in their language. But young girls often did not consummate their marriages on their wedding night. They were so much younger than their husbands that they acted indifferent and rejected the groom. This was Nisa's style. Her breasts were just beginning to develop; she was not ready to make love. And her refusal to copulate was so persistent that, after several months of waiting, her second husband, Tsaa, grew impatient and departed.

Then Nisa fell in love—with Kantla, a married man. Kantla and his wife encouraged Nisa to become a co-wife. But she refused. !Kung women do not like to share a husband; they say that the sexual jealousy, the subtle favoritism, and the quarrels outweigh the companionship and the help with domestic chores. Moreover, all three partners often share the same tiny bedroom hut, so none of them has any privacy. As a result of all these pressures, only about 5% of all !Kung men maintain a long-term relationship with two wives simultaneously. The other 95% amuse themselves endlessly, telling stories about the complications that arise in these ménages à trois.

Nisa liked her third husband; eventually she loved him—and made love to him. As she told Shostak, "We lived on and I loved him and he loved me. I loved him the way a young adult knows how to love; I just *loved* him. Whenever he went away and I stayed behind, I'd miss him. . . . I gave myself to him, gave and gave."

Nisa soon had secret lovers, though. Kantla, her teenage sweetheart, was the first of many. Sometimes she met a lover in the bush when her husband went traveling or hunting; sometimes she entertained in her hut when she was alone. If she visited relatives, she had lovers in other settlements as well.

These rendezvous were both thrilling and dangerous; often they were emotionally painful too. The !Kung believe that if you copulate with a lover while pregnant you will abort your child. Nisa did abort a fetus after a tryst with a lover. But she had more lovers anyway. And some caused her a lot of jealousy, as well as that sickening feeling of despair that jilted people suffer.

After her young husband died prematurely, Nisa became a single mother with small children. She got meat from her father and other relatives and seemed determined to raise her family without a spouse. The single parent is not a phenomenon unique to Western family life.

Then one of Nisa's three paramours, Besa, persevered, and she married for the fourth time. Nisa and Besa argued continually, usually about sex. As she said to anthropologist Shostak, he was "like a young man, almost a child, who lies with his wife day after day after day. Don't her genitals get sore after a while?" "You're just like a rooster," she shouted at Besa, "At night, once is good; once is enough; . . . in one night you'd screw a woman to death!"[2] And the arguments would escalate from there.

But Nisa and Besa lived together for several years, and they both had extramarital affairs. Once Besa followed Nisa's tracks. Nisa had gone out to collect firewood, and her footprints joined those of a man. Soon Besa found his wife relaxing with her paramour beneath a tree. The lovers began to tremble when they saw Besa's face. And after a lot of bitter words an irate Besa ushered the couple back to camp where the headman ordered beatings for both Nisa and her boyfriend. Nisa refused hers, impudently offering to be shot with a bullet instead. Then she stalked off. Her partner took his punishment, four hard whacks.

⁕

Here, then, are patterns of human sexuality among the !Kung that are common in Western cultures too: childhood frolic, teenage crushes, youthful experiments at pairing, then a lattice of marriages and affairs during reproductive years. All of these patterns were probably commonplace by the time our ancestors were painting murals of stampeding beasts in the dark caves of France and Spain.

The !Kung also have all sorts of sexual codes, another fundamental element of the human mating game. Unlike the vast majority of traditional peoples, the !Kung have no fear of menstrual blood or other body fluids, though they believe a woman must refrain from joining a hunt while she bleeds. Men and women also generally avoid intercourse during the height of menses. But spouses resume copulating during its final days if they want to have a child. Menstrual blood, they believe, combines with semen to make the infant.

And the !Kung love sex. "Sex is food," they say. They think that if a girl grows up without learning to enjoy coitus, her mind doesn't develop normally and she goes around eating grass. "Hunger for sex," they are convinced, "can make you die."

Women have specific complaints about men's genitals, however. They do not like a man's penis to be too big, since this hurts, or too full of semen, since this is messy. So women discuss among themselves the contents and the fit of their men's penises. And they demand orgasms. If a man has "finished his work," he must continue until a woman's work is finished too. Women should be sexually satisfied.

Men, of course, also have opinions about what constitutes good sex. One summed up a bad rendezvous this way: "She's so wide, she's like a Herero's mouth.[3] I just flounced around inside, but I couldn't feel anything. I don't know what it was like for her, but today my back hurts and I'm exhausted." Men also worry about their performance. When they are unable to get an erection, they take medicines.

The !Kung love to kiss each other on the mouth. But they do not perform cunnilingus. "A vagina would burn a man's lips and tongue," Nisa explains. Both women and men masturbate occasionally. Everybody jokes about sex too; an afternoon sometimes becomes a theater of witticisms, puns, and bawdy banter. Sexual dreams are considered good. And women talk endlessly about their lovers while they forage with close girlfriends.

But some sexual etiquette is strict. Men and women always try to hide their love affairs from their spouses. They feel that these trysts tap into intense emotions—particularly a "burning heart." Because spouses get jealous, it is wise to hide one's passion for fear of violence at home. So paramours try to meet in safe places—away from spying eyes and tattling tongues. They say their love for their spouses is a different matter. After the torrid sexual craving of early marriage has subsided, husband and wife often become good friends, almost parents to each other.

Nisa's fifth husband plays this role. She says, "We fight and we love each other; we argue and we love each other. That's how we live." And she still sneaks into the bushes with her first love, Kantla, as well as with other men.

Did our Cro-Magnon ancestors feel Nisa's zest for sex? Did they have childhood frolics and teenage lovers as they and their parents followed reindeer across the grass of France and Spain? Did they marry after gruesome puberty rituals in caverns deep below the ground? And, like Nisa, did they divorce and remarry when things went wrong, as well as meet other lovers in secret spots to dally through an occasional afternoon?

Probably, for the sexual escapades of traditional people living far from the arid bush of southern Africa are not too different from those of Nisa and her friends. Both cultures may reflect a world of sex and romance that evolved long before contemporary times.

## Love in the Jungle

"Good fish get dull, but sex is always fun," explained Ketepe, a Mehinaku tribesman of central Brazil in the heart of Amazonia, to anthropologist Thomas Gregor. Ketepe had a wife he said was dear. He liked to take her and his children off on long fishing trips so that they could spend time by themselves. When he tried to copulate with her in his hammock after his children were asleep, someone nearby invariably got up to stoke the fire or go outdoors to relieve themselves; home was not a private, sexy place. Moreover, Ketepe rarely met his wife in the family garden to make love in the afternoon. Village life, he said, was too hectic.

Ketepe was out of his hammock by dawn. Sometimes he and his wife went to the river to bathe together, stopping along the trail to chat with other couples. But on most days he joined a fishing party that left soon after the sun came up. His wife stayed home to feed their children and do other chores, women's work. By noon Ketepe returned, gave his fish to his spouse, and joined his friends in the village "men's house," which stood in the middle of the plaza.

The men's house was forbidden to women. None had ever entered—for here the sacred flutes resided, hidden in a corner. If a woman accidentally saw these sacred objects, the men would waylay her in the forest and rape her, a practice common in several Amazonian societies.

The men's clubhouse was a jovial place. Amid the teasing, lewd jokes, and chitchat, the men made baskets, worked on their arrows, or decorated their bodies with paints in preparation for "wrestling time" in midafternoon. Then, after all the straining, grunting, dust, and cheers that the matches regularly provoked, the triumphant and the defeated all adjourned to their thatched homes which encircle the plaza playing field. Here Ketepe sat around the family fire with his wife, ate manioc bread heaped with a thick, spicy fish stew, and played with his children until they all retired to their hammocks and drifted off to sleep.

The Mehinaku were busy. Women worked as much as seven to nine hours every day processing manioc flour, weaving hammocks, spinning cotton, making twine, fetching firewood, and carrying tubs of water from the nearby stream. Men did a good deal less. Fishing, trading, helping in the family garden plot, and taking part in their many local rituals took only about three and a half hours every day—except in the dry season, when men worked hard to clear the land for the new manioc garden.

But the villagers also avidly engaged in another time-consuming activity—sex. "Sex," they said, "is the pepper that gives life and verve." For the Mehinaku, sex liberally seasoned daily life.

Soon after a traditional Mehinaku child began to walk, he or she joined other youngsters in play groups in the plaza. As the tots rolled and tussled on the ground, adults teased them, saying, "Look, look, my boy is copulating with your daughter." Children soon learned the game. As they aged, they, like !Kung children, began to play a fantasy they called "marrying."

Little boys and girls slung hammocks in the trees beyond the village, and while the girls stoked "pretend fires" or played at weaving cotton, boys gathered big leaves. These "make-believe fish" they proudly presented to their spouses to be cooked. Then, after the couple ate together, they started another fantasy, "being jealous." Either the boy or girl snuck into the bushes, followed closely by a suspicious "spouse." When he or she caught the other in a make-believe assignation, the cuckolded partner got mad.

Older children, on the other hand, had seen their parents copulating in the family garden, and they often abandoned their innocent games for more grown-up sexual sports. If parents caught their young trying to couple, however, they taunted them unmercifully, so children learned early to be prudent.

The carefree days of childhood sex ended abruptly around age eleven or twelve, when formal rules of sexual decorum demanded that a boy enter up to three years of seclusion. His father built a wall of palm wood staves and palm leaves at one end of the family house and hung his son's hammock behind this barrier. Here the teenager spent much of his time, taking medicines that ensured that he would grow. The adolescent must speak softly, follow several dietary restrictions, and, above all, avoid any sexual encounters.

Toward the end of his stay he began to sneak out and have affairs, however.

Hearing of a tryst, his father then tore down the partition. The boy had become a man—equipped to go on long fishing trips alone, ready to cut a garden and have a wife.

Then young men were free to indulge in sexual adventures, dalliances that would become a normal part of adult life. Boys met their girlfriends in the woods to copulate.[4] They took little time for foreplay, however.[5] If a couple found a spot where a thick log lay along the ground, they might make love on top of it in the missionary position, with the man on top. But comfortable logs were rare, the ground was often muddy, and insects bit. So lovers normally sat facing each other; she was on top, her legs wrapped around his hips.

In another common stance, he knelt and spread his legs, holding her thighs, buttocks, and lower back above the ground while she braced her upper body with outstretched arms. Couples also liked coitus in a pool of quiet water—chest high was best for leverage, they said. And if there was little time, lovers might copulate standing up; she wrapping one leg around her sweetheart while he raised her slightly off her feet.

Sex was over after the man had ejaculated. Although the Mehinaku had no word for female orgasm, they were well aware that the clitoris swells during intercourse and was the seat of female pleasure. They likened the female genitals to a face; the clitoris the nose that "sniffs out sexual partners." But whether women had orgasms regularly is still unknown to anthropologists.

Soon after ending coitus, lovers took different paths back home—but not without exchanging small gifts. Fish were currency for sex. After a fishing expedition, a man often stopped just prior to entering the village, selected the oiliest of his catch, and sent it by a messenger to a lover. He gave her a fish when they met too. And lovers regularly gave one another other mementos, like a spindle of cotton, a basket, or some shell jewelry. This teenage sexuality was so common that when a girl walked into the central plaza smeared with a boyfriend's body paint, no one blinked. The Mehinaku saw nothing wrong with premarital coitus in the woods.

But parents got exceedingly upset if their unmarried daughter got pregnant. So soon after a girl emerged from her period of seclusion, which began at her first menses and lasted a year or more, she wed. This was a special day. The new husband moved his hammock into his wife's home and presented her with an abundant catch of fish. She made a particularly sweet batch of manioc bread. And over the course of several days friends and kin exchanged more gifts and sentiments.

The Mehinaku thought a display of romantic love was silly, in poor taste, so newlyweds were supposed to be reserved. Excessive thoughts of a loved one, they believed, could attract deadly snakes, jaguars, and malevolent spirits. Yet newlyweds slept in the same large hammock and spent their days together bathing, talking, and making love in the woods outside the village. Young married people got jealous too, particularly if they caught a mate in an affair.

These dalliances generally began soon after marriage. Central to the rendezvous was something the Mehinaku called "alligatoring." A man who had established a liaison with a woman lay in wait for her in an "alligator place," either in the woods behind her house, along one of the trails that radiated from the village plaza, or near the gardens or bathing spots. As a paramour walked by, her would-be lover smacked his lips to beckon her, then propositioned her as she drew near. She might oblige or make a later date. Men said women were "stingy with their genitals," although one might not agree. Tamalu, the most promiscuous woman in the village, had fourteen lovers. On average, Mehinaku men had four separate affairs at any given time.

These extramarital liaisons, Gregor reported, had a valuable social function: village cohesion. The Mehinaku thought that semen made a baby and that many copulations were needed to form a child. As men reported, baby making was a "collective labor project," something like a fishing expedition. Thus every lover was convinced that a woman's forthcoming infant was partly his. Occasionally a man publicly recognized the infant of a lover as his own and helped raise the child.[6] But spouses got jealous. As they said, they "prize each other's genitals." So the real father of an infant rarely revealed himself. This belief about baby making, however, silently linked men and women in an elaborate web of kinship ties.

Probably as a result of all these veiled sexual connections, adulterers rarely got fined or beaten. In Mehinaku myths philanderers were hit, dismembered, even put to death. But in real life only newlyweds made a fuss or confronted a spouse about infidelity—for an understandable reason. Villagers often jeered a jealous husband, calling him a "kingfisher," because these birds flap about aimlessly, screeching and scolding. Rarely did a man put aside his dignity to invite this scorn.

This is not to say that men and women with roving spouses did not suffer; sexual tensions often led to divorce. Marital discord was most easily measured by where a couple slept. If spouses strung their hammocks inches from one another, they probably were relatively happy. These couples tended to talk about the events of the day after their children were asleep, even copulate in one or the other's hammock. As their quarrels escalated, however, they strung their hammocks farther apart, sometimes even sleeping on opposite sides of the fireplace. And if a wife became enraged, she might take a machete and cut down her husband's bed. This often initiated divorce.

Although some single women with small children lived in the village when Gregor was there, the vast majority of adults remarried. As far as the Mehinaku were concerned, a man needed a wife to carry firewood, make manioc, and mend his hammock, as well as for companionship and sex. Like the !Kung and many other peoples, the Mehinaku regularly pursued the mixed human reproductive strategy of marriage, adultery, divorce, and remarriage.

Also like the !Kung, the Mehinaku loved sex—a preoccupation that was evident in their myriad beliefs. Fish and manioc, their staples, both had sexual connotations. When women grated manioc tubers, something they did most of the day, villagers said they were having sex. Sex was the fabric of the daily litany of jokes. Men and women frequently teased each other sexually. Women painted their bodies, plucked their pubic hair, and wore a G-string through their vulvar lips and buttocks to accentuate their genitals. The Mehinaku's myths, their songs, their rituals, their politics, their dress, and their daily activities were all saturated with sexual symbolism.

Yet their sexuality had a macabre undercurrent of fear. Gregor thought that Mehinaku men had rampant castration anxieties. In a study of Mehinaku dreams, he discovered that 35% of the men worried about the amputation or mangling of their genitals, a rate much higher than that among American men. The Mehinaku were also scared of impotence, for good reason. Gossip was endemic in this village of only eighty-five people, and the extent of a man's sexual prowess quickly became common knowledge. Hence dysfunction in the morning could turn into performance anxiety by night.

Men were also terrified of women's menstrual blood. This dark, "foul-smelling" secretion, they said, "races" into the water containers, the fish stew, the manioc drinks, and the bread the moment a woman begins to bleed. If this poison got under a man's skin, they said, it turned into a foreign body that caused pain until a shaman magically removed it. So it was not unusual for a wife to throw a whole day's manioc flour into the jungle if one woman in the house began to menstruate in late afternoon.

Moreover, sex, the Mehinaku believed, stunted growth, weakened a man, inhibited his wrestling and fishing ability, and attracted evil spirits. Even thinking about coitus while traveling could be dangerous to one's health.

A few men were cowed into abstention or impotence by these beliefs; many others tried to moderate their trysts; and some cast caution to the wind and sowed their seed whenever and wherever possible. But all the Mehinaku, Gregor thought, were troubled. They believed that too much sex, sex at prohibited times, or sex with a partner in the wrong kin relationship could cause disease, injury, even death. "Anxious pleasures," as Gregor called their dalliances, may have been an understated description of these people's sexual escapades.

## Blueprint of Human Sexuality

Are Ketepe's sojourns in the woods beside the Amazon any different from Nisa's rendezvous with Kantla on the Kalahari? Surely our Cro-Magnon forebears grew up with sex around them, played at coitus when they were children, went through ceremonies in teenage to announce their adult sexual status,[7] and then entered a labyrinth of marriages and affairs drenched with passion, rules, and superstition.

Cro-Magnon children almost certainly huddled in mammoth-bone huts on bear rugs in the middle of the night, listening to their parents' jostling and heavy breathing. In the morning they saw their parents smile at each other. Occasionally after their father had left camp to hunt, they saw mother vanish beyond the meadow with a man who admired her and gave her gifts. And like their counterparts in many other cultures, the more astute children knew what their parents were up to and could rattle off the names of clandestine lovers for most of the grownups in their band. They probably didn't tattle, though.

By age ten, Cro-Magnon youngsters must have begun their own journeys into sex and love.[8] Little girls may have slipped off to a river to bathe and play at "marrying" and "being jealous" with the boys. They probably roamed in gangs, and by early teenage some had started to play seriously at sex—long before puberty.[9] A few may have loved one boy and then another, while others had a constant "puppy love" for a single mate.

As teenagers they spent hours decorating themselves—as adolescents do in many cultures—plaiting their hair, donning garlands of flowers in order to smell sweet, wearing bracelets and pendants, and decorating their tunics and leggings with fur, feathers, beads, and red and yellow ocher. Then they strutted, preened, and showed off for one another in the fire's glow.

Sometime before puberty our Cro-Magnon juveniles must have begun the important rituals for adulthood that culminated in the caverns beneath the earth. Here they entered the spirit world and danced and sang in ceremonies designed to teach them to be brave and smart. And as girls matured, they wed older boys who had established their hunting skills.

When the reindeer started their annual migration in the spring, a "newly married" couple and their friends must have set brushfires that drove the giant beasts stampeding to their death in a steep ravine, then butchered these creatures and carted home great hunks of meat. Around a roaring blaze they reenacted the high points of the hunt. Then some vanished from the firelight to hug and nuzzle in the dark.

During the summer months a wife probably tanned the hide of a bear her husband had trapped; she roasted the fish he had caught in the teeming streams; and she came home from gathering expeditions to tell him where the horses were feeding and where the bees were making honey. Her husband showed his wife new nutting groves and fishing pools. Together they collected raspberries and blueberries. And together they lay in secret spots on lazy afternoons.

Then in autumn, they may have gone together on trading expeditions to where the waves pounded on the shore. Here they exchanged fox hides for purple shells and golden stones and saw old friends and relatives. Then, as winter began to rage, they probably spent hours in the house, drilling beads, carving figurines, and telling tales.

Some men and women married more than once. Some had extra lovers. But they all had hopes and fears and sweethearts. For in their souls they carried an ancient script—a template for human bonding: "The family face," as Thomas Hardy called it, "the eternal thing in man that heeds no call to die."

⌒

This basic human nature would be sorely challenged by what happened next. By 10,000 years ago, the most recent ice age had passed into the present interglacial thaw. The land began to warm. Glaciers that had gripped the earth as far south as modern London retreated north, and the vast grasslands that stretched across Eurasia from Europe to the South China Sea turned into miles and miles of deep, thick woods. The woolly mammoth, the woolly rhino, and many other large mammals died out, replaced by red deer, roe deer, boar, and all the other modern creatures that still roam the European forests. Now men and women were forced to hunt smaller game, catch more fish, fell more birds, and collect lots of forest vegetables.[10]

Soon some would settle down, domesticate wild seeds, and tame wild beasts. With this, our farming forebears would change the face of marriage with two new ideas: honor thy husband; and till death us do part.

# 15

## "Till Death Us Do Part"

### Birth of Sexual Double Standards

> To have and to hold from this day forward,
>
> for better for worse,
>
> for richer for poorer,
>
> in sickness and in health,
>
> to love and to cherish,
>
> till death us do part.
>
> —*BOOK OF COMMON PRAYER*, 1549

Thwack, thwack, thwack. A giant willow crackled, swayed, then thundered down beside the lake. Trout, perch, pike, chub, and catfish sped below the lily pads and darted among the bulrushes that lined the lake with marsh. A forest boar dashed, stricken, from the underbrush. Ducks and geese and mud hens lifted, flapping, from the reeds. Two otters froze, listening, among the cattails. Someone new was in the woods.

By 3,000 B.C., central Europe was strewn with ponds and lakes and streams, signatures of massive glaciers that had retreated north some 5,000 years earlier. Surrounding these glacial footprints were deep, thick forests. First birches and pines had spread across the grass. Then oaks, elms, spruce, and fir trees appeared. And beech trees, chestnut trees, ashes, and maples cloaked the river valleys. Where oak trees spread their limbs, light bathed the forest floor. Here thistles, stinging nettles, and other underbrush could thrive, providing luxuriant hotels for teeming forest life. But where beech trees took root, their thick leaves drank the sunlight, and only ferns, wild onions, garlic, and grasses grew.

No more did mammoths and mastodons trumpet in the morning air. Gone the open plains, the swaying grasses, low shrubs, and early-morning chill. Instead, the August light danced off crystal lakes and dew on leaves and bark. Solitary creatures like red deer, boars, elk, and badgers picked among the forest browse. Roe deer and brown bears hung along the rims of meadows where the hazel, raspberry, strawberry, and elderberry bushes grew. And wildcats stalked rabbits in fields of dandelions. The modern landscape and all the fauna that now live in Europe had appeared.[1]

New people lived here too: farmers.

Along the river valleys of Germany, Austria, the Czech Republic, Slovakia, Poland, Belgium, the Netherlands, and Luxembourg, men and women had begun to fell the trees and till the soil. In some clearings only a single farmstead stood. Elsewhere, four to ten squat, rugged wooden buildings comprised a tiny hamlet. In small kitchen gardens just outside their doors, these first European cultivators grew peas, lentils, poppy plants, and flax. They housed domesticated cattle, pigs, sheep, and goats in barns attached to their homes. Dogs slept at their feet. And behind their houses lay scattered fields of planted wheat.

How the first farmers in southwestern Germany got along with the local hunter-gatherers we may never know. But archaeologist Susan Gregg has a hypothesis based on ingenious data.[2]

To reconstruct daily life along these riverbanks, she chose a hypothetical village consisting of six households, with thirty-four women, men, and children. Then, by meticulously studying the landscape, the artifacts of this period, and the life cycles of wheat, peas, pigs, and other plants and animals that lived here, Gregg pieced together these first farmers' work schedule, their cultivating and herding practices, and their estimated production and consumption of meat, milk, grains, and vegetables per individual per year.

Included in her calculations were the precise amount of time needed to plant each hectare of ancient wheat, the most suitable size for each field and garden plot, and the crop losses due to snails, mice, birds, and winter storage. To the equation she added the straw yield of each harvest

and the amount of pastureland, forest browse, and winter fodder necessary to maintain the optimal number of cattle, sheep, goats, and pigs. She
also weighed the lifespan of these species, the number of baby animals
born each year, the abundance of wild berries, greens, and condiments,
the time spent to cut wood, and many other factors in order to establish
the most efficient way these farmers might have lived.

Her conclusion: they planted wheat in spring; and they employed the
local foragers to help them seed their crop.

In exchange, she theorized, the farmers gave these hired hands surplus meat—ewes, calves and piglets that had expired just after birth in
early spring, the leanest time of year for nomads. Then, in August when
the wheat ripened, Gregg thinks the farmers hired the local wanderers
again to help cut the grain and carry straw to storage bins—this time in
exchange for milk. They may also have bartered with the foragers for wild
game, special flint, and volcanic rocks for making axes. Most important,
they got information—news of other farmers that these wanderers collected as they roamed.

The foragers, Gregg thinks, welcomed the farmers not only for their
meat, milk, and grain but also for their abandoned fields. These clearings
made gaps in the thick woods where new shrubs, herbs, and grasses took
hold and attracted wild deer and forest swine. So around these fallow
fields hunting may have been particularly good. More important, with
farm produce at hand, the foragers could forgo some of their arduous
long-distance fishing expeditions. They too could begin to settle down.

No doubt these early contacts between farmers and foragers were not
all as friendly or as symbiotic as Gregg reports. Surely hunters and plant-
ers sometimes fought. But eventually the latter prevailed. These settlers
would fundamentally alter ancient gender roles, initiating sexual codes
and attitudes regarding women that have been passed down the centuries
to us.

## The Gentrification of Europe

How and why farming took root in Europe has been avidly debated. But
Western agriculture had its origins on hillsides that stretch like a horse-

shoe from Jordan north through Israel, Lebanon, Syria, and Turkey, then south through Iraq and Iran—the Fertile Crescent. Here, by 10,000 B.C., in clearings among the pistachio and olive trees, the cedars, junipers, oaks, and pines, wild grasses grew and feral cattle, pigs, sheep, and goats all grazed.

Our nomadic ancestors had probably visited these meadows to hunt and collect grains for millennia. As the hot, dry summers got even hotter and drier, however, and as people clustered around the few remaining freshwater lakes, food supplies grew short. And with time these people began to store the grain they had collected and plant seeds in an effort to intensify their harvest of these wild cereals. The earliest farmers may have lived in the Jordan valley. But by 8000 B.C., many more hamlets had taken root and early villagers of the Fertile Crescent had begun to sow wild wheat, rye, and barley and herd sheep and goats.[3]

The hearth of Western civilization had been laid.

Agriculture then spread north and west. And as the custom of planting grains and vegetables seeped into Europe along the riverbanks from Asia Minor, farming gradually became a way of life. For millions of years our ancestors had meandered across the ancient world in a constant search for food. Now nomadism was becoming a thing of the past. As archaeologist Kent Flannery summed it up, "Where can you go with a metric ton of wheat?"

## The Plow

There is probably no single tool in human history that wreaked such havoc between women and men or stimulated so many changes in human patterns of sex and love as the plow. Exactly when the plow appeared remains unknown. The first farmers used the hoe or digging stick. Then sometime around 6000 B.C. someone invented the ard, a primitive plow with a stone blade and a handle like a plow's. And by 3000 B.C., the plow was widely used.

What a difference this made.

In cultures where people garden with a hoe, women do the bulk of the cultivating; in many of these societies women are relatively powerful as well.[4]

But with the introduction of the plow—which required much more strength—much of the essential farm labor became men's work. Moreover, no longer could women wander off the land to collect the evening meal. Women lost their ancient, honored roles as independent gatherers and providers. And soon after the plow became crucial to farming, a sexual double standard emerged among farming folk. Women were judged inferior to men.

## Honor Thy Husband

The first written evidence of women's subjugation in farming communities comes from law codes of ancient Mesopotamia dating from about 1780 B.C., in which women were described as chattels, possessions.[5] One code indicated that a wife could be killed for fornication, but her husband was permitted to copulate outside of wedlock—as long as he did not violate another man's property, his neighbor's wife. Matrimony was primarily for procreation so abortion was forbidden.[6] And if a woman produced no children, she could be divorced.

The treatment of women as child-producing property and subservient beings was not singular to people in the Middle East. These mores sprang up among many farming folk.[7]

In traditional agrarian India, an honorable wife was supposed to throw herself on the burning funeral pyre of her husband—a custom known as suttee. In China an upper-class girl's toes (all but the big toe) were curled underneath her foot and tightly bound when she was about age four, making it terribly painful to walk, impossible to run away from her husband's home. During the golden age of ancient Greece, upper-class girls were married off by age fourteen, ensuring that they were chaste until their wedding night. Among the Germanic peoples who invaded classical Rome, women could be bought and sold.[8]

"Wives, be subject to your husbands, as is fitting in the Lord," the New Testament bid.[9] This credo was not just a Christian view. In ancient

Sumeria, Babylonia, Assyria, Egypt, classical Greece and Rome, across preindustrial Europe, in India, China, Japan, and the farming communities of North Africa, men became the priests, political leaders, warriors, traders, diplomats, and heads of household. A woman's sovereign was first her father and her brother, then her husband, then her son.

As the fifth-century B.C. Greek historian Xenophon encapsulated a wife's duties to her spouse, "Be therefore diligent, virtuous, and modest, and give your necessary attendance on me, your children, and your house, and your name shall be honorably esteemed even after your death."[10]

~

I do not wish to imply that the sexual double standard was unique to farmers. Among some gardeners of Amazonia (who use the digging stick rather than the plow) and some herding peoples of East Africa, women were largely subservient to men in most arenas of social life. But a codified sexual and social double standard was not common to all peoples who herded, who gardened with a hoe, or who hunted and gathered for a living, whereas it prevailed in societies with the plow.[11]

I also do not wish to suggest that *all* women in farm societies experienced the same degree of sexual restriction and social inferiority. Women's status changed from century to century. Class, age, and economic and social station affected women's position too.

Hatshepsut, for example, ruled Egypt in the fifteenth century B.C., and she was only one of several powerful Egyptian queens. Unlike the cloistered housewives of classical Greece, courtesans were educated and highly independent. Some urban, upper-class Roman women of the first and second centuries A.D. became literary figures; others were politicians. During the Middle Ages a number of nuns were educated power brokers in the Church; others wielded enormous influence in the marketplace. In the 1400s some Islamic women of the Ottoman Empire owned land and ships. And a sizable number of Renaissance women of England and the Continent were as well read as any man.

Moreover, even where the sexual double standard is rigorously maintained, it does not always guarantee informal power, day-to-day influence.

As we all know, the most insipid woman of a higher class or a more prestigious ethnic group can sometimes dominate a man from a lower social
rung. Older women often control younger men. Young, sexy women can
manipulate much more influential men. Sisters can rule brothers. And
certainly wives can govern husbands. Even where the sexual double standard has been extreme, men have never universally dominated women—
not in agricultural America, not in the little farmhouses that hugged the
Danube several thousand years ago.

These exceptions notwithstanding, there is no question that during
our long European farming ancestry women were largely second-class citizens.[12] Unlike women in nomadic foraging societies, who left camp regularly to work and brought home precious goods and valuable information,
who traveled freely to visit friends and relatives and ran their own love
lives, a farming woman took her place in the garden or the house—her
duty to raise children and serve a man.

With plow agriculture came general female subordination, setting in
motion the entire panorama of agrarian sexual and social life, including
the rise of the sexual double standard.

Exactly how the plow and farm life led to changes in agrarian sexuality has been debated for at least a hundred years.[13] I will propose that
sedentary living, the need for *lifelong* monogamy, the rise of ranked societies, a peculiar property of testosterone (the largely male sex hormone),
and the escalation of warfare all played important roles.

## Seeping Inequality

"All thought is a feat of association," poet Robert Frost once said. So, to
begin, then, with what we know:

Foremost, the vast majority of hunting-gathering peoples are—and
probably always were—relatively egalitarian. No extant hunting-gathering
society has a rigid, codified sexual double standard. And, generally speaking, women did have an inferior status in all traditional societies that used
the plow for agriculture. So a *relative equality* between the sexes was the
rule in most (if not all) of ancient, pre-agricultural societies. And this bal-

ance of power between the sexes became *pronounced inequality* sometime soon after the plow was introduced and spread around the globe.

## Permanent Monogamy

Equally important, I have marshaled a great deal of data to propose that monogamy, or pair-bonding, emerged long before the plow—indeed, millions of years ago. Monogamy did not first emerge with farming life. However, it is highly likely that *permanent* monogamy became the rule with the emergence of sedentary living. With the advent of plow agriculture, neither husband nor wife could divorce. They had become tied to their mutual real estate and to each other. This certainly could compromise a woman's sexual expression and curtail her ability to leave an unhappy partnership.

Another factor that must have contributed to the decline of women's position was a simple reality: a plow is heavy; it needs to be pulled by a large animal; it requires the strength of men.

As hunters, husbands had supplied the luxuries that made life thrilling, as well as some of the daily fare. But as tillers of the soil, men's farm labor became critical to survival. Women's vital role as gatherers, on the other hand, was undermined as our farming ancestors began to rely less on wild plants for food and more on domesticated crops. Long the providers of at least 50% of the daily fare, women now assumed the secondary tasks of weeding, picking, and preparing the evening meal.

This single ecological factor—men's rising control of the vital economic resources—is sufficient to explain the decline of women's social and sexual power. Those who own the purse strings rule the world.

## Big Men

Other factors conjoined to create women's fall. Among them, an insidious phenomenon of farming peoples: rank. For millennia, "big men," as some hunter-gatherers call their leaders, must have arisen among our nomadic ancestors during hunting, foraging, and trading expeditions. But for the vast majority of our human heritage, *formal* ranks did not exist. No one

could accumulate enough spare goods to gain higher rank. Not coincidentally, hunter-gatherers have strong traditions of equality and sharing.

To organize the yearly farming harvest, however, and store grain and
fodder, distribute surplus food, oversee long-distance, systematic trade,
and speak for the community at regional gatherings, chiefs arose.

There is some evidence of rank in the European archaeological
record as early as 15,000 years ago; some graves contained much fancier
goods than others. Thus, village headmen had probably gained power
with the rise of the first seasonal, nonagricultural communities. Moreover, along the Danube by 3000 B.C. one home in a hamlet was often
larger than the rest; so social stratification had surely begun by then.
Then with the spread of plow agriculture and village life, political organization grew more and more complex—and undoubtedly more hierarchical as well.[14]

So now we have sedentary living, permanent monogamy, dependence
on the plow, the rise of male economic power, and the emergence of stratified societies. This rise of ranked individuals was most likely another
death knell for women—because in every single society where ranks are
prevalent, men hold the majority of the authoritative roles. In fact, in 88%
of ninety-three societies canvassed in the 1970s, *all* local and intermedi-
ate political leaders were men; in 84% of these cultures men held *all* of
the top leadership positions in the kin group too.[15]

This was not always because women were barred from these positions. In many of these cultures—such as the United States—women
have been permitted, often even encouraged, to seek influential positions in government. And today greater numbers of women worldwide
are indeed running for office. But even now women in America and many
other cultures do not seek or acquire political leadership positions with
the regularity that men do—*until after their childbearing years are over.*
There certainly are cultural reasons for this. Released from the constant
chores of rearing young, post-menopausal women are liberated to pursue
activities outside the home. But biology may contribute: with menopause,
levels of estrogen decline—unmasking levels of testosterone.

And testosterone has been directly linked with the drive for rank in
many species, from fish and doves to monkeys, chimps and men.[16]

In one study of 350 women, for example, those who had been subject to high levels of testosterone in the womb were less likely to marry, had fewer children, regarded career as more important than family, pursued more male-dominated occupations, and achieved higher-status jobs. And women in professional, technical, and managerial jobs tend to have higher levels of testosterone than do female clerical workers, housewives, and women in service occupations.[17]

Nature isn't tidy. There is no simple correlation among hormones, aggressiveness, and status. For example, professional men tend to have lower levels of male hormones than do blue-collar and unemployed men. Bodily testosterone needs to be at a specific level to correlate with high rank.[18] Moreover, other chemical systems are certainly involved. And your social maturity, who you know, how long you have lived in the community, how you conduct yourself and a host of other cultural and psychological phenomena contribute to the creation of your rank.

Nevertheless, young men have at least seven times more testosterone than young women. And like males of many other species, men everywhere in the world are much more likely to compete aggressively for rank[19]—sacrificing their time, pleasure, health, safety, affection, relaxation, and family life to attain positions of rank, authority, and power.

## Warfare

Sedentary living, couples obliged to remain together on their mutual home range (lifelong monogamy), men's more important economic roles as farmers, the rise of stratified societies, men's drive for rank: what a volatile mixture. Here was a perfect opportunity for one sex to gain authority over the other.

But a last factor surely played a role in the decline of women's social power: warfare. As villages proliferated and population density increased, people were obliged to defend their property, even extend their landholdings when they could. Warriors became invaluable to social life. And as anthropologist Robert Carneiro has pointed out, everywhere in the world where fighting enemies is important to daily living, men come to increase their power over women.

Indeed, that's just what happened. Patriarchy sprang up across Eurasia and seeded deep into the soil.

## Paradise Lost

So our European ancestors settled down to farm. They paired for life. They plowed and warred and traded. And gradually men's new jobs as plowmen, traders, and warriors became crucial to survival, while women's vital role as gatherers dwindled in importance. Then, as ranks emerged and men scrambled for these positions, women's formal power declined. For every farmer's foot was now sown into the soil. A mixture of immobility, skewed economic roles, permanent monogamy, stratified societies, the burgeoning of warfare, and, quite possibly, a peculiarity of testosterone and other physiological mechanisms set in motion systems of patriarchy seen in traditional agrarian societies around the world.

And with patriarchy, women became possessions to be coveted, guarded, and exploited—spawning social precepts known collectively as the sexual double standard. These credos were then passed across the centuries to us. The belief that men have a higher sex drive than women, the conviction that men are more adulterous, the tradition of female chastity at marriage, and the long-held assumption that women are often weak, stupid, and dependent became rooted deep in the plowman's dirt.

Of all the social changes that farm life produced, however, the most dramatic were our patterns of divorce.

## Till Death Us Do Part

Divorce rates were very low through much of our agrarian past. In the ancient lands of Israel, for example, divorce was rare.[20] The classical Greeks reveled in almost any sexual experiment, but they prohibited sexual practices (like bringing a courtesan into the home) that threatened the stability of the family.[21] Among the Greeks of the Homeric age, divorce was permitted but uncommon. Marital dissolution was low in Rome's early days, when the vast majority of citizens were farmers. Only as cities bloomed and some women became wealthy and independent did divorce rates soar among the urban upper classes.[22]

Early Christian fathers regarded marriage as a necessary remedy for fornication; to them bachelors and spinsters, celibates and virgins in honor of the Lord were far more pure. On the subject of divorce they were divided. "What therefore God has joined together, let no man put asunder," Jesus had advised.[23] Yet different passages of the Bible sent conflicting messages and some scholars think early Christian men had both the legal and religious right to divorce a wife for adultery or for being a nonbeliever. Regardless, divorce was never common among farming Christians, either before or after the decline of Rome.[24]

When Teutonic peoples overran Roman soil, they brought customs of their own. Divorce and polygyny were permitted among the ruling classes of pre-feudal Germany. Pre-Christian Celtic and Anglo-Saxon peoples also allowed divorce and remarriage. Given the genetic payoffs of polygyny for men, it is no surprise that those with money took several wives. But what evidence is available suggests that the rate of divorce was low among European peasant farmers during the dark centuries following the fall of Rome.[25]

During the ninth century, feudalism spread across Europe from its birthplace in France. As was customary in this system, feudal lords granted land to their vassals in exchange for allegiance and military duty. Each vassal then sub-granted his lands to tenants in return for special services. Theoretically, vassals and tenants "held" these homesteads rather than owning them; but in actuality vassals and tenants passed these land grants—and the land—from generation to generation within their families. Under feudalism, therefore, marriage continued to be the only way most men and women could acquire soil and secure it for their heirs.

European couples could have a marriage annulled on grounds of adultery, impotence, leprosy, or consanguinity—which the rich and the well-connected indeed did.[26] A spouse could also leave a mate if a properly constituted court pronounced a judicial separation that ordered partners to live apart. But this agreement carried a restriction: neither party was permitted to remarry.[27] In that case, who was to look after the goods, the lands, the animals, the house? Without a mate, a farmer could not make ends meet. In feudal Europe only the rich could afford to divorce a spouse.

～

Till death us do part. What economics had prescribed for plowmen, Christian leaders sanctified.

Augustine is generally thought to be the earliest Church leader to regard marriage as a holy sacrament; but as the centuries passed, most Christian authorities came to agree with him. Divorce became impossible under any circumstances for members of the Roman Catholic Church.[28] Although Catholic doctrine continued to make provisions for annulment and separation, lifelong marriage—a requisite of farm living—became a mandate straight from God.

With the rise of cities and trade in Europe in the tenth and eleventh centuries, women entered all sorts of occupations. In medieval London in the 1300s women were textile dealers, grocers, barber-surgeons, silk workers, bakers, beer makers, servants, embroiderers, shoemakers, jewelers, hat makers, and craftsmen of many other kinds. Not surprisingly, some women, like the Wife of Bath, Chaucer's bawdy entrepreneur, married five husbands in succession.

But she was exceptional. A woman normally worked alongside her spouse; she was socially subservient to him too. In fact, a woman's business debts were her husband's responsibility—a woman was not "a free and lawful person."[29] Predictably, divorce was uncommon in medieval European cities.

This pattern of low divorce persisted. After the Reformation marriage became a civil contract, rather than a sacrament, for Protestants. So beginning in the 1600s women in non-Catholic countries could obtain a divorce from civil authorities.[30] In fact, divorce rates fluctuated throughout the centuries following Christ's call for permanent monogamy. Where married men and women *could* leave each other, they did. But divorce rates remained notably low in Scandinavia and the British Isles, across the farmlands of Germany, France, the Low Countries, Spain, and Italy, through Hungary and the other eastern European cultures, in Russia, Japan, China, and India, and in the Muslim farm societies of North Africa—until the Industrial Revolution began to erode farm life.[31]

And when a spouse died (and where remarriage was permitted), a farmer took a new bride. Widowers who owned land often wed a few days after the mourning period ended. Remarriage by widows was widely discouraged in preindustrial European farming cultures, perhaps because this jeopardized the pattern of inheritance. But a great many women took a new husband anyway.

The realities of farm life required pairing.

Not all of our farming ancestors believed in God. Not all of these men and women were happily wed. Not all were excited about remarriage either. But the vast majority of these people lived by the sun and by the soil. These farming men and women were tethered to their land and to one another—forever.

Not until factories emerged behind the barns of the agricultural world did men and women start to regain their independence. Now patterns of sex and love and marriage would begin to swing forward to our ancient past.

# 16

## Future Sex

### Slow Love and Forward to the Past

And the end of all our exploring
Will be to arrive where we started
And know the place for the first time.
—T. S. ELIOT, *FOUR QUARTETS*

"Thus the sum of things is ever being replenished and mortals live one and all by give and take. Some races wax and others wane, and in a short space the tribes of living things are changed, and like runners hand on the torch of life."[1] Lucretius, the Roman poet, spoke of the unbrokenness of human nature—those dispositions that emerged with our nativity and can be seen in men and women around the world today. Among them is our human reproductive strategy, the way we mate and reproduce.

Day by decade by century our ancestors fell in love and paired; some philandered; some abandoned their partners; some paired again; most settled down as they got older or had more young—selecting for this complex, flexible, yet distinct blueprint of human romantic life. Not everyone conformed to this multipart mating script. Individuals differed in the past as they do today and will millennia from now. We can triumph over our predispositions. But these natural patterns prevail around the world. Stomp as culture may, she does not wipe them out.

Culture can, however, affect the frequency of adultery and divorce, the *number* of people who play out this ancient text. Farm living, for example, produced permanent monogamy for many in our elastic tribe. Where are we headed now?

## Working Women

As you know, all sorts of sociological, psychological, and demographic forces contribute to divorce rates.[2] "Nomadism" is one. Many of us have moved away from home; our parents live in different cities, often with new partners. So the wide network of family and community support that couples need when times are tough is vanishing, increasing the likelihood of divorce. Urbanism, secularism, and migration are associated with marital dissolution. Those who choose partners with different habits, different values, different interests, and different leisure activities are more likely to divorce. The contemporary emphasis on individualism and self-fulfillment has also contributed to the rising incidence of divorce.

But of all the major factors that contribute to marital instability, perhaps the most powerful in America today (and around the world) can be summed up in two words: working women.[3] Money spells freedom. Working women have more of it than those who mind the house. And demographers regularly cite this correlation between women working and high divorce (and remarriage) rates.

This is not to blame working wives for the American divorce rate. Although two-thirds of today's divorces are filed by women,[4] demographers will never know who actually leaves whom. But when women work outside the home and bring back staples, luxuries, or money, spouses caught in violent or desperately unhappy and unhealthy relationships have the option to leave each other.

They do because they can.

## The Road to Modern Divorce

The Industrial Revolution launched this trend of more women in the workplace. Tracing this single phenomenon in the United States explains much about the pulse of modern family life.[5]

As soon as hamlets of European settlers began to dot the Atlantic coast, American women began to make money outside the home by selling their surplus soap, their jars of raspberry preserves, their scented candles and home-baked pies. A few spinsters set up shops to sell books or imported clothes. Some widows became innkeepers or land agents. But the vast majority of women worked on a farm and kept a home.

By 1815, however, textile mills and other factories had begun to rise behind the apple trees and chicken yards and some young women had begun to leave home for factory work. They sought regular pay and shorter work hours—time and money to spend thumbing through catalogs for store-bought clothes. Even married women began to take home piecework for extra cash. America was turning industrial. And soon the divorce rate began to increase by fits and starts.[6]

In the mid-1800s cheap labor—immigrant men—appeared. This vast new workforce, the flight of American men from the farm into the factory, the belief that working women drove men's wages down, and the conviction that more children produce a larger tax base, a stronger military, a larger consumer market, and more bodies in church on Sunday popularized the dictum "A woman's place is in the home."[7] By 1900 only about 20% of women were in the labor force, most of them immigrants, youths, and singles.

Nevertheless, more married women worked than in preceding decades—and the divorce rate continued to increase.

The twentieth century saw a periodic escalation of these social trends launched by the industrial age: more working women; more divorce.[8] With one exception: America's emergence as a superpower after World War II brought an era of marital stability some think of as a golden age.

Actually the 1950s was the most unusual decade of that century.[9] Millions of women left the labor market as war veterans returned home and claimed their jobs in industry. Tuition loans, cheap life insurance for servicemen, government-guaranteed mortgages, tax advantages for married couples, and the expanding economy provided economic opportunities for postwar husbands and their families. These young men and women had also grown up during the Great Depression, when family life was particularly turbulent. They valued a stable home.

So in the 1950s Americans settled down. Adlai Stevenson summed up the times in 1955, advising graduating women of Smith College to "influence man and boy" through the "humble role of housewife."[10]

America took Stevenson's advice. Homemaking became fashionable. Women's magazines warned brides of the dangers of mixing work with motherhood. Psychiatrists described women with careers as struggling with "penis envy." And social critics proclaimed that mothering and keeping house were women's natural roles. Anthropologist Ashley Montagu delivered the coup de grace, saying, "No woman with a husband and small children can hold a full-time job and be a good homemaker at one and the same time."[11]

Not surprisingly, men and women married younger in the 1950s than in any other twentieth-century decade; 20.2 was the median age for women; 22.6 for men.[12] The divorce rate remained unusually steady. Remarriage rates declined. And the birthrate rose to its twentieth-century high: the baby boom. In 1957 the bumper crop of infants peaked.

The spreading suburbs became a cradle.

## Sleeping Beauties

"Clap hands, clap hands until Daddy comes home, because Daddy's got money and Mommy's got none." This nursery rhyme became obsolete in the early 1960s, when historic trends sparked by the Industrial Revolution resumed: more working women; more divorce. The wide use of new kinds of contraceptives, including the Pill, as well as several other forces played a role.[13] But demographers point to wives as a key factor in increasing rates of marital instability.

Many of these women, however, were not looking for careers. They wanted pink-collar jobs, positions that would supplement the family income and buy a dishwasher, a washing machine and dryer, an automobile, a TV set. Their goal: the good life.

American employers embraced them. Here were women who spoke English, women who could read and write, women willing to take part-time, go-nowhere, dead-end jobs. Anthropologist Marvin Harris summed up the times, saying that with the generation of immigrant

Chinese fading from the scene, "the dormant white American house-wife was the service-and-information employer's sleeping beauty."[14]

You know what happened next; the women's movement erupted. More important to our story, America resumed its modern course: between 1960 and 1983 the number of working women doubled.[15] Between 1966 and 1976 the divorce rate doubled too.[16] In 1981 the divorce rate hit an all-time high.[17] And today it has stabilized, indeed declined somewhat, although current estimates range from a rate of 41% (Divorcesource.com) to almost 50%.[18]

Yet most Americans will remarry.[19] And, remarkably, they will do it in a familiar pattern: Most will rewed between the *third and fourth* year after divorcing.[20] Most will also remarry between the ages of twenty-five and forty-four, largely during their reproductive years.[21] These patterns have remained stable for decades, if not millions of years.[22]

We are creatures living in a sea of currents that pull and stretch our family lives. Upon the ancient blueprint for serial monogamy and, for some, clandestine adultery, our culture casts its own design. Yet, after many centuries of permanent monogamy among our farming forebears, the primordial human pattern of serial pairing has emerged again.

## Through the Looking Glass of Prehistory

"If you can look into the seeds of time and say, which grain will grow, and which will not, speak then to me," Shakespeare wrote. Predicting the future is dangerous. But the human animal has been built to think, feel, and act in certain ways. What can our deep history say about the future of women, men, sex, and love?

Foremost, we are heading forward to the past.

Today most men and women work; the double-income family is the rule. Few of us still live in the house we grew up in. Instead, we have several places we call home: our parents' house, our office, our residence, and perhaps a vacation spot. We migrate between them. We no longer grow our own food. We hunt and gather in the grocery store and other shops. And we have a loose network of friends and relatives, many of whom live far away. All are returns to our prehistoric roots.

Even *how* we wed and *whom* we wed are returns to our deep history.

For the past several thousand years, most farming women had only three options: to be uneducated housewives, cloistered nuns, or courtesans and concubines. Most chose to wed. Moreover, a wedding marked a merger of property and an alliance between extended families. So marriages had to be permanent. This necessity is gone. On the farm, a woman had to be a virgin on her wedding night. Virginity at marriage is gone. Arranged marriages were common in our farming days. These are now largely out of style in most postindustrial societies. Our farming forebears had a double standard for adultery. This credo is gone. And they celebrated the marital mottos: "Honor thy husband" and "Till death us do part." These too are becoming history.

Of all of our returning marital habits, however, perhaps none is more profound than our current drive to marry for love.

⁐

Ever since someone invented the plow, our agrarian forebears were obliged to choose the "right" girl or boy, with the "right" kin connections, the "right" ethnic background, and the "right" religious beliefs. And a girl's only way to get ahead was to "marry up"—hypergamy. Farming men and women expected perks at the altar too, such as land, livestock, and community connections. Few dared to jeopardize their livelihood and their future for something as fickle as romantic passion.[23]

Today only 14% of single Americans would marry for financial security, while 86% seek a "committed partner to share my life with" instead. Over 90% also want someone who "respects" them, someone they can "trust and confide in," someone who "makes them laugh," and someone who "makes enough time" for them.[24] Contemporary singles seek a soul mate "first and foremost."[25] Moreover, over 54% of single Americans believe in love at first sight; 56% believe laws should be changed to make it easier to wed; and 89% believe you can stay married to the same person forever.

And, most will wed.

I do. I do. I do. "Marriage," Voltaire reportedly said, "is the only adventure open to the cowardly." Despite changing times, Americans participate with gusto. Today some 84% of American men and women are projected to wed their beloved by age forty, with women first marrying at age twenty-six and men at age twenty-seven.[26] Even those who don't want to marry say their primary reason is that they "don't think you need a marriage to prove you love someone."[27] Most remarkable, in 2014, 33% of men and women believed it is acceptable to leave a satisfactory marriage if they were not longer passionately in love.[28] In America, as in much of the postindustrial world, romantic love is in full bloom.

We are not alone. In a study of thirty-seven societies, men and women ranked love, or mutual attraction, as the first criterion for choosing a spouse.[29] This reflects ancient times. In a study of 190 historical and extant hunting and gathering societies,[30] 88% of *first* marriages were typically arranged by parents or close kin. But these arrangements were regularly casual and the marriages were fragile. Moreover, in these cultures, parents played a minor role in the second and third marriages of their young. People wed for love.

We are returning to this antique habit—seeking passionate romance within our partnerships. I think this is good news. There is more.

## Singles in America

As I have mentioned, I am the Chief Scientific Advisor to Match.com. Since 2010 we have annually conducted a national study, "Singles in America." We don't poll the Match.com population. Instead, we query a representative sample of over 5,000 Americans each year, based on the United States census. To date we have queried over 25,000 men and women—the largest national study of singles. And the results say much about today—and tomorrow.

Foremost, singles may be leading the way to a less prejudiced society.

In our 2014 "Singles in America" survey, 75% of singles reported that they would make a long-term commitment to someone of a different ethnic background, and 73% said they would commit to someone of a different faith. (Most singles will still wed someone of the same racial and spiritual tradition, but *attitudes* are changing.) Most also approve of same-sex marriage, as well as those who marry without having children and those who have children without marrying. Most singles are not concerned about a partner's past divorces either, or even the number of their past sex partners.

But singles care deeply about commitment. They don't approve of commuter marriages, sexually open relationships, or partners sleeping in separate homes. Americans are also more disapproving of adultery "for any reason" than in former decades.[31]

Today, however, marriage is becoming optional. On the farm, women and men needed a spouse to help work the land. Even in hunting-gathering societies, people believe one must marry to be considered fully adult. Marriage—the making of a formal social and reproductive alliance—was central to daily life throughout deep history. But now, some 67% of American cohabiting couples say they are scared of the social, legal, emotional, and economic consequences of divorce.[32] Divorce, they wanly joke, is in the drinking water. Indeed, between 43% and 50% of U.S. marriages will fail, what sociologist Andrew Cherlin calls the "marriage-go-round."[33]

*So I have come to believe that today's singles are ushering into vogue a long pre-commitment courtship process, what I call slow love.* And I am optimistic about this trend too.

## Slow Love

You may regard "hooking up" and "friends with benefits" as utterly irresponsible. Certainly those who engage in these behaviors risk sexually transmitted infections, unwanted pregnancy, and/or emotional trauma. In spite of these real dangers, many men and women are having casual sex.[34]

Take hooking up—a no-strings-attached, uncommitted sexual encounter between two people who are not currently in a romantic relationship with each other. In 2014, 58% of American singles in our SIA study had had a one-night stand—66% of men and 50% of women.

Hooking up isn't just for the young, either. When sociologists Monto and Carey compared the weekly uncommitted sexual capers of some 1,800 men and women in two age cohorts, those in their forties had had *more* sex with *more* partners than those in their twenties.[35] In fact, across our SIA studies, men and women in their sixties had engaged in just as many fleeting sexual encounters as those in their twenties and thirties.

But hooking up isn't new—it's another trend forward to the past.

Nisa, who, as you know, grew up in a hunting-gathering community in the Kalahari Desert, had her share of casual sex (as well as several husbands). Ketepe and his friends living along the Amazon River regularly slipped into the jungle for an afternoon's casual rendezvous. The Neanderthals had trysts with Cro-Magnon men or women. And if Lucy's bones could speak, this ancient relative could probably rattle off an impressive list of assignations over three million years ago. Even on the farm, men and women must have occasionally slipped behind the barn for casual sex—a strict taboo for women.

Today this taboo on uncommitted sex is vanishing. Once again, hooking up is commonplace—I suspect because *today's singles want to know every detail about a potential partner before they tie the knot, slow love.* This may be adaptive behavior in an age when many of us have too much property, making divorce potentially devastating, and most of us know how to protect ourselves from pregnancy and disease.

## Hooking Up . . . For Love?

Singles may even hope that casual sex will trigger romance and lead to a committed partnership.

I say this because when biologist Justin Garcia and anthropologist Chris Reiber asked college students why they had had a recent hookup, 51% said they had hoped it would initiate a traditional romantic relationship.[36] Psychologists Meston and Buss corroborate this finding. The U.S. college students they queried gave 237 reasons for hooking up. Among the top five were: "I was attracted to the person" and "I wanted to show my affection to the person."[37]

Many may win this new partner too—because nature has laid a trap. Any stimulation of the genitals promotes dopamine activity, which can potentially push you over the threshold into falling in love. And at orgasm, oxytocin and vasopressin—neurochemicals linked with feelings of attachment—spike.[38]

So unless you are so drunk that you can't remember the event, casual sex can trigger feelings of romance and/or attachment to this sex partner. Our 2012 "Singles in America" participants were no exception. When asked, "Have you ever had a one-night-stand that turned into a long-term, committed partnership," 33% said yes.

With just one night of casual sex, risky as it is, you may win life's greatest prize—a committed mating partner.

Nevertheless, today few hookups proceed quickly into commitment. Instead, caution reigns: *slow love*.

## Commitment-Lite

Perhaps there is no greater evidence of this caution than the current practice of friends with benefits. In this sexual arrangement, pairs have coitus when convenient, but they do not appear in public as a couple. These arrangements are popular. In 2013, 58% of men and 50% of women in our "Singles in America" study reported that they had had a friends-with-benefits relationship, including one in three people in their seventies.

But friends with benefits isn't new either. All kinds of creatures create ongoing sexual relationships devoid of long-term obligations. Among common chimps, males give females meat in exchange for sex—creating uncommitted sexual relationships that can persist for years.

The current popularity of friends with benefits is most likely due to its twenty-first-century purpose, however: to learn a great deal about a potential mate before one makes a formal commitment, marries, and possibly falls victim to divorce: slow love.

Indeed, you learn a lot between the sheets. You vividly see, hear, taste, feel, and smell your partner. In fact, in a study of 1,000-plus men and women, over 50% reported that the first kiss was the kiss of death, immediately ending a potential alliance.[39] But if you pass this breaking point and other crucial barriers that precede coitus, you can gather reams of data about a person during sex—including their health, patience, and ability to change their style to accommodate your needs.

Moreover, just like hooking up, a friends-with-benefits relationship can lead to romance and attachment. When we asked participants in our 2012 "Singles in America" study if they had ever had a friends-with-benefits relationship turn into a long-term partnership, 44% said yes. Mother Nature has her schemes for pair-bonding and procreation—regardless of our caution.

I suspect this form of *commitment-lite* will become more and more popular in a world where marriages are often fragile and divorce looms large; it's another stage of slow love.

## "Trial Marriages"

In her famous *Redbook* article of July 1966, anthropologist Margaret Mead proposed that Americans should forge a seemingly unconventional pair-bonding plan: marriage "in two steps."[40] Mead suggested that a young couple with no immediate plans to reproduce should first make an "individual marriage," a legal tie that excluded bearing children, did not imply a lifelong commitment, and had no economic consequences should the couple part. Then, when the couple decided to procreate, Mead recommended that they enter a "parental marriage," a legal relationship that confirmed a long-term bond and made formal provisions for children should they divorce.

Living together, a version of the first step of this two-step marriage, erupted in the 1970s; and today what was once scandalous has become routine. In 2012, 58% of U.S. singles reported that they have lived with one to five partners outside of wedlock.

Yet 64% of Americans believe this living arrangement is a step toward formal wedding[41]—another credo of our prehistoric past. Among hunting-gathering peoples, living together is often viewed as a "trial marriage."

Today, however, caution reigns even after partners have agreed to wed: 36% of singles want a prenuptial agreement.

I suspect that these "prenups" will soon become the norm—because our forebears had *natural* prenups. In hunting-gathering societies, a child was born into a specific clan; his or her living arrangements were not open to negotiation at divorce. A man's bows and arrows were his property; a woman's digging stick, shawls, and baskets belonged to her. Spouses probably argued bitterly before parting, but no one's possessions were up for grabs. Prenuptial agreements are our heritage; they will be our future too.

∽

One-night stands, hooking up, friends with benefits, living together; prenups: these arrangements bespeak the caution prevailing in our modern world. For the past 10,000 years, marriage was the beginning of a partnership; today it's the finale.[42]

And these long pre-commitment stages of slow love may be paying off. Foremost, be you in your first, second, or third marriage, most Americans appear to be in happy partnerships.

In 2012, with Match.com, I surveyed 1,095 married American men and women (not, of course, on this Internet dating site). Among our many questions was: "Knowing what you now know about your spouse, would you marry the same person again?" A resounding 81% said: "yes." Moreover, 76% of the men and 73% of the women said they were still "very much in love." The only thing they envied about the single life was "having my own independent schedule."

In another current study of marital happiness, scientists phoned 166 women and 149 men in their fifties who were married or living with a long-term mate.[43] A whopping 86% said they were either "very intensely in love," "intensely in love" or "very in love." The obsession of first infatuation had waned, but, as the authors concluded, the "intensity, engagement and sexual interest" had remained. Interestingly, level of income, amount of education, and length of the relationship made no significant difference in their romantic passion. And men were just as likely as women to be "very much in love."

These happily married American men and women are apparently not unusual. A 2013 survey of 12,000+ adults in fifteen countries established that 78% of married men and women were "happy"[44]—most likely because, due to the long pre-commitment stage of current partnerships, many unhappy relationships end before partners tie the knot.

We even stumbled on some of the neural ingredients of this marital bliss—data that may help partners survive the bumps and sustain their relationship long-term.

## Positive Illusions

For centuries, psychologists, clergy, family, and friends have offered advice on how to keep a partnership happy. Our research adds to this collection—with data directly on brain activity.

As discussed in Chapter Two, my brain scanning partners and I put seventeen men and women in their fifties and sixties into the brain scanner. On average, these participants had been married twenty-one years, and all maintained that they were still madly in love with their wedded mate. But we also gave each of the participants a questionnaire on marital satisfaction, a series of queries that either Bianca Acevedo, the lead author of the study, or I administered on the morning of the scan. Interestingly, those who scored high on this "marital satisfaction" questionnaire also showed more activity in brain regions linked with *empathy* and *controlling one's emotions*.

My colleagues stumbled on more of nature's blueprint for partner happiness in China.

Psychologist Mona Xu and her colleagues used my original research design to collect data on seventeen young Chinese men and women who were newly and passionately in love. These Chinese subjects responded just like our Americans: the same basic brain regions associated with romantic love became active when they looked at their beloved's face.

More intriguing, Xu went back to China almost four years later to see whether any of these participants were still in love with the same partner. Eight were. And when Xu and her colleagues compared their brain scans with the brain scans of those who had broken up, they found the difference: men and women who were still in love showed specific activity in a brain region associated with the ability to *suspend negative judgment* and *over-evaluate a partner*, what psychologists call "positive illusions."[45] As the old tune goes: "accentuate the positive; eliminate the negative."

Empathy, controlling your emotions, positive illusions: we are beginning to map the brain's pathways for long-term romantic bliss.

As scientists learn more about the brain in love and more bad relationships end during the long pre-commitment stage of courtship, more happy partnerships are likely to emerge as the twenty-first century proceeds.

Yet even this is not new. Because men and women were *not* economically sewn to one another across deep history, and bad relationships could end, it is likely that our forebears spent most of their years in happy partnerships. We are moving forward to the past in this way too.

## "Big Data" on Love

How is the Internet changing love and marriage?

Perhaps most remarkable is the proliferation of Internet dating sites. These services are cheap, easy to navigate, and safe—as long as you follow some obvious rules of where to meet and how to conduct yourself. They are also effective. In 2014, some 36% of singles met their last first date through the Internet, while only 25% met through a friend, 8% met at work, and 6% met at a bar, club, or social event. Moreover, 37% of relationships now start online, as do 20% of marriages.

Academics quibble about these services. But I don't think they understand them. Internet dating services are not *dating* services; they are *introducing* services. Internet algorithms can weed out obviously inappropriate mates and thus help you kiss fewer frogs. But the only true algorithm for sizing up a potential partner is your own brain. And the basic physiology of the human brain has not changed in over 200,000 years.

So when you meet a potential partner, your ancient mind springs into action—and you court by its prehistoric rules. IPhones and social media sites can't stamp this process out.

The Internet is changing *how* we court, however.[46] Foremost, courtship communication is now short and "in real time." Text messaging and emailing to set a date are prime examples. And in an age of time constraints, this is most likely adaptive too.

## The Age of Transparency

A curious twist of our modern era is our craving for privacy in conjunction with our urge to be known and heard. Hunting-gathering men and women did not struggle with this conflict. Everybody knew almost everything about everybody else. Theirs was a true age of transparency; privacy was scarce. Moreover, in deep history, gossip served as the local newspaper, as well as the way to set rules and ostracize offenders.

This heritage, I suspect, is the root cause of our remarkable impulse to share our lives and whisper about others. All this was fine a million years ago—but it can be lethal on the Internet today.

Take sexting. Today some 33% of American singles have sent a sexy photo of themselves to a potential partner via the Internet; while 49% have received a sexy photo. Moreover, 25% of those who have received a spicy picture have shared it with one or more friends.[47] And today these racy photos can tear around the globe.

So to see if people even grasp the possible consequences of sexting, I asked participants in our "Singles in America" studies whether they believed that sending sexy photos could jeopardize their lives. Indeed, 75% thought that sexting could endanger their reputation, and over 60% believed it could damage their career, friendships, and self-esteem. Singles sent these sexy photos anyway.

Men and women are apparently willing to risk personal and professional disaster to pursue primal human goals: romance and attachment. They always have; they always will.

## Researching a Date . . . Like the Old Days

Many other emerging Internet dating habits come from our deep history. Among them, today 38% of men and 53% of women research a new date on Facebook, and 32% of singles use Google.

Our forebears researched potential partners too. In former times, however, singles had relatives and friends who easily did this research for them. Communities were close-knit, word spread, and everyone knew someone who could find out anything about anybody else. Today singles do this research by themselves.

We will see more of this Internet investigation in coming years, because we have only so much time and metabolic energy to mate and breed. False starts aren't adaptive.

We'll see new taboos as well. Among them, being secretive about texts and phone calls. Today over 53% of singles would not consider dating someone who is cagey about their correspondence. Transparency is becoming important—in step with the conviction that a deep, loving connection is the core of life, and in step with our ancient past.

I am also happy to report that some 60% of singles now believe it's rude to text "too frequently" while on a dinner date.[48] Maybe our Wild West attitude toward cell phone use will wane, replaced with the intimate repartee that our hunting-gathering forebears enjoyed as they whispered to each other over a steak and salad dinner a million years ago.

## Sexy Women

With this sea change forward to the past and our new trend towards slow love, I think we may finally come to realize that women are just as sexual as men.

In a revealing study, when men and women were asked about their sex lives, men admitted to far more sex partners than women. However, when the sexes were hooked up to a lie detector, women admitted to just as many coital mates.[49] This is not new. Although little known to any but anthropologists, men and women in seventy-two of ninety-three traditional societies have maintained that both sexes demonstrate a roughly equal sex drive.[50]

The strong human female sex drive mirrors behavior in the animal kingdom. All female mammals come into heat; and as estrus emerges they actively solicit males—behavior known as female proceptivity.

A wild female chimpanzee in estrus, for instance, will stroll up to a male, tip her buttocks toward his nose, and pull him to his feet to copulate. When he has finished, she copulates with almost every other male in the community except her sons. In one laboratory environment, captive female chimps initiated up to 85% of all matings. Captive male orangutans tend to fall asleep after coitus, but at the height of estrus a female will pester a male to stay awake for a second round. And if you have not seen the aggressive sexuality of female apes, surely you have observed the antics of female dogs. You have to bar the door if you want a bitch in heat to remain chaste.

This female sexual persistence makes biological sense. As Darwin pointed out, those who seek sex and breed, survive.

⌒

Women express their sexuality somewhat differently, however.[51]

Men think about sex more regularly; and men are more consistently motivated to initiate and engage in sex.[52] But women's sexuality is more intense; women have more contractions per orgasm, and women are far more likely to orgasm several times in one sex event.

Women also tend to embed sex in a broader context. A fancy dinner, candlelight, sexy words, flowers, and soft sheets: all are part of the experience for most women. Women are more sexually flexible, responding to cues in their environment. Men, on the other hand, tend to focus more narrowly on orgasm.[53] Women express more bisexuality; men tend to be either gay or straight. And while men are more likely to seek their partner's satisfaction in bed, women are more likely to try to please themselves.[54]

The ancient Greeks told the story of Zeus and Hera debating which gender had more pleasure during coitus. Zeus held that it was women; Hera believed it was men. So they asked Tiresias, a man who was transformed into a woman for several years as punishment for having interrupted some snakes during intercourse. He responded, saying, "Of ten parts a man enjoys one only, but a woman enjoys the full ten parts in her heart."[55]

Tiresias had it wrong. Current studies suggest that women and men have, on average, exactly the same degree of sexual response and pleasure.[56]

⌒

Women's sexual attitudes differ from those of men, however. Women are the custodians of the egg; they must bring the fetus to term; and women spend more time caring for the very young. As a result, women are the picky sex. Women are far less inclined to approve of sex on the first date. Women have fewer one-night stands. And women are more discriminating about their partners.[57]

This was evident in our "Singles in America" studies. Women are considerably more likely than men to want a partner who makes at least as much money, and who has a similar level of education, belongs to the same political party, and shares their ethnic and religious background. Women are also more likely than men to want their own bank account, regular nights out with girlfriends, their "own personal space," and a mate who will help in child-rearing and household duties.[58]

Today's women believe they can have a successful career *and* a happy relationship. And men approve. In our 2011 SIA study, over 45% of men of all ethnic groups reported that they were turned off by a woman who "doesn't care about her career." Coming decades should see more powerful women in the office and more expressive women in the bedroom. For when women have an independent income, live in an urban setting, have access to contraception and abortion, and are healthy and educated, they express their *natural* libido.

## The New Prehistoric Man

Scientists and laymen have spent the last fifty years dispelling myths about women. It's time to dispel the lore about men. I'll begin by proposing that with time, we will come to understand that men are just as romantic as women.

Foremost, in our brain scanning study (using fMRI) of young happy lovers, *men showed just as much activity in neural pathways for romantic love as women did*.

Moreover, all men aren't "players." When Match.com queried singles about their approach to dating, only 3% replied, "I just want to meet a lot of people."[59] And on the site OKCupid, only 6% of men said they were "explicitly looking for sex."[60] In fact, in 2014, more men were actively seeking a relationship than women were. Moreover, 87% of men were willing to make a commitment to a woman who was "considerably" better educated, "considerably" more intellectual, and made "considerably" more money; and 39% of men would even date a woman ten or more years older than themselves.

Men fall in love faster and more often than women too.[61] Men are more eager to kiss a new partner in public, faster to introduce a new mate to friends and family, and quicker to want to live together. Men have more intimate conversations with their partners—because women have their intimate conversations with their girlfriends. Men suffer just as much from loneliness,[62] and when asked why they want to marry, men are equally likely to say "love."[63] Moreover, men are just as likely to believe you can stay married to the same person forever (89%). And after a breakup, men are 2.5 times more likely to kill themselves.[64]

Trumping romance, however, is men's desire to make a commitment to an appropriate reproductive partner—illustrated by men's remarkable response to a particular question we ask American singles annually: "Would you make a long-term commitment to someone who has everything you are looking for, but with whom you are not in love?" In our 2014 "Singles in America" study, 36% of men (versus 29% of women) said they were "somewhat likely"; and men in their twenties and thirties (the peak years of reproduction) were just as likely as older men and women to forgo romantic passion to make an appropriate long-term partnership.

Why would a young man forfeit romantic passion to make a long-term partnership?

It's the call of the wild, I suspect. Bob is a good example. Bob had lived with Julia for three years. Julia was beautiful, educated, happy, athletic, established in her career, popular with his friends and family, and madly in love with Bob. She urgently wanted to marry him. But Bob had secretly fallen in love with a barmaid who had little education, no career plans, and an accent that would have made his parents cringe. He married Julia. Years later, he told me he had made the right decision. Julia had been enormously helpful to his business, and, as he said, "she is a great mother to our child."

When the "almost right" woman came along, Bob's unconscious drive to pass on his DNA trumped his passion for a less appropriate mate.

≈

Fathering is human—it evolved over four million years ago.

In fact, in a different Match.com survey of 1,500 American married men, 68% reported that they bonded with their baby as fast as the mother did. Moreover, 48% said they were equally busy in the laundry room; 46% did just as many dishes; 34% prepared just as many family meals; and 43% spent equal time with the mop and vacuum cleaner. These men also did the yard work, auto care, and household repair. Some 59% believed they were better dads than their fathers were. Their own fathers were better at providing financially, they said; but they spent more time caring for and educating their young. And when asked what men want women to know about them, one of the top three replies was that they are "compassionate."[65]

In 1989, sociologist Arlie Hochschild wrote her highly popular book *The Second Shift*, about the struggles of working women who also did the vast majority of childcare and housework. Will men begin to struggle with the second shift as well? Some 48% of these dads reported that they became more stressed with fatherhood. We may see more. As women's business roles expand, men's parenting roles are expanding too. Men are reacquiring parental roles they assumed millions of years ago.

## Our Time: Senior Love

We may also come to realize that the elderly are not as old as they look.

In our Match.com surveys, over 50% of people over sixty had had a one-night stand.[66] Seniors were the most likely to experience orgasm 91–100% of the time; and people over sixty were also the happiest, least anxious, least lonely, and least desperate to find love.[67] In fact, when asked, "Would you make a long-term commitment to someone who had everything you were looking for, but with whom you were not in love," men and women in their sixties were the *least* likely to say yes. The quest for romance never dies.

Most seniors were also *un*willing to make a long-term commitment to someone whom they didn't find sexually attractive, even if this person had everything else they were looking for in a partner.[68] And seniors were just as intolerant as younger people of a potential mate who talked too much, watched too much television, or who was lazy, stubborn, or humorless.

Moreover, seniors were far less interested in marrying than men and women of any other age cohort. Some 80% would not move in with their children to assume daily grandparenting roles, either.[69] Instead, some 62% of American widows and widowers choose to live alone[70]—perhaps to search for love.

Indeed, Our Time, a dating site that currently serves fifty-plus men and women, is the third largest paid dating site in America, with millions of unique visitors each year. The future will see even more seniors engaged in the marriage-go-round—just as they most likely did a million years ago.

## Gay Love

In his timeless epic *The Iliad*, Homer called love "Magic to make the sanest man go mad." This brain system lives deep in the human brain. Gays and lesbians are no exception. Brain regions associated with intense romantic passion are just as active in gays and lesbians as in heterosexuals.[71]

Moreover, our "Singles in America" data clearly show that gays and lesbians are equally inclined to believe in love at first sight. They fall in love just as often. They are just as likely to regard sex with a familiar partner as "extremely intimate,"[72] and just as likely to make a long-term commitment to a partner.[73] Some 41% of gays and 43% of lesbians want to marry, and 95% of married gays and 87% of married lesbians would *remarry* their current spouse.

Just about everyone feels the magic of romance. So I suspect we will come to see how similar to heterosexuals these men and women are.

## Going Solo

This marriage-go-round has contributed to one thoroughly modern social phenomenon, however: the large number of singles living alone.[74]

Today almost 50% of American adults are single, and 27% of American households have only one occupant, up from 9% in 1950.[75] Even more singles live alone in Japan, France, Germany, Sweden, and several other countries.[76] This is new. Even in 1900, when 46% of all Americans over age fifteen were single, they did not live alone. In the city; on the farm; in all hunting-gathering, horticultural, and herding societies: throughout human history, most young singles, single parents, and single widows and widowers lived with relatives.

Émile Durkheim traced this "cult of the individual," as he called it, back to the days when our agrarian forebears left their rural roots to live in cities.[77] And many still worry that this "individualism" has left us fragmented and cut off.

I don't agree. Today an American sends, on average, some 15,000 emails every year. Many connect with thousands more through their personal blogs, Twitter messages, homemade videos, and social networking sites. Facebook members have, on average, over three hundred "friends." And in any public place, people relentlessly yammer and tap on their cell phones, suggesting vast networks of attachment.

We are hyperconnected, immersed in a worldwide web of huge and diverse social networks.[78] Far from tuning out, men, women, and children are constantly tuning in.

Even this isn't new. Our forebears were also hyperconnected. A few years ago I had the opportunity to travel briefly with the Hadza hunter-gatherers of Tanzania, pitching my tiny tent near their cluster of grass huts by night, following them by day. One morning I joined fourteen women as they set out through the grass to gather berries. They bantered constantly. In camp, men and women relaxed in separate groups, just out of earshot of each other, where both sexes continued to talk constantly. Traditionally, all also met during the dry season at permanent water holes where men and women mingled with about five hundred other friends and relatives.

The human drive to establish and maintain kin, social, and business relationships is natural. Today we just connect more and more through technology instead. In fact, this is spurring into existence a new family form: *the association*. Associations are composed of unrelated friends who talk regularly; assemble for minor holidays, like birthdays; and help one another when one is sick—a mesh of kin based on companionship instead of blood.

And "going solo," as sociologist Eric Klinenberg calls it, is likely to enable more men and women to find true love too—unless they succumb to a subtle, possibly sinister, new phenomenon: antidepressant drugs.

## The Numbing of the World?

Nothing in the brain works alone. As one chemical system increases its activity, others adjust in myriad different ways. And it is well known that drugs that boost the serotonin system in the brain tend to suppress dopamine circuits—the circuits associated with feelings of intense romantic love.[79]

So it is my hypothesis that *when an antidepressant jeopardizes the activity of these dopamine pathways, it can also imperil feeling of intense romantic passion.* Among these drugs are Prozac, Zoloft, and Paxil (selective serotonin reuptake inhibitors, or SSRIs) and their descendants, Celexa and Lexapro.

Much scientific work needs to be done to substantiate my premise. I certainly welcome it, because ever since psychiatrist Andy Thomson and I wrote an article on this possible relationship,[80] I have been receiving unsolicited emails from strangers on this topic.

One wrote that she had been dating her boyfriend for eight months before starting Paxil, and six weeks later she lost that loving feeling for him. Another wrote that Lexapro had ruined his marriage, keeping his wife from feeling love. Another wrote that her boyfriend abruptly dumped her four weeks after starting Celexa, saying that he had lost that spark. Another wrote that soon after his wife began Effexor, she became cold and distant toward him, with almost no visible emotion. And one vivid epistle came from a woman who said that soon after her husband began an SSRI, he became totally emotionless, that the pills reminded her of the film *Invasion of the Body Snatchers.*

It's important to remember that some people need these antidepressants to get out of bed in the morning. One woman wrote that she hadn't felt any romantic passion for over ten years, but even though the pills had crippled her love life, her former depressions had made it almost impossible to go on living at all. Another used an SSRI to kill an infatuation to a woman in the office—enabling him to stay with his family and be a good dad.

A world without love?

No one has done systematic studies of the relationship between serotonin-boosting antidepressants and the brain systems for romantic love and attachment. But dozens of studies show that these drugs curb obsessive thinking and blunt the emotions—central characteristics of romantic passion. They can affect the brain's attachment system too.[81]

Today over 150 million prescriptions for these drugs are written annually in America. And generic versions are now available in countries around the world. *These medications can save lives and marriages*. But Harvard Medical School psychiatrist Joseph Glenmullen estimates that 75% of all patients on antidepressants, largely SSRIs, are "needlessly on these drugs."[82]

A vaccine against love? Perhaps.

## Love Potion #9

But can we trigger love with chemistry?

Humankind has been concocting love potions for centuries, most likely millennia. And several of my colleagues are convinced we will eventually be able to offer sophisticated medications to generate feelings of romance.[83] Among them is neuroscientist Larry Young, who recently wrote in *Nature*: "Recent advances in the biology of pair-bonding mean it won't be long before an unscrupulous suitor could slip a pharmaceutical love potion in our drink."[84]

But I suspect that Young and others are overlooking a major component of romance: your love map. You may recall that, as you grow up, you build a conscious (and unconscious) list of traits you are looking for in a mate; then, with time and experiences, this vision of an ideal partner crystallizes. Drugs can't change these memories, these experiences, this mental template.

Such was the experience of an American psychology graduate student attending a conference in Beijing. He was madly in love with another graduate student who was not in love with him. So he invited her to take a rickshaw ride. He knew that novelty and danger can trigger the dopamine system—potentially pushing one over the threshold into falling in love. He hoped this would happen to her. Off they sped, hurtling through busy streets, dodging buses, pushcarts, bicycles, and pedestrians as the driver madly pedaled. She squealed with joy and clung to him affectionately. His heart pounded with hope. Yet when they arrived back at the hotel she bounded from the rickshaw seat, threw her arms up and exclaimed, "Wasn't that wonderful! And wasn't that rickshaw driver handsome!"

Altering brain chemistry can change your basic feelings. But it can't *direct* those feelings. Mate choice is governed by complex interactions between our myriad experiences, as well as our biology. In short, if someone set you up with Hitler or some other monster, no "slipped pharmaceutical love potion" is going to make you love them.

## Future Sex

"O love is the crooked thing," wrote poet William Butler Yeats. I have proposed that some time around 4.4 million years ago our ancestors developed a *dual* human reproductive strategy: serial monogamy and clandestine adultery. So I suspect the single greatest twenty-first-century issue in relationships will be how each of us handles these conflicting appetites: our ancient drive to fall in love and build a partnership and our drives to seek autonomy and fresh features.

Much has changed, of course. We have come to regard love as the core of our social lives. Many now get into a relationship slowly, extending the pre-commitment stages of romance. And with self-help books and magazines, blogs, TV and radio talk shows, and therapists of many stripes, we are working harder on our relationships than at any time in history or prehistory. Furthermore, peer marriages—weddings between equals—have become the norm and more marriages are happy because bad marriages can end. And many of us have a long middle age, as well as access to new technologies—from Internet introductions to Viagra—to find, make, and keep the love we want.

Perhaps most important, although marriage has become optional, love has not. Ardi loved. Lucy loved. Twiggy loved. *Homo erectus* men and women loved. Neanderthal peoples loved. You and I love. Everywhere in the world people fall in love and make attachments to one another. Women and men are like two feet; we need each other to get ahead. And if we survive as a species, our descendants will fall in love and form pair-bonds a million years from now.

Is the family an endangered species?

Absolutely not. As anthropologist Paul Bohannan summed it up, "The family is the most adaptable of all human institutions, changing with every social demand. The family does not break in a storm as oak or pine trees do, but bends before the wind like the bamboo tree in Oriental tales and springs up again."[85]

So I will conclude with this. Any prediction about future relationships must take into account the most important determinant of the future: the unquenchable, adaptable, and primordial human drive to love.

# Fisher Romantic Love Scale

This questionnaire is about "being in love,": the feelings of being passionately in love, infatuated, or strongly romantically attracted to someone. If you are not currently in love, but felt very passionate about someone in the past, please answer the questions with that person in mind.

1. I have a hard time sleeping because I am thinking about _____.

   | 1 | 2 | 3 | 4 | 5 | 6 | 7 |

   strongly disagree · · · · · · strongly agree

2. When someone tells me something funny, I want to share it with _____.

   | 1 | 2 | 3 | 4 | 5 | 6 | 7 |

   strongly disagree · · · · · · strongly agree

3. _____ has some faults but they don't really bother me.

   | 1 | 2 | 3 | 4 | 5 | 6 | 7 |

   strongly disagree · · · · · · strongly agree

4. It is never good to be out of touch with _____ for a few days.

   | 1 | 2 | 3 | 4 | 5 | 6 | 7 |

   strongly disagree · · · · · · strongly agree

5. _____ has a distinctive voice.

   | 1 | 2 | 3 | 4 | 5 | 6 | 7 |

   strongly disagree · · · · · · strongly agree

6. When the relationship with _____ has a setback, I just try harder to get things going right.

| 1 | 2 | 3 | 4 | 5 | 6 | 7 |

strongly disagree                                                       strongly agree

7. I try to look my best for _____.

| 1 | 2 | 3 | 4 | 5 | 6 | 7 |

strongly disagree                                                       strongly agree

8. When I am with _____, my mind never wanders to other loves I have had.

| 1 | 2 | 3 | 4 | 5 | 6 | 7 |

strongly disagree                                                       strongly agree

9. My heart races when I hear _____'s voice on the phone.

| 1 | 2 | 3 | 4 | 5 | 6 | 7 |

strongly disagree                                                       strongly agree

10. I love everything about _____.

| 1 | 2 | 3 | 4 | 5 | 6 | 7 |

strongly disagree                                                       strongly agree

11. I feel happy when _____ is happy and sad when he/she is sad.

| 1 | 2 | 3 | 4 | 5 | 6 | 7 |

strongly disagree                                                       strongly agree

12. I feel preoccupied by my feelings for _____.

| 1 | 2 | 3 | 4 | 5 | 6 | 7 |

strongly disagree                                                       strongly agree

13. When I am talking to _____ , I am often afraid I will say the wrong thing.

    1       2       3       4       5       6       7
    strongly disagree                           strongly agree

14. The last person I think of each day as I fall asleep is _____.

    1       2       3       4       5       6       7
    strongly disagree                           strongly agree

15. Sex is not the most important part of my relationship with _____.

    1       2       3       4       5       6       7
    strongly disagree                           strongly agree

16. It upsets me when _____ is not being treated fairly.

    1       2       3       4       5       6       7
    strongly disagree                           strongly agree

17. I have more energy when I am with _____.

    1       2       3       4       5       6       7
    strongly disagree                           strongly agree

18. It really bothers me when _____ is having a bad day.

    1       2       3       4       5       6       7
    strongly disagree                           strongly agree

19. If _____ is unavailable, I don't go out on romantic dates with other men/women.

    1       2       3       4       5       6       7
    strongly disagree                           strongly agree

20. _____ is the center of my life.

        1        2        3        4        5        6        7

strongly disagree                                       strongly agree

21. I interpret _____'s actions, looking for clues about his/her feelings toward me.

        1        2        3        4        5        6        7

strongly disagree                                         strongly agree

22. My feelings for _____ are never overshadowed by passionate romantic feelings for another person.

        1        2        3        4        5        6        7

strongly disagree                                         strongly agree

23. I will never forget our first kiss.

        1        2        3        4        5        6        7

strongly disagree                                         strongly agree

24. When I'm in class/at work my mind wanders to _____.

        1        2        3        4        5        6        7

strongly disagree                                         strongly agree

25. The best thing about love has never been the sex.

        1        2        3        4        5        6        7

strongly disagree                                         strongly agree

26. I never give up loving _____, even when things are going poorly.

        1        2        3        4        5        6        7

strongly disagree                                         strongly agree

27. I often wonder whether _____ is as passionate about me as I am about him/her.

   1        2        3        4        5        6        7
   strongly disagree                              strongly agree

28. Sometimes I search for alternative meanings to _____'s words and gestures.

   1        2        3        4        5        6        7
   strongly disagree                              strongly agree

29. Sometimes I feel awkward, shy, and inhibited when I am around _____.

   1        2        3        4        5        6        7
   strongly disagree                              strongly agree

30. I deeply hope _____ is as attracted to me as I am to him/her.

   1        2        3        4        5        6        7
   strongly disagree                              strongly agree

31. I eat less when I am infatuated.

   1        2        3        4        5        6        7
   strongly disagree                              strongly agree

32. When I feel certain that _____ is passionate about me, I feel lighter than air.

   1        2        3        4        5        6        7
   strongly disagree                              strongly agree

33. Having a good relationship with _____ is more important to me than having a good relationship with my family.

   1        2        3        4        5        6        7
   strongly disagree                              strongly agree

34. My daydreams about _____ include making love/sexual contact.

    1        2        3        4        5        6        7
    strongly disagree                              strongly agree

35. I never feel totally self-confident when I am with _____.

    1        2        3        4        5        6        7
    strongly disagree                              strongly agree

36. No matter where it starts, my mind always seems to end up thinking about _____.

    1        2        3        4        5        6        7
    strongly disagree                              strongly agree

37. My emotional state depends on how _____ feels about me.

    1        2        3        4        5        6        7
    strongly disagree                              strongly agree

38. My relationships with my closest friends are less important to me than my relationship with _____.

    1        2        3        4        5        6        7
    strongly disagree                              strongly agree

39. _____ has special smells that I would recognize anywhere.

    1        2        3        4        5        6        7
    strongly disagree                              strongly agree

40. I save the cards and letters that _____ sends me.

    1        2        3        4        5        6        7
    strongly disagree                              strongly agree

41. _____'s behavior always seems to affect my emotional well-being.

    1      2      3      4      5      6      7

strongly disagree                      strongly agree

42. Being sexually faithful is important when you are in love.

    1      2      3      4      5      6      7

strongly disagree                      strongly agree

43. When _____ does well, I feel so happy for him/her.

    1      2      3      4      5      6      7

strongly disagree                      strongly agree

44. Being infatuated rarely helps me to concentrate on my work.

    1      2      3      4      5      6      7

strongly disagree                      strongly agree

45. When I think about _____ I feel excited, rather than calm and serene.

    1      2      3      4      5      6      7

strongly disagree                      strongly agree

46. I remember trivial things _____ says and does.

    1      2      3      4      5      6      7

strongly disagree                      strongly agree

47. I like to keep my schedule open so that if _____ is free, we can see each other.

    1      2      3      4      5      6      7

strongly disagree                      strongly agree

48. _____'s eyes are like nobody else's.

      1     2     3     4     5     6     7

strongly disagree             strongly agree

49. Falling in love was not really a choice; it just struck me.

      1     2     3     4     5     6     7

strongly disagree             strongly agree

50. Knowing that _____ is in love with me is more important to me than having sex with my partner.

      1     2     3     4     5     6     7

strongly disagree             strongly agree

51. My passion for _____ can overcome any obstacle.

      1     2     3     4     5     6     7

strongly disagree             strongly agree

52. I like to think about tiny moments that I have spent with _____.

      1     2     3     4     5     6     7

strongly disagree             strongly agree

53. I go through periods of despair when I think _____ might not love me.

      1     2     3     4     5     6     7

strongly disagree             strongly agree

54. I spend hours imagining romantic episodes with _____.

      1     2     3     4     5     6     7

strongly disagree             strongly agree

SCORING: The higher your score, the more intensely you are in love (378 is the highest score). The questionnaire is also available in my book *Why We Love* (2009) and on our website, TheAnatomyOfLove.com)

NOTE: We have done two brain scanning experiments to validate this questionnaire (unpublished data). We began by administering the questionnaire to two groups of participants: seventeen participants who had just fallen madly in love, and fourteen who were still in love with their long-term partner. In both experiments, those who scored high on the Fisher Romantic Love Scale showed specific brain activities, indicating that these men and women were exhibiting "positive illusions"—the ability to overlook what they didn't like about their partner to focus on what they adored.

# FISHER TEMPERAMENT INVENTORY

Circle your answer next to each question:
SD = Strongly disagree  D = disagree  A = agree  SA = strongly agree
*See scoring directions at end of test, after you have filled out all four sections.*

SCALE 1

1.  I find unpredictable situations exhilarating.  SD  D  A  SA

2.  I do things on the spur of the moment.  SD  D  A  SA

3.  I get bored when I have to do the same familiar things.  SD  D  A  SA

4.  I have a very wide range of interests.  SD  D  A  SA

5.  I am more optimistic than most people.  SD  D  A  SA

6.  I am more creative than most people.  SD  D  A  SA

7.  I am always looking for new experiences.  SD  D  A  SA

8.  I am always doing new things.  SD  D  A  SA

9.  I am more enthusiastic than most people.  SD  D  A  SA

10.  I am willing to take risks to do what I want to do.  SD  D  A  SA

11.  I get restless if I have to stay home for any length of time.  SD  D  A  SA

12.  My friends would say I am very curious.  SD  D  A  SA

13.  I have more energy than most people.  SD  D  A  SA

14.  On my time off, I like to be free to do whatever looks fun.  SD  D  A  SA

TOTAL_____

## SCALE 2

1. I think consistent routines keep life orderly and relaxing.  SD  D  A  SA

2. I consider (and reconsider) every option thoroughly before making a plan.  SD  D  A  SA

3. People should behave according to established standards of proper conduct.  SD  D  A  SA

4. I enjoy planning way ahead.  SD  D  A  SA

5. In general, I think it is important to follow rules.  SD  D  A  SA

6. Taking care of my possessions is a high priority for me.  SD  D  A  SA

7. My friends and family would say I have traditional values.  SD  D  A  SA

8. I tend to be meticulous in my duties.  SD  D  A  SA

9. I tend to be cautious, but not fearful.  SD  D  A  SA

10. People should behave in ways that are morally correct.  SD  D  A  SA

11. It is important to respect authority.  SD  D  A  SA

12. I would rather have loyal friends than interesting friends.  SD  D  A  SA

13. Long-established customs need to be respected and preserved.  SD  D  A  SA

14. I like to work in a straightforward path toward completing the task.  SD  D  A  SA

TOTAL_____

## SCALE 3

1.  I understand complex machines easily.  SD   D   A   SA

2.  I enjoy competitive conversations.  SD   D   A   SA

3.  I am intrigued by rules and patterns that govern systems.  SD   D   A   SA

4.  I am more analytical and logical than most people.  SD   D   A   SA

5.  I pursue intellectual topics thoroughly and regularly.  SD   D   A   SA

6.  I am able to solve problems without letting emotion get in the way.
    SD   D   A   SA

7.  I like to figure out how things work.  SD   D   A   SA

8.  I am tough-minded.  SD   D   A   SA

9.  Debating is a good way to match my wits with others.  SD   D   A   SA

10. I have no trouble making a choice, even when several alternatives seem
    equally good at first.  SD   D   A   SA

11. When I buy a new machine (like a camera, computer, or car), I want to
    know all of its technical features.  SD   D   A   SA

12. I like to avoid the nuances and say exactly what I mean.  SD   D   A   SA

13. I think it is important to be direct.  SD   D   A   SA

14. When making a decision, I like to stick to the facts rather than be swayed
    by people's feelings.  SD   D   A   SA

TOTAL_____

## SCALE 4

1. I like to get to know my friends' deepest needs and feelings.
SD  D  A  SA

2. I highly value deep emotional intimacy in my relationships.
SD  D  A  SA

3. Regardless of what is logical, I generally listen to my heart when making important decisions.  SD  D  A  SA

4. I frequently catch myself daydreaming.  SD  D  A  SA

5. I can change my mind easily.  SD  D  A  SA

6. After watching an emotional film I often still feel moved by it several hours later.  SD  D  A  SA

7. I vividly imagine both wonderful and horrible things happening to me.
SD  D  A  SA

8. I am very sensitive to people's feelings and needs.  SD  D  A  SA

9. I often find myself getting lost in my thoughts during the day.
SD  D  A  SA

10. I feel emotions more deeply than most people.  SD  D  A  SA

11. I have a vivid imagination.  SD  D  A  SA

12. When I wake up from a vivid dream, it takes me a few seconds to return to reality.  SD  D  A  SA

13. When reading, I enjoy it when the writer takes a sidetrack to say something beautiful or meaningful.  SD  D  A  SA

14. I am very empathetic.  SD  D  A  SA

TOTAL_____

SCORING: To Score the test, give yourself:

0 points for each answer of "strongly disagree"
1 point for each answer of "disagree"
2 points for each answer of "agree"

3 points for each answer of "strongly agree."

Then add up the points in *each* of the four scales; *do not* add together all points on all scales.

Scale 1 measures the degree to which you express the traits linked with the dopamine system (Explorer: curious and creative).

Scale 2 measures the degree to which you express the traits linked with the serotonin system (Builder: cautious and social norm-conforming)

Scale 3 measures the degree to which you express the traits linked with the testosterone system (Director: analytical and tough-minded).

Scale 4 measures the degree to which you express the traits linked with the estrogen/oxytocin system (Negotiator: prosocial and empathetic).

NOTE: *We are all different combinations of these four trait constellations, but we express some trait suites more than others. It is not unusual to score equally on two (sometimes three) temperament dimensions. This happens when you express an equal number of traits in two or more of these four brain systems. Also pay attention to the brain systems you do not predominantly express, as it is important to know who you are not as well as who you are. See my book* Why Him? Why Her? *(2009) for full description of these personality dimensions.*

## Divorce charts

*Figure 1:* FINLAND DIVORCE PROFILES, 1950–87

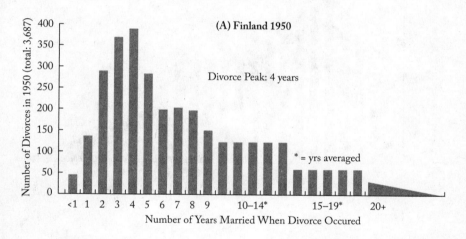

(A) Finland 1950

Divorce Peak: 4 years

\* = yrs averaged

Number of Divorces in 1950 (total: 3,687)

Number of Years Married When Divorce Occured

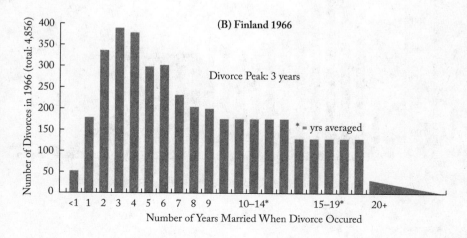

(B) Finland 1966

Divorce Peak: 3 years

\* = yrs averaged

Number of Divorces in 1966 (total: 4,856)

Number of Years Married When Divorce Occured

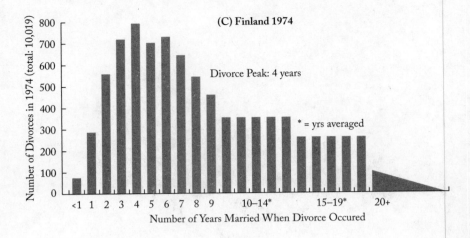

**(C) Finland 1974**

Divorce Peak: 4 years

* = yrs averaged

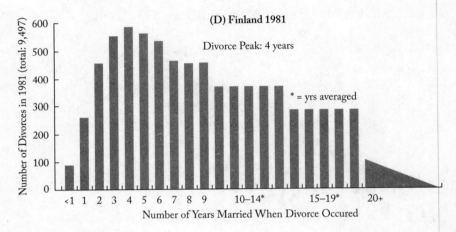

**(D) Finland 1981**

Divorce Peak: 4 years

* = yrs averaged

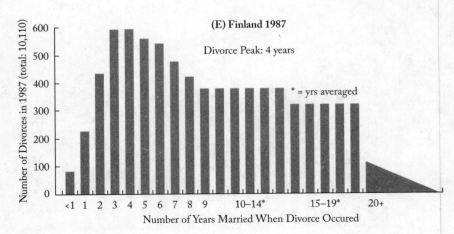

**(E) Finland 1987**

Divorce Peak: 4 years

* = yrs averaged

Figures A–E show the divorce profiles for Finland in five years as shown in the demographic yearbooks of the United Nations. In 1981, most divorces occurred during the fourth year of marriage. Data on divorces occurring between 10 and 14 years of marriage and between 15 and 19 years of marriage were averaged because the raw data lumped them together. Divorces in the 20+ category were designated 20–40 years married and averaged as well. In actuality, divorces steadily declined with increasing number of years married. As can be seen in these histograms, divorces in Finland cluster around a three- to four-year peak, and this pattern shows little change despite steadily increasing divorce *rates* during these decades.

*Figure 2:* THE THREE- TO FOUR-YEAR ITCH: DIVORCE PEAKS, 62 SOCIETIES, ALL AVAILABLE YEARS, 1947–89 (188 CASES)

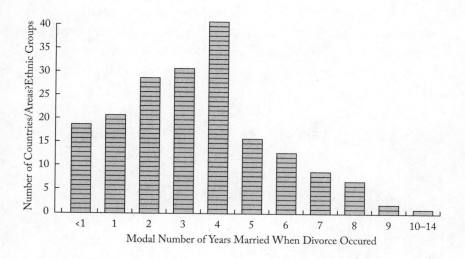

Figure 2. The divorce profiles for 62 countries, areas, and ethnic groups in specific years between 1947 and 1989 were drawn (188 cases). Then the divorce peak (the mode) for each of these histograms was marked as a box on the master chart. Finland 1981, for example, is represented as one box in the column marked "4." Thus human beings in a variety of societies tend to divorce between the second and fourth years of marriage, with a divorce peak during the fourth year.

*Figure 3:* EGYPT 1978 DIVORCE PROFILE

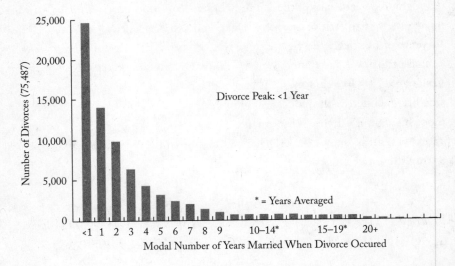

Figure 3. In Egypt in 1978, as well as in almost all other Muslim countries for which the United Nations has data between 1947 and 2012, most divorces occurred in the first year of marriage, and the longer a couple remained married the more likely they were to stay together. Explanations for this variation are given in chapter 5.

*Figure 4:* THE UNITED STATES 1986 DIVORCE PROFILE

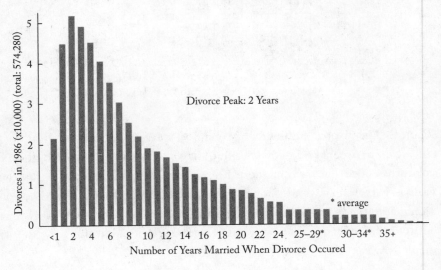

Figure 4. The divorce profile for the United States in 1986 as taken from the

*Vital Statistics of the United States.* Data on divorces occurring between 25 and 29 years of marriage, between 30 and 34 years of marriage, and in the the 35+ years category were average because the raw data lumped them together. Most divorces occurred between the second and third year of marriage—as in all other years I examined between 1960 and 1989. An explanation for this consistant divorce peak appears in chapter 5.

*Figure 5:* DIVORCE PEAK PER COUNTRY BETWEEN 2003–2012; 85 CASES

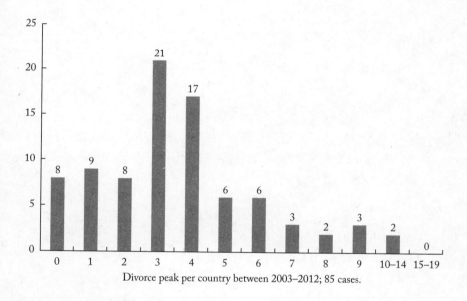

Divorce peak per country between 2003–2012; 85 cases.

Figure 5. The three- to four-year itch: DIVORCE PEAKS, 79 COUNTRIES, ALL AVAILABLE YEARS, 2003 TO 2012 (85 CASES). The divorce profiles for 79 countries for all available years between 2003 and 2012 were analyzed (85 cases). Then the divorce peak (the mode) for each of these histograms was added on the master chart. Divorce peaks (modes) have barely changed since data were collected on previous decades. Human beings in a variety of societies still tend to divorce during the third and fourth year of marriage, regardless of enormous societal changes due to the rise of the Internet and global networking.

## ACKNOWLEDGMENTS

Thank you, Hillary DelPrete, for your superb research help on this book. Thank you, John Gurche, for your fascinating depiction of an ancestral couple. I am indebted to Mandy Ginsberg, Amy Canaday, and everyone else at Match.com for providing me with my data on singles in America, and to Justin Garcia for helping me share this material with a wide academic and lay audience. I am grateful to Amy Cherry at W. W. Norton, who invited me to do this rewrite, to Allegra Huston for your copyediting, to Remy Cawley and all the Norton staff for your efforts on behalf of this book, and to Amanda Urban, my agent, for your guidance. Thank you Lucy Brown for our collaboration on many intellectual projects and for your continual work on our website (TheAnatomyOfLove.com), which features some of the ideas in this book. Thank you, Lee Silver, for doing complex mathematical analyses of my personality data presented here. Thank you to my friend Fletcher Hodges for your wisdom and encouragement; to my friends at the Royce Carlton lecture agency and the TED conferences for helping me broadcast some of these ideas; to Dave Labno for working with me to apply these data on personality to business consulting; and to Gerry Ohrstrom, Thomas Campbell Jackson, Elizabeth Eiss, and Dyan Daley for enabling these ideas to reach broader business and medical communities. Thank you, Christian Frei, for your documentary *Sleepless in New York*, featuring some of the ideas in this book. I thank Lorna, Audrey, and the rest of my family and friends for your patience and good humor during this odyssey. Last, I deeply thank Ray Carroll, my deceased friend, for all he did for the original version of *Anatomy of Love*.

# NOTES

Complete details for all sources can be found in the bibliography.

## PROLOGUE: HERE'S TO LOVE!

1. All "Singles in America" data is the property of Match.com and is, to date, unpublished. It is presented in this book courtesy of Match.com and me, Helen Fisher, the company's Chief Scientific Advisor.

## CHAPTER 1: GAMES PEOPLE PLAY

1. The word *ethology* comes from the Greek *ethos*, meaning "manner" or "behavior." Ethology is generally considered to be the observation and analysis of animal behavior in the natural environment. It is based on the premise that characteristic behavior patterns of a species evolved in the same way that physical traits evolved, through selection. Darwin laid the groundwork for the science of ethology with his examination of motor patterns, such as snarling and other facial gestures, in different species (see Darwin [1872] 1965).
2. For cross-species similarities in body language and facial expressions, see Givens 1986, 1983; Goodall 1986; Darwin [1872] 1965.
3. Eibl-Eibesfeldt 1989.
4. De Waal 1987.
5. Smuts 1985, 1987.
6. Ekman 1985.
7. Darwin [1872] 1965.
8. Ekman et al. 1969; Ekman 1980, 1985; Goleman 1981. Cartography of the face: Using anatomy texts, cameras, and a mirror, psychologist Paul Ekman and his colleagues learned to contract several individual facial muscles at will. When they were unsure which muscles they were using, they inserted specially wired needles into specific muscles to isolate the activity of each. Ekman reports that the human "open smile" is among the least complicated facial expressions. It takes only the "lip corner puller," the "dimpler," and the "cheek raiser" to make our wide, inviting grin. The ninety-six major variations of anger use several hundred different muscle combinations, depending on their intensity. See Ekman 1985.
9. Field et al. 1982; Trevathan 1987.
10. Givens 1983; Perper 1985.
11. Human spatial territories: People divide space into four distinct types. For Americans "intimate space" is generally about eighteen inches around the head. You permit only intimate companions and pets into this private territory for any length

of time. "Personal space" is the two to four feet surrounding you; you allow friends to enter here. "Social space," about four to eight feet away, you use when you interact with others during work or social gatherings. "Public spaces" are all the areas beyond nine to ten feet from you. Different societies measure the territory around the body differently, but they all have a code for proximity. See Hall 1966.

12. Hughes et al., 2004.

13. Apicella et al. 2007.

14. Conversational courting tactics: As a couple begin to talk, they search for common interests and try to establish compatibility. They may test each other by disagreeing, then watch how the other handles this adversity. The goal is trust. One may reveal a weakness, yet wrap it in a positive self-image. And early in the courtship they may ask a minor favor—another test. Vital to these interactions are three subtle undercurrents. People strive to "make a good impression"; they seek the attention of the other; and they revert to cooing and other babylike behaviors. All the while they try to convey a panoply of assets, including stability, self-control, intelligence, kindness, caring, acceptance, competence, reliability, bravery, humor, and, most important, availability. See Eibl-Eibesfeldt 1989.

15. Touch: Our ancestors were held constantly as babies and slept next to their mother's breast, so human beings are designed to live in skin contact with others. In some cultures, infants are held so continually that they never crawl; their first solo exploration of the world comes when they try to walk. As a result, we naturally like to touch and be touched unless we are trained otherwise. See Hall 1959; Montagu 1971; Henley 1977.

16. Givens 1983.

17. Eibl-Eibesfeldt 1989.

18. Hall 1976.

19. Douglas 1987.

20. Annually from 2010 to 2014, I have conducted a national survey of singles, in collaboration with Match.com, the Internet dating service. Together we design a questionnaire with some 150 queries and poll over 5,000 single men and women. We do not sample the Match members; instead, we collect data on a national representative sample based on the U.S. census. Blacks, Whites, Latinos, Asians; gays, lesbians, and heterosexuals; people aged 21 to 70+; those in rural, suburban, and urban areas; men and women in every region of the country: all are polled. None of these 25,000-plus single men and women was engaged, living with a partner, or in a serious relationship. First, we ask participants several general questions: their religious affiliation, political membership, sexual orientation, where they live, their household income, their employment status, their occupation and level of education, even how many hours of sleep they get per night. Then we get to the essentials. What "must you have" in a partner? Have you ever experienced love at first sight? (More than one out of three have.) Have you ever fallen in love with someone you didn't initially find attractive? (35% say yes.) Would you date a Democrat? A Republican? Who should pay at a dinner date? What do you lie about when courting? What percentage of time do you achieve orgasm with a familiar partner? (Republicans have more orgasms per sexual event, but less sex!) Have you ever imagined a future together while on the first date? (56% of men and 48% of women have.) To my knowledge, this is the most comprehensive scientific survey of singles in America or anywhere in the world.

21. Courtship feeding: It is possible that courtship feeding mimics feeding between mother and infant, triggering feelings of caring and protection by the man and childlike acceptance by the woman that enhance the bonding process. See Eibl-Eibesfeldt 1989.

22. Goodall 1986; Teleki 1973a.

23. Ford and Beach 1951.
24. Ibid.
25. Jespersen [1922] 1950.


CHAPTER 2: WHY HIM? WHY HER?

1. Liebowitz 1983; Fisher 1998; 2004; Hatfield 1988; Hatfield and Sprecher 1986; Harris 1995; Tennov 1979.
2. Tennov 1979.
3. Van Steenberger et al. 2013.
4. Fisher 2004.
5. Stendhal [1822] 1975.
6. Buss 2000.
7. Tennov 1979.
8. Fisher 2004, 2006, appendix A.
9. Hatfield and Rapson 1987.
10. Ackerman 1990; Russell 1976; Hopson 1979.
11. The term *pheromone*, coined in 1959, can be applied to any chemical substance that a creature excretes as a signal that elicits a specific, unlearned response in other creatures. Although creatures give off pheromones as repellants and for other uses, the term *pheromone* is generally used to describe sex attractants. See Shorey 1976.
12. Hopson 1979.
13. Gregersen 1982.
14. Fisher 1998; 2004.
15. Eibl-Eibesfeldt 1989.
16. Givens 1983.
17. Fisher 2004; Zentner 2005.
18. Feinman and Gill 1978.
19. Bower 1990.
20. Ford and Beach 1951; Frayser 1985.
21. Buss 1989.
22. Shepher 1971; Spiro 1958.
23. Fisher 2004.
24. Tennov 1979.
25. See Pfaff and Fisher 2012.
26. Aron and Aron 1996.
27. Fisher 2009; see Pfaff and Fisher 2012.
28. Fisher 2009, 2010; L. L. Brown et al. 2013.
29. L. L. Brown et al. 2013. In this study, the Fisher Temperament Inventory (FTI) was administered to participants in two brain scanning studies (fMRI). High questionnaire scores for the Curious/Energetic temperament dimension co-varied with activation in a region of the substantia nigra, consistent with the prediction that this temperament dimension reflects activity in the dopamine system. High questionnaire scores for the Cautious/Social Norm Compliant temperament dimension correlated with activation in the ventrolateral prefrontal cortex in a region associated with social norm compliance, a trait linked with the serotonin system. High questionnaire scores on the Analytical/Tough-Minded scale co-varied with activity in regions of the occipital and parietal cortices associated with visual acuity and mathematical thinking, traits linked with testosterone; testosterone also contributes to the construction of brain architecture in these areas. High questionnaire scores on the Prosocial/Empa-

thetic scale correlated with activity in regions of the inferior frontal gyrus, anterior insula and fusiform gyrus, regions associated with mirror neurons and empathy, a trait linked with the estrogen/oxytocin system and regions where estrogen contributes to brain architecture. These findings, replicated across two studies, indicate that the FTI measures the influences of four broad neural systems, and that these temperament dimensions and neural systems could constitute foundational mechanisms in personality structure and play a role in romantic attraction and partnership formation.

30. Fisher, 2009; Fisher, Rich, Island, et al. 2010; Fisher 2012.
31. Fisher 1999.
32. In a recent study, researchers scanned the brains of men and women (using fMRI) as they looked at photos of unfamiliar potential partners, individuals whom they would soon meet at a "speed dating" event. The brain regions that became active showed that these men and women were rapidly judging the photos on two criteria: physical attractiveness and perceived personality, particularly likability (Cooper et al. 2012).
33. Capellanus 1959.
34. Jankowiak 1992.
35. Ibid.
36. Jankowiak and Fischer 1992.
37. There are many forms of homosexuality. Some people experiment in college; others are in prison; some male immigrants in the 1900s practiced same-sex sex until they could bring their wives to America from the "old country." But among gays and lesbians who knew in childhood or early teenage that they were homosexual, genetic factors appear to be involved. Gay genes? There is some evidence that gay men have a somewhat different structure in part of the hypothalamus (LeVay 1991). And in 1993 geneticist Dean Hamer and his colleagues reported that they had located a gene (or genes) on the X chromosome likely to be involved in male sexual orientation (Hamer et al. 1993). New data on 400 gay brothers also suggests that these genes on the X chromosome are involved (Sanders et al. 2015). Moreover, homosexuality occurs in roughly the same proportions in societies that permit it and those that have traditionally been homophobic (Posner 1992); and homosexuality runs in families (Hamer et al. 1993).

Today, however, some scientists regard the "gay gene" as a cluster of "male-loving genes" instead. As the reasoning goes, men who carry these genes love other men. But women who inherit this gene assemblage start at sex and romance earlier than most women; they also have more children because they are *hyper*-sexual. In fact, female relatives of gay men have 1.3% more children than women who have only heterosexual male kin. (Camperio-Ciani et al. 2004; Camperio-Ciani and Pellizzari 2012). These women have a reproductive advantage, explaining how "gay genes" could be favored during evolution. There may be some "female loving genes," too, although there is no proof as yet. Perhaps when men inherit this package of DNA, they also start mating sooner and have more children, while women with this array of DNA fall in love with other women. Hence the genes for lesbianism could be passed on through *hyper*-sexual men.

Life in the womb also plays a role in homosexuality, due to the effect of hormones on the growing brain. During the first trimester, fetal androgens and estrogens begin to sculpt the male and female genitals, as well as the fetal brain. Alterations in this hormonal bath may change one's sexual orientation in later life.

Stress and birth order may also play a role in male sexuality. If mother was highly stressed during pregnancy, or if she has borne several boys previously, her male fetus is more likely to grow up to be gay. In fact, with every older brother that a boy has, his chances of becoming gay increase by one-third. One theory for this is that the mother's body creates an immune response to proteins that influence the development of the male brain in the womb. Less is known about lesbians. But it is well known that if a female embryo is exposed to high levels of fetal testosterone, the girl is more likely to become a lesbian.

Some researchers and laymen still believe that male homosexuals more regularly come from homes where the father was absent, cold, or detached, mother was domineering or smothering, or the household was all-female. But a classic study has shown that the family life of homosexuals and heterosexuals is basically the same (Bell and Weinberger 1978). Even children growing up in a lesbian household are not likely to become lesbians as adults (Golombok and Tasker 1996).

An enormous amount has been written on homosexuality, largely investigating how and why it evolved. But I think the most parsimonious answer in humans is through *direct selection*. In our "Singles in America" questionnaire, we asked gays and lesbians if they had ever had a sexual experience with someone of the opposite gender: 34% of gay men and 47% of lesbian women said yes. Moreover, in the United States today, some 37% of lesbian, gay, bisexual, and transsexual people have a child; and about 60% of these are their own biological offspring. In past millennia, homosexuals could have had even more children, because few came "out of the closet" in most societies. Instead, they married and bred.

I will add that homosexuality is common in nature. Some mice are gay. Female cats housed separately from males display all of the behavior patterns of homosexual arousal. Wild female gulls sometimes mate as a lesbian couple. Male gorillas band together and exhibit homosexuality. Female pygmy chimps have regular lesbian interactions. Some male fruit flies that buzz around your peaches in the kitchen on a summer morning are gay (Bailey and Zuk 2009). Homosexuality has been recorded in over 60 species; in fact, it is so common in other creatures that human homosexuality is striking not in its prevalence, but in its rarity.

38. Zeki and Romaya 2010.
39. Jankowiak and Fischer 1992; Fisher 1998; Hatfield and Rapson 1996.
40. Fisher 2004.
41. Givens 1983.
42. Fehrenbacker 1988.
43. Fisher 2004.
44. Fisher et al. 2002; Fisher 2004; Fisher et al. 2006.
45. Darwin 1871, 745.
46. Thomas 1993, 46.
47. Galdikas 1995, 144–45.
48. Fisher et al. 2005; Aron et al. 2005.
49. Fisher 1998.
50. Fisher 1998, 2004.
51. Fisher 2005; Aron 2005.
52. Group activation occurred in several regions of the brain's reward system, including the ventral tegmental area (VTA) and caudate nucleus (Fisher et al. 2003; Fisher et al. 2005; Aron et al. 2005), regions associated with pleasure, general arousal, focused attention, and motivation to pursue and acquire rewards, and mediated primarily by dopamine system activity (Schultz 2000; Delgado et al. 2000; Elliot et al. 2003), as well as the insula, a brain region associated with anxiety. Moreover, in a principal component analysis on these 17 men and women, we found evidence of activity in the nucleus accumbens (unpublished data). These regions of the reward system are directly associated with addiction in many studies of drugs of abuse (see Fisher 2014).
53. Xu et al. 2011.
54. Fisher 1998.

55. Gingrich et al. 2000.
56. Fabre-Nys 1998.
57. Fisher 1998, 2004.
58. Acevedo et al. 2011.
59. Fisher and Thomson 2007.
60. Marazziti et al. 1999.
61. SIA 2012 (unpublished data).
62. Liebowitz 1983, 200; Bowlby 1969.
63. Acevedo et al. 2011.
64. O'Leary et al. 2011.

## CHAPTER 3: IS MONOGAMY NATURAL?

1. Daly 1978.
2. Van Valen 1973.
3. Hamilton 1980; Hamilton et al. 1981.
4. Dougherty 1955.
5. Parker et al. 1972.
6. Origin of two sexes: There are several theories for why *two* sexes evolved. Some primitive blue-green algae have two mating types, designated + and - because the gender of neither is distinguishable. One theory holds that these algae evolved two mating types to avoid inbreeding (see Daly and Wilson 1983). The "genetic repair" theory proposes that with sexual reproduction new combinations could repair the mutational damage to DNA material that had occurred during preceding cell divisions (see Michod 1989). Another theory is known as the parasitism hypothesis. The sexes arose in the same fashion that modern viruses parasitize host cells: the virus incorporates its own DNA into the host cell; then, as the host cell reproduces itself, it replicates the DNA of the virus too. Thus the precursors of males were tiny gametes that parasitized larger female gametes. For an overview of the advantages of asexual and sexual reproduction, the costs of sexual reproduction, and theories on the origin of sexual reproduction, see Daly and Wilson 1983; Gray and Garcia 2013.
7. Hamilton 1964.
8. "Inclusive fitness" and altruism: The theory of inclusive fitness was first suggested by Darwin (1859) when he noted that natural selection may operate on the level of the family rather than on that of the individual. Inclusive fitness was anticipated again in the 1930s by the British geneticist J. B. S. Haldane. But the theory was formally proposed in 1964 by the British population geneticist William D. Hamilton, to explain the evolution of altruism: if an ancestral man sacrificed himself to save his drowning brother, he was actually saving half of his own DNA and, thereby, some of his altruistic nature. Hence one's fitness is measured by the number of one's own genes and those of one's relatives who survive. With Hamilton's concept of inclusive fitness many other social behaviors became explicable: creatures defend a common territory; animals share and cooperate; people are nationalistic because when they help their relatives they further their own DNA (see Wilson 1975). Today inclusive fitness and the related concept of kin selection are standard means for explaining some patterns of animal behavior. See Barish 1977; Hamilton 1964; Gray and Garcia 2013.
9. Reproductive strategies: This adaptation of terms has been incomplete; the two variants of monogamy—monogyny and monandry—are not used to describe human marriage systems. As a result, the *separate* reproductive tactics of men and

women are largely overlooked. For example, we are told that the Afikpo Ibo of eastern Nigeria are "polygynous." Thus some Afikpo Ibo men have several wives. But Afikpo Ibo women marry only one man at a time, monandry. So two marriage patterns occur, polygyny and monandry, depending on whether you are describing men or women. When social scientists describe a society as polygynous, they ignore the reproductive tactics of women.

10. See Trivers 1985; Mock and Fujioka 1990; Westneat et al. 1990; Hiatt 1989.
11. Bray et al. 1975.
12. Gibbs et al. 1990.
13. Mock and Fujioka 1990; Wittenberger and Tilson 1980.
14. Mock and Fujioka 1990; Wittenberger and Tilson 1980.
15. Birkhead and Moller 1998.
16. Laumann et al. 1994; Tafoya and Spitzberg 2007.
17. Allen and Baucom 2006.
18. Buss 2000.
19. Schmitt and Buss 2001.
20. Definitions of marriage: Many anthropologists have defined marriage. Suzanne Frayser's version is a good one: "Marriage is a relationship within which a group socially approves and encourages sexual intercourse and the birth of children" (Frayser 1985, 248). Anthropologist Ward Goodenough defines the three essential components of marriage as the jural or legal dimension, the priority of sexual access, and the eligibility to reproduce (Goodenough 1970, 12).
21. United Nations Statistical Office 2012.
22. Cherlin 2009.
23. United Nations Statistical Office 2012.
24. Murdock 1967; van den Berghe 1979; Betzig 1986.
25. Betzig 1982, 1986.
26. Tiwi marriages and the role of women: Traditional Tiwi women were not pawns in the marriage wars of men. On the contrary, women played crucial roles in negotiating marriages. Every son-in-law had to cater to the needs of the woman who would bear his bride, and a mother-in-law could break this contract if his gifts and work were paltry. So Tiwi women were powerful nodes in the marriage system, as well as powerful in other aspects of society. See Goodale 1971; Berndt 1981.
27. Verner and Wilson 1966; Orians 1969; Borgerhoff Mulder 1990.
28. Polygyny and women: Women living with co-wives are generally less fertile than women in monogamous marriages (Daly and Wilson 1978). However, among women living with polygynous husbands, the first wife often bears more children then junior co-wives do, probably because she does less strenuous work and has access to more food (Isaac and Feinberg 1982). Polygyny also creates more intra-household abuse, neglect, and homicide; co-wife conflict is endemic in polygynous households (Henrich et al. 2012)
29. Bohannan 1985; Mealey 1985.
30. Forms of polygyny: Males in the animal community acquire harems in at least four ways; each has parallels in humankind (Flinn and Low 1986). Polygyny is frequently found in species where the food supply, hiding places, nesting spots, or mating grounds are located in clusters. Females tend to gather at these places to feed or breed, and if a male can succeed in becoming the sole proprietor of one of these rich locations, he may acquire a harem simply by driving off other males and waiting for the females to arrive. This tactic is known as *resource-defense polygyny* (Emlen and Oring 1977). Among the Kipsigis of Kenya, women traditionally choose to marry polygynous men with large pieces of real estate (Borgerhoff Mulder 1990).

Males of some species round up a group of females and then forcibly prevent other males from courting them; this is known as *female-defense polygyny*. If a Tiwi husband of Australia suspected a young wife of adultery, he sometimes beat her or complained to the girl's natal family. If a boy eloped with an adolescent married woman and refused to repent, an irate husband might kill the thief (Goodale 1971). This guarding behavior is reminiscent of female-defense polygyny seen in other species (Flinn and Low 1986).

Another strategy is known as *male-dominance polygyny*. Male sage grouse maneuver among themselves to acquire "mating stations" on a lek (see chapter 1), from which they can be easily seen by passing females. Females then walk among them and rest in their mating stations to mate. Older, more vigorous males tend to attract most of the passing females (De Vos 1983). Among the !Kung San of the Kalahari Desert of southern Africa some men are charismatic, strong, and healthy, and they occasionally acquire two wives not with resources but with their personalities (Shostak 1981).

Orangutans, moose, and bumblebees persistently seek out receptive females, mate, and move on; this is known as *search polygyny*. A variation of this form of harem building is characteristic of truck drivers, traveling salesmen, international businessmen, and sailors who have "a wife in every port." See Flinn and Low 1986; Dickemann 1979.

31. Frayser 1985; van den Berghe 1979; Murdock and White 1969.
32. Marlowe 2000; Sefcek et al. 2006.
33. Murdock 1949, 27–8.
34. Daly and Wilson 1983.
35. Murdock 1967; van den Berghe 1979.
36. Klein 1980.
37. Alexander 1974; Finn and Low 1986; Goldizen 1987; Jenni 1974.
38. Lancaster and Lancaster 1983.
39. Nayar marriage customs: The Nayar of India's Malabar Coast in Kerala have a marriage form that defies classification. These people live in households consisting of siblings and mother. The head of household is a man. A woman's first marriage is a brief ceremony; after this ritual, she does not need to socialize or even have sex with her husband. If a wife wishes to take other lovers, she is free to do so. Her husband and lovers call on her only at night; thus they are called visiting husbands. Women have anywhere from three to twelve lovers at any one time. A marriage ends when a husband no longer gives his wife gifts at annual festivals. It is essential that one or more men of the proper social group claim paternity when a "wife" becomes pregnant, although the biological father often does little more than observe the incest taboo in later life—if he knows the child is his. For the Nayar, marriage provides nothing but legitimacy for children. See Gough 1968; Fuller 1976.
40. "Free love" communes: Studies of six American communes indicate that their members do not actually practice "free love"; instead, rules about copulation are rigid and sexual and social roles are hierarchical and highly structured. See Wagner 1982; Stoehr 1979; Constantine and Constantine 1973.
41. See van den Berghe 1979.
42. Bohannan 1985.
43. Polygyny and polyandry are secondary human reproductive strategies: Because polygyny provides males with genetic advantages and polyandry provides females with extra resources, some anthropologists argue that these reproductive strategies are primary reproductive tactics of humankind, that men and women endure monogamy only because men are unable to gain the resources they need to acquire harems, and that women endure monogamy only because they are unable to entice several males to provide resources. Supporting this view is the ample evidence

for polygyny among powerful men (Betzig 1986). But the *variant* reproductive strategy of monogamy in conjunction with adultery provides similar reproductive advantages; males have the opportunity to inseminate multiple partners; females can garner extra resources. Moreover, many human beings exhibit monogamy in conjunction with adultery. So I think the primary reproductive strategy of *Homo sapiens* is serial social monogamy in conjunction with clandestine adultery, while polygyny and polyandry are opportunistic, secondary reproductive tactics.

44. Whyte 1978, 74; Frayser 1985, 269.
45. Mace and Mace 1959.

## CHAPTER 4: WHY ADULTERY?

1. Diana, n.d.
2. Carneiro 1958.
3. Tsapelas et al. 2010. World patterns of adultery: Of 139 societies surveyed in the 1940s, 39% permitted men and women to have extramarital affairs either during certain holidays or festivals, with particular kinfolk, such as one's wife's sister or husband's brother, or under other special circumstances. Extramarital relations were extremely common in 17 of the remaining 85 cultures, and offenders were rarely punished (see Ford and Beach 1951). In a different study in the 1940s, anthropologist George Murdock surveyed 148 societies, past and then current, and found that 120 had taboos against adultery, 5 freely allowed adultery, 19 allowed philandering under some conditions, and 4 disapproved of but did not strictly forbid sex outside of marriage (Murdock 1949). In all cases, however, Murdock was measuring adultery as sexual activity with distantly related or unrelated people. This distinction is important. He supported Ford and Beach's (1951) finding that a substantial majority of societies allow extramarital relations with individuals in certain kin relationships. Suzanne Frayser (1985) later confirmed the widespread taboo against adultery with unrelated individuals too: she reported that 74% of 58 cultures forbade adultery either for the woman or for both sexes. She noted that punishments for adultery vary. In 83% of 48 societies, both partners received penalties for adultery; in 40% of them men and women got the same degree of chastisement; in 31% of them the man's punishment was more severe that that of his female lover. No society tolerated a female's dalliances while punishing males; and significantly more cultures had restrictions on women than on men. Societies with few prohibitions against extramarital liaisons of any kind and with a high degree of extramarital sexual behavior for both sexes included the Dieri of Australia, the Gilyak of northeast Asia, the Hidatsa Indians of North Dakota, the Lesu of New Ireland, the Masai of East Africa, the Toda of India, the Kaingang of Brazil, and the Yapese of the Pacific (Ford and Beach 1951). Stephens (1963) reported, however, that even in those cultures where adultery was condoned, men and women suffered from jealousy. Yet, in 72% of 56 societies surveyed in the 1970s, female adultery was moderate to common (van den Berghe 1979).
4. Schneider 1971.
5. Gove 1989.
6. Westermarck 1922.
7. *People* 1986.
8. Glass and Wright 1992.
9. Bullough 1976.
10. Ibid.
11. Lampe 1987; Bullough 1976.
12. Bullough 1976.

13. Song of Solomon 3:16.
14. Lawrence 1989; Foucault 1985.
15. Bullough 1976.
16. Origin of sexual terms: By the fourth century A.D. adultery was so commonplace in Rome that officials began to fine offenders. The revenue from this taxation was apparently so great that the state built a temple to Venus with it (Bardis 1963). The terms *cunnilingus, fellatio, masturbation,* and *prostitute* all come from ancient Roman vernacular (Bullough 1976).
17. Bullough 1976; Lawrence 1989.
18. See Bullough 1976; Lawrence 1989; Brown 1988; Pagels 1988.
19. Bullough 1976, 192.
20. Lampe 1987, 26; Lawrence 1989, 125; Pagels 1988.
21. Burns 1990.
22. Lawrence 1989, 169.
23. Kinsey et al. 1948; Kinsey et al. 1953.
24. Hunt 1974, 263.
25. Blumstein and Schwartz 1983.
26. Laumann et al. 1994.
27. Greeley 1994; Laumann et al. 1994; Tafoya and Spitzberg 2007.
28. Gangestad and Thornhill 1997.
29. Schmitt and Buss 2001.
30. Schmitt 2004.
31. See Tsapelas et al. 2010.
32. E. S. Allen et al. 2008.
33. Aron et al. 2001.
34. Fraley and Shaver 2000; Hazan and Diamond 2000.
35. Schmitt 2004.
36. Shackelford et al. 2008.
37. Orzeck and Lung 2005.
38. Schmitt 2004.
39. Tsapelas et al. 2010.
40. Lim et al. 2004; Lim and Young 2004; Carter 1992.
41. Hammock and Young 2002.
42. Ophir et al. 2008.
43. Walum et al. 2008.
44. Garcia, J. R., J. Mackillop, E. L. Aller et al. 2010.
45. Wedekind et al. 1995.
46. Garver-Apgar et al. 2006.
47. Ibid.
48. Fisher 1998.
49. Fisher 2004.
50. Ibid.
51. See Bateman 1948; Trivers 1972; Symons 1979.
52. Shostak 1981, 271.
53. Fisher 1992; Buss 2000.
54. Hrdy 1981, 1986.
55. Many American laymen and academics cling to the supposition that men are more adulterous than women, and it is an old axiom in science that what you are looking for, you tend to find. This may well have become the case in the scientific examination of adultery. In a now classic study of adultery, scientists asked 415 college students whether they would have sex with an anonymous student of the opposite gender. In this imaginary scenario, participants were told that all risk of pregnancy, discovery, and disease would be absent. The results were those you would expect.

Males were consistently more likely to say "yes," confirming the going credo that men are more interested in sexual variety than women (Symons and Ellis 1989). But here's the glitch. This study takes into consideration the primary genetic motive for *male* philandering (to fertilize young women). But it does not take into account the primary Darwinian motive for *female* philandering—the acquisition of resources.

What if these researchers had asked these same male participants a different question: "Would you be willing to have a one-night stand with a woman from the nearby old age home?" I doubt these male college students would have expressed such enthusiasm for this kind of sexual variety. And what if the scientists had also asked these young coeds a different question: "Would you be willing to have a one-night stand with a movie star if he also gave you a brand new Porsche or paid for your college education?" Just about all would say yes. Evolutionary logic holds that women sleep around for goods and services. And until scientists take into account the underlying genetic motivations of *both* genders, we will never know which sex is more interested in sexual variety.

56. Ford and Beach 1951, 118.
57. Gregor 1985.
58. Reichard 1950.
59. Bullough and Bullough 1987.
60. Nimuendaju 1946.
61. Beals 1946.
62. Nadel 1942.
63. Wiederman 1997; Brand et al. 2007.
64. Lampe 1987, 199.


## CHAPTER 5: BLUEPRINT FOR DIVORCE

1. Abu-Lughod 1987, 24.
2. Abu-Lughod 1986.
3. Farah 1984.
4. Ibid.
5. Ibid., 26.
6. Ibid., 20.
7. Murdock 1965.
8. Weisman 1988.
9. Male/female rights to divorce: In 30 of 40 traditional societies surveyed by George Peter Murdock in 1950, men and women had equal rights in initiating divorce; in 10% of these cultures women had superior privileges regarding divorce. He concluded that divorce was generally equally accessible to both sexes (Murdock 1965). In a study of 93 societies Whyte confirmed this, concluding, "We find equal divorce rights by far the most common pattern" (Whyte 1978). Suzanne Frayser reported that, of 45 societies she surveyed, 38% allowed both husband and wife to obtain a divorce; one or both partners had a difficult time securing a divorce in 62% of these cultures. In many insular Pacific societies divorce was easy to obtain for both men and women. In circum-Mediterranean societies it was more difficult for women to obtain a divorce, but in many African societies it was generally harder for men to do so. See Frayser 1985.
10. Murdock 1965, 319.
11. Betzig 1989.
12. Marriage as a reproductive strategy: Murdock (1949) argued that because sex and reproduction could be obtained outside of marriage, economic cooperation and the

division of labor between the sexes were the primary reasons for marriage. But in the 40 traditional societies he surveyed in 1950, he noted that reproductive issues were prominent reasons for divorce (Murdock 1965). A survey by Frayser confirms the important role that reproduction plays in divorce—and thus in marriage. In a sample of 56 cultures, men divorced their wives first for reproductive problems, second for incompatibility, third for illicit sex on the wife's part. In a sample of 48 cultures, women abandoned their husbands most frequently because of incompatibility; second, because of failure to meet economic and domestic responsibilities; third, because of physical violence. See Frayser 1985.

13. Remarriage: A survey of 37 traditional peoples found that remarriage was openly allowed in 78% of these societies; where remarriage was difficult to obtain (in 22% of these cultures), it was generally harder for the woman to remarry than for the man (Frayser 1985). Remarriage occurred in preindustrial western European societies, but it was regularly associated with the death of a spouse rather than divorce, since divorce was banned by the Roman Catholic Church. Common to several of these peoples was the charivari tradition, the belief that it was unethical for widows to remarry. Underlying this precept were the complex property transactions and mechanics of inheritance that widow remarriage threatened (Dupâquier et al. 1981). The disapproval of remarriage by widows (and sometimes widowers) among the European peasantry of past centuries notwithstanding, remarriage was both frequent and widespread (Dupâquier et al. 1981; Goody 1983). Remarriage by widows was difficult in preindustrial India, China, Japan, and other agrarian peoples as well (Dupâquier et al. 1981; Goody 1983, 40). *In all societies for which records are available, however, remarriage rates were highest for women of reproductive age.* See Dupâquier et al. 1981; Furstenberg and Spanier 1984; also see chapter 16 of this book.
14. Kreider 2006.
15. Howell 1979; Shostak 1981.
16. Howell 1979.
17. Female autonomy and high divorce rates: Cultures that have a high degree of female autonomy and high divorce rates include those of the Semang of the Malay Peninsula (Sanday 1981; Murdock 1965; Textor 1967); several Caribbean populations (Flinn and Low 1986); the Dobu, who live on an island off the eastern tip of New Guinea (Fortune 1963); the Fort Jameson Ngoni, the Yao, and the Lozi of southern Africa (Barnes 1967); the Turu of Tanzania (Schneider 1971); the Samoans of Oceania (Textor 1967); the Gururumba of New Guinea (Friedl 1975); the Trobriand Islanders of Papua New Guinea (Weiner 1976); the natives of Mangaia, Polynesia (Suggs and Marshall 1971); the Tlingit of southern Alaska (Laura Klein, personal communication); the Kaingang of southern Brazil, the Crow of Montana, and the Iroquois of New York (Murdock 1965).
18. Lloyd 1968, 79.
19. Friedl 1975.
20. Van den Berghe 1979.
21. Le Clercq 1910, 262.
22. Dupâquier et al. 1981.
23. Mark 10:11–12; Lawrence 1989, 63.
24. Fisher 1987, 1989.
25. Cherlin 2009.
26. Cherlin 1981; Levitan et al. 1988; Glick 1975; Espenshade 1985; Whyte 1990.
27. The rising autonomy of Roman women: Historians do not agree on the reasons or the timing for the increased emancipation and self-assertion of women in ancient Rome. Some point to the defeat of Hannibal in 202 B.C.; others, to the defeat of Macedonia in 168 B.C.; still others, to the destruction of Carthage in 146 B.C. As a

result of a series of historical developments, however, Rome experienced rising opulence in the centuries preceding Christ, a concomitant rise in women's economic, political, and social power, and a rise in rates of divorce. See Balsdon 1973; Carcopino 1973; Rawson 1986; Hunt 1959.

28. Burgess and Cottrell 1939; Ackerman 1963; Lewis and Spanier 1979; Bohannan 1985; London and Wilson 1988.

29. Whyte 1990, 201.

30. Guttentag and Secord 1983.

31. Fisher 1989.

32. Divorce data in the Human Relations Area File: Cross-cultural data on divorce can be found in the Human Relations Area File. This file, known as the HRAF, was started in the 1950s by George Peter Murdock, who collected "ethnographies" (anthropological descriptions of specific cultures) and then cross-indexed these books and articles. Today over 850 cultures are cataloged. But the divorce data in this file present several problems. As Charles Ackerman (1963) reports, "For the most part, ethnographers have stated only that divorce is 'low,' 'common,' 'infrequent,' etc. Rarely has any ethnographer justified his assessment of the rate by any statement of the actual incidence of divorce." Ackerman also notes that HRAF data make it impossible to compare divorce rates *between* societies; one cannot tell whether a "low" divorce rate in one culture is equivalent to a "low" divorce rate in the next. In addition, the researcher does not know whether the "low" divorce rate of one community represents divorce rates in neighboring villages or in the same community in other decades. Synchronic and diachronic data on divorce are lacking. Moreover, different ethnographers of the same culture report different frequencies of divorce, and data in some of the entries conflict with reports by social scientists in other books and articles (Textor 1967). Last, few ethnographers tabulate the duration of the marriage that ends in divorce, the age at divorce, the number of children per divorce, and other data that could be used to make comparisons with Western peoples.

33. Ackerman 1963; Murdock 1965; Friedl 1975.

34. Cohen 1971.

35. Avery 1989, 31.

36. Barnes 1967; Murdock 1965; Textor 1967; Friedl 1975.

37. Fisher 1989, 1991, United Nations Statistical Office 2012.

38. The seven-year itch: The American concept of the seven-year itch stems from the demographic use of the *median* to establish marriage duration. The median is the middle number of a group of numbers; 50% of the incidents occur before the median and 50% after the median. In the United States between 1960 and 1982 the median duration of marriage that ended in divorce ranged between 7.2 and 6.5; thus 50% of all marriages had terminated by about seven years (U.S. Bureau of the Census 1986, chart 124). But I am interested in establishing what *most* people do, the divorce *peak* or *mode*. Across the United Nations sample from 1947 to 1989, an average of 48% of all divorces occur within seven years of marriage—the median—but divorces clustered around a four-year *peak* (Fisher 1989).

39. Chute 1949.

40. United Nations Statistical Office 2012.

41. Bullough 1976, 217.

42. Fisher 1989.

43. *Vital Statistics of the United States* 1981.

44. Ibid. 1964, 1974, 1984, 1985, 1987, 1990.

45. Cherlin 1981.

46. Procedural matters that skew the U.N. data: The time from the petition of divorce to the granting of the decree generally ranges, skewing these divorce data. Several

other technicalities tend to skew these divorce statistics: some countries include annulments, which decrease the duration of marriage; some include legal separations, which increase the duration of marriage; some include certain grounds for divorce, such as "separation for two years," that extend the divorce process; some base their statistics on "petitions for divorce" rather than on final divorce decrees; and so on. Procedural problems such as the overloading of court cases and the hearing of cases near the end of the calendar year also skew the data. Fortunately the incidences of annulments and legal separations are few. Because of the imprecision of these data on the legal duration of marriage, I would prefer to examine the duration of human pair-bonds—measured from the moment a man and woman begin to court and behave like a couple to the moment they decide to end the tie. But these numbers are not available.

47. Johnson 1983, 1.
48. Klinenberg 2012; Kreider 2006.
49. Cherlin 2009.
50. Klinenberg 2012, 88.
51. Divorce risk by number of dependent children—an important problem: To establish the risk of divorcing with any specific number of children in the family, one needs data not available in the yearbooks of the United Nations. For example, to establish the risk of divorcing with one dependent child, one must compare the number of couples who divorce with one dependent child with the number of couples who remain married with one dependent child. I have been unable to find the appropriate correlating census data to establish the divorce risk by number of dependent young for any year in any foreign country or for any year in the United States. Thus, the above data on divorce with dependent children *suggest* that the presence of "issue" stabilizes a marriage—but they do not prove it.
52. Kreider 2006.
53. Relationship between these divorce profiles: Because these data from the demographic yearbooks of the United Nations on the duration of marriage that ends in divorce, on the age at divorce, and on divorce with dependent children are not available in multivariate form, they cannot show the relationships between these three divorce profiles. The divorce peak among couples with one or no children, for example, may be an artifact of the divorce peak during and around the fourth year of marriage.
54. Dorius 2010.
55. Chagnon 1982.
56. Barnes 1967.
57. Betzig 1989.
58. Beardsley et al. 1959.
59. Radcliffe-Brown 1922.
60. East 1939.
61. World patterns of child custody and property division following divorce: The most common constraints on divorce stem from decisions about the custody of children and about the allocation of property and other resources. A survey of 41 cultures showed that 44% granted the custody of children according to the circumstances that precipitated the separation or according to the wishes or ages of the "issue." In 22% of 41 societies surveyed, children were placed in the custody of the husband; in 20% of them they became the property of the wife. The circumstances of the divorce governed property allocation in 41% of 39 societies. In 29% of 39 cultures, economic resources were divided equitably between spouses; in 23% of them the wife incurred greater financial loss, and the husband and his relatives saw greater economic devastation in 15% of them (Frayser 1985).
62. Henry 1941.

63. Cohen 1971, 135.
64. Howell 1979.

## CHAPTER 6: "WHEN WILD IN WOODS THE NOBLE SAVAGE RAN"

1. The fauna and flora mentioned here and in subsequent sections of the book are ancient varieties of species and families that are now extinct.
2. Chesters 1957; Andrews and Van Couvering 1975; Bonnefille 1985; Van Couvering 1980.
3. Corruccini et al. 1976; Rose 1983.
4. Andrews 1981.
5. Smuts 1985, 16.
6. Nadler 1988.
7. Goodall 1986; Fossey 1983; Galdikas 1979.
8. Tutin and McGinnis 1981; Fossey 1979; Veit 1982; Galdikas 1979.
9. Pygmy chimpanzee sexual behavior: Pygmy chimps, also known as bonobos, have sex lives quite different from those of the other apes. They engage in a great deal of homosexuality, and although homosexual activities peak during estrus, these contacts occur during other parts of the menstrual cycle (de Waal 1987; Thompson-Handler et al. 1984). Bonobo heterosexual activities also occur throughout most of the menstrual cycle (ibid.). And female bonobos resume sexual behavior within a year of parturition (Badrian and Badrian 1984). Because pygmy chimps exhibit these extremes of primate sexuality and because biochemical data suggest that pygmy chimps emerged as recently as two million years ago (Zihlman et al. 1987), I do not feel they make a suitable model for life as it was among prehominoids 21 million years ago.
10. Hrdy 1981; Goodall 1986; de Waal 1982.
11. Conoway and Koford 1964; Goodall 1986; Rowell 1972; Harcourt 1979; Veit 1982; Fossey 1983; Goodall 1986; MacKinnon 1979.
12. Fossey 1983.
13. Veit 1982; Fossey 1983; de Waal 1982, 1987.
14. Rape in other species: During several free-access tests (FATs), a single female common chimp, gorilla, or orangutan was housed with a single male of the same species in a common cage; each animal had continual access to the other. In some cases in all three species the male dominated the female and forced copulation—regardless of the female's sexual status or her preference (Nadler 1988). The most frequent and conspicuous examples of rape were offered by male orangutans. Rape occurred every day a couple were housed together, regardless of the stage of the female's estrus cycle or her interest in sex. In a second test a doorway was installed that divided the cage in half and was so designed that the female could pass freely to join the male but the male could not pass freely to join the female. Under these conditions, females of all three species sought copulations only during a restricted period associated with mid-cycle estrus (ibid.). Hence when females were able to control mating, sex was markedly periodic (ibid.).

    Rape does occur among free-ranging apes. In two incidences of forced copulation among chimpanzees (Tutin and McGinnis 1981), a male trapped a female in a tree and forced intercourse. On a few occasions a male gorilla was observed expressing aggressive gestures toward a female during courtship, but in no instance was copulation forced (Harcourt 1979). Rape may be among the primary reproductive strategies of subadult male orangutans. Dominant, fully adult males establish a consortship with a female during her period of sexual receptivity; they do not coerce a female into copulation (Galdikas 1979). But subadults often accost a female and try to copulate by force (MacKinnon 1979). This "sneak rape" behavior is now considered a "stable alternative strategy" for reproduction among orangutans (Rodman 1988). Rape has also been observed in other species such as ducks, gulls, herons, albatrosses, and bank swallows. In monogamous, colonially nesting bank swallows, for example, a male mated to one female will attempt to knock another mated female out of the sky and force copulation (see Daly and Wilson 1983).

15. Van Couvering 1980.
16. Berggren and Hollister 1977.
17. Van Couvering and Van Couvering 1975; Berggren and Hollister 1977; Thomas 1985.
18. Axelrod and Raven 1977.
19. Andrews and Van Couvering 1975, 65.
20. Van Couvering 1980; Axelrod and Raven 1977.
21. Andrews and Van Couvering 1975.
22. A savanna is a "well-drained grassy vegetation with 10% to 40% cover by trees" (Retallack et al. 1990).
23. Andrews and Van Couvering 1975; Van Couvering 1980; Retallack et al. 1990.
24. Andrews and Van Couvering 1975; Van Couvering 1980; Axelrod and Raven 1977; Maglio 1978; Bernor 1985; Vrba 1985.
25. Klein 2009.
26. Wolpoff 1982; Ciochon and Fleagle 1987. Dating the divergence of humankind: Data from DNA and other biochemical, anatomical, and genetic analyses of differences between humankind and the African apes suggest somewhat different dates for the divergence of the human line. Estimates range from 10 to 4 million years ago. See Sarich and Wilson 1967a, 1967b; Cronin 1983; Sibley and Ahlquist 1984; Andrews and Cronin 1982. Data now suggest that human beings are most closely related to chimpanzees; that gorillas diverged earlier (Miyamoto et al. 1987); and that humankind first diverged from this basal stock between 8–5 million years ago (Klein 2009).
27. Veit 1982.
28. Nadler 1975.
29. Veit 1982.
30. Fossey 1983.
31. Darwin 1871; Freud 1918; Engels [1884] 1954.
32. Lucretius 1965, 162–3.
33. Klein 2009.
34. Kano 1979; Kano and Mulavwa 1984.
35. Kano 1979; Badrian and Malenky 1984.
36. De Waal 1987; Thompson-Handler et al. 1984; Kano and Mulavwa 1984.
37. Kuroda 1984; de Waal 1987; Savage-Rumbaugh and Wilkerson 1978.
38. De Waal 1987.
39. Ibid.
40. Kano 1980.
41. Face-to-face coitus in nature: Several animals copulate face-to-face on some occasions, including gorillas (Nadler 1975), orangutans (Galdikas 1979), siamangs (Chivers 1978), and whales and porpoises (Harrison 1969).
42. Coolidge 1933; Zihlman et al. 1987; Zihlman 1979; Susman 1984.
43. Ellen Ingmanson, anthropologist, personal communication.
44. McGinnis 1979; Goodall 1986.
45. Tutin 1979; McGinnis 1979; McGrew 1981; Goodall 1986.
46. McGrew 1981; Goodall 1986; de Waal 1982; McGinnis 1979.
47. McGinnis 1979; Tutin 1979; Goodall 1986; McGrew 1981.

48. Pusey 1980.
49. McGinnis 1979; Tutin 1979; Goodall 1986.
50. Tutin and McGinnis 1981.
51. Bygott 1979; Goodall et al. 1979; Wrangham 1979b; Goodall 1986.
52. Goodall et al. 1979.
53. Bygott 1974, 1979; Goodall et al. 1979; Goodall 1986.
54. Teleki 1973a, 1973b; Goodall 1986.
55. Teleki 1973a; McGrew 1981.
56. Plooij 1978.
57. Goodall 1968, 1970, 1986; McGrew 1981.
58. De Waal 1989.
59. McGrew 1979, 1981; also see Boesch and Boesch 1984.
60. Goodall 1970, 1986; McGrew 1974, 1981.
61. Goodall 1986.
62. Fouts 1983.
63. Moss 1988.
64. Tanner 1981; McGrew 1981; Fisher 1982; Mansperger 1990; Foley and Lee 1989.
65. Klein 2009.
66. White et al. 2009.
67. Ibid.; Plavcan 2012, 51.
68. See Chapter 7, n. 6.
69. Harrison 2010.

## CHAPTER 7: OUT OF EDEN

1. Hay and Leakey 1982.
2. Leakey and Hay 1979; Hay and Leakey 1982.
3. Leakey et al. 1976; White 1977, 1980.
4. Johanson and Edey 1981; Johnston 1982; Lewin 1983a.
5. Johanson and White 1979; see Johanson 1982; Susman et al. 1985; Jungers 1988; McHenry 1986; Klein 2009.
6. Plavcan 2012. A large difference in body size between males and females of a species, known as sexual dimorphism, has traditionally been used as an indicator of a species' mating system. In species that bond for life, males and females tend to have similar body sizes, whereas in those species in which males form harems, males tend to be considerably larger than females—the result of male–male competition for mates. Lucy and her chums most likely exhibited considerable body size dimorphism (Plavcan 2012), suggesting to some academics that the mating strategy of pair-bonding had not yet evolved. Reno et al. (2003, 2010) and Nelson et al. (2011) disagree, proposing that A. afarensis exhibits less bodily sexual dimorphism, most likely within the human range. Several have questioned these analyses, however (see Plavcan 2012).

In response to this issue, I propose that A. afarensis had evolved the mating strategy of serial social monogamy: making *temporary* pair-bonds in conjunction with infant rearing, and *serial* pair-bonds across the life course as they bore additional young; moreover, these temporary pairs traveled within larger multi-male/multi-female groups, much as hunter-gatherer pairs do today. A mating strategy of serial monogamy within a large multi-male/multi-female group could have generated considerable competition between males for females—sustaining selection for a high degree of body dimorphism. More important to my argument, the skeletal and dental material of *Ardipithecus ramidis* (living over a million years *earlier* than A. *afarensis*) shows no evidence of substantial body size dimorphism (White et al. 2009), suggesting that some form of monogamy may have evolved by then. Moreover Gordon (2006), White et al. (2009), and Lovejoy (2009) argue that the bodily sexual dimorphisms seen in the later species, including *A. afarensis*, occurred *due to a reduction of female body size from earlier forms* for reasons other than male–male competition for mates. These data support my hypothesis that hominin serial social monogamy had occurred prior to the emergence of *A. afarensis*.

Another issue must be considered, however. Lucy and her *A. afarensis* relatives exhibit reduced dimorphism in their canine teeth—traditionally regarded as an indicator of pair-bonding in many species. Yet Dixson (2009) suggests that with the extensive development of bipedalism in *A. afarensis*, these male forebears could have fought one another with their fists or weapons, suggesting that reduced canine dimorphism in this species is not an indicator of pair-bonding. But if bipedalism and *serial* pairing (in conjunction with rearing infants) evolved long *before* the emergence of *A. afarensis*, indeed soon after our first forebears began to walk bipedally at least 4.4 million years ago, males were most likely still inefficient at bipedal walking and weapon use. In this scenario, reduced canine dimorphism (White et al. 2009) could have been an indicator of serial social monogamy (Lovejoy 2009).

Perhaps most important to this issue, Plavcan (2012, 45) writes that "The causes of human sexual size dimorphism are uncertain, and could involve several non-mutually-exclusive mechanisms, such as mate competition, resource competition, intergroup violence, and female choice." For example, scavenging and hunting (as well as serial monogamy) may have selected for large males, whereas Lucy's diminutive frame may have been a compensation for the demands of bearing young. Because of pregnancy and lactation, female mammals need extra calories; they must eat for two and then nurse a child, so the smaller Lucy was, the less she needed to feed herself. The many ecological factors *other than mating strategy* that can affect bodily and canine sexual dimorphisms (see Frayer and Wolpoff 1985; Mock and Fujioka 1990; Plavcan 2012) suggest that bodily and canine sexual dimorphisms are *not* good indicators of early hominin reproductive strategies.

7. Alemseged et al. 2006.
8. Van Couvering 1980; Vrba 1985; Axelrod and Raven 1977; Bernor 1985.
9. Binford 1981, 1985; Blumenschine 1986, 1987, 1989; Shipman 1986; Potts 1988; Sinclair et al. 1986; Lewin 1987b.
10. Tunnell 1990; Schaller and Lowther 1969; Blumenschine 1986.
11. Scavenging among nonhuman primates: Goodall has reported scavenging among the chimps at the Gombe Stream Reserve, Tanzania, on several occasions. On most of them, a chimp returned to eat meat left behind after a group of chimps had made a kill earlier in the day. In one case, a chimp stole the limb of a dead monkey as Goodall was photographing it. Gombe chimps ignored the fresh meat of a dead bushbuck fawn and guinea fowl. But on four occasions chimps in the nearby research site at the Mahale Mountains scavenged the carcasses of blue duikers or bushbucks (Goodall 1986). Savanna baboons also scavenge (Strum 1990; Cavallo and Blumenschine 1989).
12. Cavallo 1990; Cavallo and Blumenschine 1989.
13. McHenry 1986; Ryan and Johanson 1989.
14. Wrangham 2009.
15. Darwin 1871, 434.
16. Watson et al. 2008.
17. Fatherhood across species: Males of many species exhibit parental behavior, although most are not monogamous. Male parental investment occurs in two

forms: *(a)* direct care, such as feeding young, carrying infants, babysitting, sleeping in contact with young, grooming young, retrieving, and/or playing with young; and *(b)* indirect care, such as defending resources, stockpiling food for infants, building shelters for young, helping pregnant or nursing females, marking and/or maintaining a territory, defending and patrolling borders of a range, expelling intruders, and/or calling to drive competitors away (Kleiman and Malcolm 1981; also see Hewlett 1992).

18. Wittenberger and Tilson 1980; Kleiman 1977; Orians 1969; Lack 1968; Mock and Fujioka 1990.

19. Monogamy in cross-species perspective: Several circumstances operate together to produce monogamy, and researchers provide alternative explanations for the evolution of monogamy in different creatures. I am particularly influenced by the work of Devra Kleiman—specifically by her contention that monogamy occurs "whenever more than a single individual (the female) is needed to rear the young" (Kleiman 1977, 51). This was said differently by Ember and Ember (1979): "Heterosexual partnerships develop wherever the need of the mother to obtain her nutrition interferes with the care of the young. The duration of this bond is dependent upon the parental care time." I think this factor was critical to the evolution of monogamy in hominins. For discussions of monogamy in birds and mammals, see Kleiman 1977; Wittenberger and Tilson 1980; Lack 1968; Orians 1969; Rutberg 1983; Peck and Feldman 1988; Mock and Fujioka 1990.

20. Precocial young: Creatures that deliver their young in a state of relative maturity, as opposed to immaturity, are said to deliver *precocial* young. Horses provide a good example; a foal can see and walk a few hours after birth.

21. Trivers 1972; Emlen and Oring 1977.

22. Henry 1985; Lloyd 1980; Zimen 1980; Gage 1979; Rue 1969.

23. Orians 1969; Mock and Fujioka 1990.

24. Eugene Morton, Dept. of Ornithology, Smithsonian Institution, personal communication.

25. Hewlett 1991; Kelly 1995; Marlowe 2010; Cohen 1980; Hassan 1980; Lee 1980; Short 1976, 1984; Konner and Worthman 1980; Simpson-Hebert and Huffman 1981; Lancaster and Lancaster 1983; Frisch 1978.

26. Birdsell 1979.

27. Galdikas and Wood 1990.

28. Raymond Hames, Dept. of Anthropology, Univ. of Nebraska, personal communication.

29. Briggs 1970.

30. Gorer 1938.

31. Heider 1976.

32. Lancaster and Lancaster 1983; Marlowe 2005; Quinlan and Quinlan 2008; Dediu and Levinson 2013; Gray and Garcia 2013; Hewlett 1991; Kelly 1995; Marlowe 2010.

Four-year human birthing cycle—modern variations, ape origins: Modern living has changed this general three- to four-year human birthing cycle. Even continually breast-feeding women in India, Bangladesh, the United States, and Scotland begin to ovulate about five to eighteen months after delivering a child (Simpson-Hebert and Huffman 1981; Short 1984). Thus modern birth spacing can be as short as two years or even less. This has traditionally been explained by the "critical fatness" hypothesis. In the 1970s Rose Frisch and colleagues proposed that a woman needs adequate stores of body fat to trigger ovulation (Frisch and Revelle 1970; Frisch 1978, 1989). Today not all academics accept this hypothesis (see Gray and Garcia 2013). But most believe that our modern diet high in calories, lack of exercise, and limited nursing frequency can initiate ovulation and produce pregnancy a few months after childbirth.

However, when our ancestors walked miles to collect dinner, when they ate fruit and lean meat, and women nursed their infants continually, women probably bore their young about three to four years apart (Lancaster and Lancaster 1983). Data on birth spacing among the apes support the antiquity of this reproductive pattern. Among chimpanzees and gorillas, birth spacing is generally four to five years, whereas birth intervals among orangutans are often about eight years (L. L. Allen et al. 1982; Galdikas and Wood 1990).

33. Adaptive reasons for males to "remarry": Among apes males tend to seek copulation with older, more mature females rather than with adolescents—presumably because females with young have a good reproductive track record. This raises the question: why would ancestral hominin males seek to form pair-bonds with young females rather than with more mature ones? The answer, I think, lies in the ecology of monogamy. In monogamous species the male will invest time and energy rearing his offspring himself. Hence the values of youth—such as fresh eggs, a supple body, a resilient personality, and a long reproductive future—may be more important to a male than the female's reproductive track record.

34. Adaptive reasons for females to "remarry": Psychologist David Buss has argued that once a woman produced a child, her reproductive value went down, making her less attractive to prime males. Hence as a woman aged, her subsequent pair-bonds were with men of lower reproductive worth. Thus serial monogamy was not an adaptive strategy for ancestral females. This argument is logical. But several practical variables must be considered: *(a)* Band size and infrequency of interband contact may have reduced opportunities for a female to acquire a prime mate on her first mateship, providing her with the opportunity to "marry up" on her second try. *(b)* The female's first mate's reproductive value might go down dramatically as a result of injury; hence, although her second mate might not be prime, he would be of higher reproductive value than the first. *(c)* A young male was probably strong and quick but inexperienced at hunting and protecting, whereas an older male was undoubtedly more experienced at hunting, scavenging, and fathering (as well as economically burdened by previous wives and children). The reproductive value of males thus probably varied enormously with factors other than age. *(d)* A female's reproductive value may have gone up with age if she became a more proficient provider and remained fertile, thereby attracting more prime males in subsequent mateships. I suspect the reproductive value of each male and female rose or fell according to several variables; the vicissitudes of the environment added more variables as well. Hence a reproductive strategy of flexible *opportunistic* serial monogamy would have been adaptive for females.

35. Bertram 1975; Schaller 1972; Hausfater and Hrdy 1984.

36. Daly and Wilson 1988.

37. Tylor 1889, 267–8.

38. Friedl 1975.

39. Laura Betzig, Evolution and Human Behavior Program, Univ. of Michigan, personal communication.

40. Tanner 1981; McGrew 1981; Fisher 1982; Foley and Lee 1989; Mansperger 1990.

41. Strum 1990; Smuts 1985, 1992.

42. Palombit et al. 1997.

43. Early hominin group size: Birdsell (1968) proposed that early hominin bands were composed of about 25 individuals, half of whom were adults. I think this standard model is a reasonable one for early hominin social groups. (Also see Foley and Lee 1989.)

CHAPTER 8: THE TYRANNY OF LOVE

1. Hatfield 1988, 191.
2. Bell 1995, 158.
3. Rebhun 1995, 252.
4. McCullough 2001.
5. Shostak 1981, 268.
6. Bowlby 1969, 1973.
7. Ainsworth et al. 1978.
8. Fraley and Shaver 2000; Panksepp 2003; Tucker et al. 2005; MacDonald and Leary 2005; Eisenberger et al. 2003.
9. Hazan and Diamond 2000; Hazan and Shaver 1987.
10. Lim et al. 2004; Carter 1992; Lim and Young 2004.
11. Wang et al. 1994.
12. Pitkow et al. 2001; Lim and Young 2004; Lim et al. 2004; see Young 1999. Genetic studies further suggest that attachment behaviors are orchestrated by DNA in mammals. Promiscuous white-footed mice and promiscuous rhesus monkeys do not form pair-bonds or express attachment behaviors toward a specific mate; and the males of these species do not express the same distribution of V1a (vasopressin) receptors in the ventral pallidum as is seen in pair-bonding prairie voles (Bester-Meredith et al. 1999; Wang et al. 1997; Young 1999; Young et al. 1997). Moreover, when scientists (Pitkow et al. 2001; Lim and Young 2004; Lim et al. 2004) transgenically inserted the genetic variant in the vasopressin system associated with pair-bonding in male prairie voles into the ventral pallidum of male meadow voles, an asocial promiscuous species, vasopressin receptors were up-regulated. These males also began to fixate on a particular female and mate exclusively with her, even when other females were available (Lim et al. 2004). When this gene was inserted into non-monogamous male mice, these creatures also began to exhibit attachment behaviors (Young et al. 1999).
13. Walum et al. 2008.
14. Pedersen et al. 1992.
15. Lim et al. 2004; Carter 1992; Lim and Young 2004; Zak et al. 2005; Zak 2012; Young et al. 1998; Young 1999.
16. Young et al. 1998; Carmichael et al. 1987; Zak 2008.
17. Jankowiak and Hardgrave 2007; Meloy and Fisher 2005.
18. Meloy 1998; Meloy and Fisher 2005; Buss 2000.
19. Symons 1979.
20. Buss 2000.
21. Rancourt-Laferriere 1983.
22. Barash 1977.
23. Young et al. 1998.
24. Peele 1975; Halpern 1982; Tennov 1979; Hunter et al. 1981; Mellody et al. 1992; Griffin-Shelley 1991; Schaef 1989.
25. Fisher 2004, 2014.
26. Many professionals define addiction as a pathological, problematic disorder (Reynaud et al. 2010). And because romantic love is a positive experience under many circumstances (i.e. not harmful), researchers remain largely unwilling to officially categorize romantic love as an addiction. But love addiction is just as real as any other addiction, in terms of its behavior patterns and brain mechanisms. Even when romantic love isn't harmful, it is associated with intense craving and anxiety and can impel the lover to believe, say, and do dangerous and inappropriate things. Moreover, all forms of substance abuse, including alcohol, opioids, cocaine, amphetamines, cannabis, and tobacco (as well as the non-substance addictions to

food, gambling, and sex) activate several of the same reward pathways that are activated among men and women who are *happily* in love, as well as those rejected in love. Unlike all other addictions, however, which afflict only a percentage of the population, some form of love addiction is likely to occur to almost every human being at some point during the life course. These data suggest that romantic love should be *treated* as an addiction, regardless of its lack of official diagnostic classification as an addiction (see Fisher 2013).

27. L. L. Brown, in Frascella et al. 2010, 295.
28. Fisher 1998, 2004.
29. Fisher, Brown, Aron, et al. 2010.
30. Hatfield and Sprecher 1986.
31. Fisher, Brown, Aron, et al. 2010.
32. Diana 2013; Koob and Volkow 2010; Melis et al. 2005; Frascella et al. 2010.
33. Baumeister et al. 1993.
34. T. Lewis et al. 2000; Fisher 2004.
35. Fisher 2004, 16; Fisher 2014.
36. Schultz 2000.
37. Kapit et al. 2000.
38. Meloy 2001, 1998.
39. Panksepp 1998.
40. Ibid.; Dozier 2002.
41. Fisher 2004; Meloy and Fisher 2005; Fisher 2014.
42. T. Lewis et al. 2000; Fisher 2004.
43. Panksepp 1998.
44. See Meloy 1998; Meloy and Fisher 2005.
45. T. Lewis et al. 2000.
46. Najib et al. 2004; Panksepp 1998.
47. Panksepp 1998; T. Lewis et al. 2000; Fisher 2004, 2014.
48. Mearns 1991.
49. Rosenthal 2000; Nemeroff 1998.
50. Schultz 2000.
51. Panksepp 1998.
52. Panksepp 1998; Kapit et al. 2000.
53. See Leary 2001.
54. Hagen 2011.
55. Watson and Andrews 2002.
56. Fisher 2004, 2014.
57. Weiss 1975.
58. Attachment in animals: Infant puppies, baby monkeys, chicks, and guinea pigs cry when their mother goes away—even if they are warm, comfortable, and satiated. Their heart races, their blood pressure increases, and their body temperature rises as "separation anxiety" escalates into panic. When they are administered endorphins or other natural opiates (of which heroin is one), these infants calm down. So many brain regions, pathways and neurochemicals work together to create the highs and lows of love.
59. Meloy et al. 2001.
60. Hatfield and Rapson 1996.
61. Mearns 1991; Nolen-Hoeksema et al. 1999.
62. Hatfield and Rapson 1996.
63. Davidson 1994; Panksepp 1998.
64. Donaldson 1971.
65. Mellen 1981; Donaldson 1971.
66. Walum et al. 2008.

67. Fisher 2004; Fisher et al. 2006.
68. Fisher 2004.
69. Fisher et al. 2002; Fisher 2004; Fisher et al. 2006.

## CHAPTER 9: DRESSED TO IMPRESS

1. Darwin 1859, 1871.
2. F. Darwin 1911.
3. Darwin 1871. Natural selection versus sexual selection: In terms of the transmission of genes, there is no difference between natural selection and sexual selection. The distinction lies in the type of selection and the type of adaptive results. *Sexual selection* is defined as selection for characteristics that are specifically concerned with increasing one's success at attracting and obtaining mates. The results are the evolution of traits useful to sex and reproduction rather than adaptations to the general environment. Following Darwin, it is customary to distinguish two kinds of sexual selection: *(a) intrasexual selection* is selection for traits that enable one to compete with members of the same sex for mates of the opposite sex; *(b) intersexual selection* is selection for characteristics that make one attractive to the opposite sex. See Darwin 1871; Campbell 1972; Gould and Gould 1989.
4. Gray and Garcia 2013.
5. Smith 1984; Eberhard 1985, 1990.
6. Daly and Wilson 1983.
7. Smith 1984.
8. Dixson 1999.
9. Short 1977; Moller 1988; Lewin 1988d.
10. Perhaps as little as 1% of sperm are equipped to fertilize the egg; others are known as blockers or kamikaze sperm. These sperm are of two types: Type A sperm obstruct foreign sperm that enter the vagina after themselves; Type B sperm tackle foreign sperm that entered before themselves (Baker, 1996). Interestingly, Baker (1996) reports that male ejaculate contains as much as three times more sperm if the man has been away from his partner for a long period; while men who have been in the vicinity of a partner for the same period of time, yet been sexually abstinent, show no increase in sperm volume. He proposes that this mechanism could have evolved as a biological tactic to counter possible adultery in a partner during a mate's absence.
11. Dixson 2009.
12. Gray and Garcia 2013, 183.
13. Darwin 1871; Bateman 1948; Trivers 1972.
14. Morris 1967.
15. Gallup 1982; Marlowe 1998.
16. Lancaster 1986.
17. Low et al. 1987.
18. Mascia-Lees et al. 1986.
19. Darwin 1871, 907.
20. Ibid., 881.
21. Alexander 1990.
22. Singh 1993.
23. Singh 2002.
24. Singh 1993, 2002; Swami and Furnhan 2008.
25. Hughes et al. 2004.
26. Gangestad and Thornhill 1997.
27. Langlois et al. 1987.

28. Gangestad et al. 1994; Jones and Hill 1993.
29. Hamilton and Zuk 1982; Thornhill and Gangestad 1993.
30. Gangestad and Thornhill 1997.
31. Aharon et al. 2001.
32. Buss 1994.
33. Gangestad and Thornhill 1997.
34. Thornhill et al. 1995.
35. Gangestad and Thornhill 1998.
36. Thornhill et al. 1995.
37. Solar et al. 2003.
38. Manning and Scutt 1996.
39. Manning et al. 1996.
40. Jankowiak et al. 2015.
41. Gray and Garcia 2013.
42. Dobs et al. 2004.
43. Hughes et al. 2007.
44. Wlodarski and Dunbar 2013, 2014.
45. Hughes et al. 2007.
46. Ford and Beach 1951.
47. Neoteny: Ashley Montagu (1981) proposes that the human female downward-tilted vaginal canal and face-to-face coitus evolved as a by-product of *neoteny*, or "growing young." Neoteny, meaning the extention of childlike characteristics into adulthood, is a remarkable phenomenon; we have several neotenous traits, including flat faces, rounded skulls, playfulness, curiosity, and other emotional and physical traits that nonhuman primates display in infancy but lose as they mature. The downward-tilted vagina occurs in the embryo of all mammals, but after birth the vaginal canal rotates backward and lies parallel with the spine. Women retain this embryonic vaginal orientation into old age.
48. Lloyd 2005.
49. Zietsch and Santtila 2013.
50. Lloyd 2005.
51. Symons 1979.
52. Orgasm as a means of stimulating physiological sensations of attachment: Oxytocin, a peptide secreted by the pituitary gland in the brain, is secreted during orgasm and serves to produce feelings of pleasure, sexual fulfillment and attachment.
53. Baker and Bellis 1995.
54. Ibid.
55. Smith 1984; Alcock 1987.
56. Dixson 1998.
57. Burton 1971; de Waal 1982; Whitten 1982; Lancaster 1979; Hrdy 1981; Savage-Rumbaugh and Wilkerson 1978.
58. Sex outside of estrus in other animals: Female bonobos engage in sexual behavior with other females daily. Heterosexual copulations also occur throughout most of the menstrual cycle, although not all of it (Thompson-Handler, Malenky, and Badrian 1984). Female dolphins reportedly masturbate and copulate regularly, with few signs of periodicity (Diamond 1980). Females of several primate species exhibit sexual behavior at times other than mid-cycle estrus, such as during troop upheaval, during captivity, or during pregnancy. One can cite many exceptions, but generally speaking, the vast majority of heterosexual interactions among female primates occur during mid-cycle estrus. See Fedigan 1982; Lancaster 1979; Hrdy 1981.
59. Kinsey et al. 1953; Ford and Beach 1951; Wolfe 1981.
60. Ford and Beach 1951.

61. Menopause: The complex programmed cessation of ovulation known as menopause, which occurs in all middle-aged women, does not appear to occur in other primates or other mammals, although elephants, pilot whales, and some primates exhibit some signs of menopause in advanced age (Alexander 1990; Pavelka and Fedigan 1991). Some scientists currently think menopause evolved in ancestral women as an adaptive strategy to aid existing offspring and other genetic relatives, in lieu of producing new children of their own that would require many years of investment as they aged. Hence the postmenopausal mother could become a grandmother and babysitter instead—a theory now known as the *grandmother hypothesis* (Hawkes et al. 1998). Menopause could also have evolved as the by-product of the increased human life span, known as a *pleiotropic effect* (Pavelka and Fedigan 1991). Moreover, perhaps women's high postmenopausal libido evolved to enable them to maintain their pair-bonds (and the political-social coalitions these accrued), as well as to help them continue to garner extra resources from clandestine copulations. See Alexander 1990; Dawkins 1976; Pavelka and Fedigan 1991.
62. Strassman 1981; Alexander and Noonan 1979; Turke 1984; Fisher 1975, 1982; Lovejoy 1981; Burley 1979; Small 1988; Gray and Wolfe 1983; Benshoof and Thornhill 1979; Daniels 1983; Burleson and Trevathan 1990; Hrdy 1983.
63. Fisher 1975, 1982.
64. Rosenblum 1976.
65. Natural peaks in the human female sex drive: Studies suggest that the peak of a woman's sexual activity occurs at mid-cycle (Hrdy 1981). Married women given a variety of contraceptive devices exhibited a rise in female-initiated sex drive during ovulation under most conditions; this was suppressed by the use of oral contraceptives (Adams et al. 1978). Intercourse peaked among a sample of American women soon after the end of menstruation, however (Udry and Morris 1977). Other studies indicate that American wives (as well as women in other cultures) experience a peak of excitability immediately before or after menstruation (Ford and Beach 1951; Kinsey et al. 1953). These data lead me to propose that women have two natural peaks in sex drive: one during and around ovulation and another just before or during menstruation. The peak during ovulation may be a holdover from estrus. The peak during menstruation may have evolved with bipedalism; blood pools naturally in the pelvic area prior to menstruation, and bipedalism may act to heighten tension on genital tissues at this time.
66. Daniels 1983.
67. Miller 2000.
68. Ibid., 3, 29.
69. Ibid., 7.

## CHAPTER 10: MEN AND WOMEN ARE LIKE TWO FEET: THEY NEED EACH OTHER TO GET AHEAD

1. Gould 1981; Russett 1989.
2. Mead 1935, 280.
3. Cultural determinism: The sharp swing toward "cultural determinism" in the 1920s and 1930s did not focus on gender differences alone but was part of an intellectual reaction to the eugenics movement at the time and emphasized racial and ethnic commonalities too.
4. See Gray and Garcia 2013.
5. Maccoby and Jacklin 1974; McGuinness 1976, 1979, 1985; see Fisher 1999.
6. Benderly 1987.
7. Sherman 1978.

8. McGuinness 1985, 89.
9. Rosenberg 2002.
10. Kimura 1989; Weiss 1988.
11. Baron-Cohen et al. 2005.
12. Benderly 1987, 1989.
13. Fennema and Leder 1990.
14. Maccoby and Jacklin 1974; McGuinness 1979; Fennema and Leder 1990; see Fisher 1999.
15. Benbow and Stanley 1980, 1983.
16. Leder 1990; Benderly 1987.
17. Manning 2002; Manning et al. 2001; Geschwind 1985; see Fisher 1999.
18. Kimura 1989.
19. L. L. Brown et al. 2013; Fisher, Island, Rich, et al. 2015; Fisher, Rich, Island, et al., 2010.
20. Silverman and Beals 1990.
21. Fennema and Leder 1990; Sherman 1978; Benderly 1987; Bower 1986.
22. See Fisher 1999; Fisher, Rich, Island, et al. 2010; L. L. Brown et al. 2013; Fisher, Island, Rich, et al. 2015.
23. Darwin 1871.
24. McGuinness 1979; McGuinness and Pribram 1979; Hall 1978; Hall et al. 1977; Zuckerman et al. 1976; Hall 1984.
25. Ingalhalikar et al. 2014.
26. Kimura 1983; McGuinness 1985.
27. Geschwind 1974; Springer and Deutsch 1985.
28. Baron-Cohen 2003.
29. Domes et al. 2007.
30. Fisher 1999.
31. See Fisher 1999; Baron-Cohen 2003a; Baron-Cohen et al. 2005.
32. See Fisher 1999.
33. See Fisher 1999, 2009.
34. Kimura 1989.
35. McGuinness 1979, 1985; McGuinness and Pribram 1979.
36. Whiting and Whiting 1975.
37. Konner 1982, 2015.
38. Miller 1983.
39. Rossi 1984; Frayser 1985; Konner 2015.
40. McGuinness 1979, 1985; McGuinness and Pribram 1979.
41. Knickmeyer et al. 2006.
42. Otten 1985; Moir and Jessel 1989; Money and Ehrhardt 1972.
43. Taylor 2000.
44. Knickmeyer et al. 2006.
45. Carter 1998; Zak et al. 2007; Barraza and Zak 2009; Domes et al. 2007; Fisher, Island, Rich, et al. 2015; L. L. Brown et al. 2013.
46. L. L. Brown et al. 2013.
47. McGrew 1981.
48. McGuinness 1979.
49. Leakey 1971.
50. Behrensmeyer and Hill 1980; Brain 1981.
51. Bunn and Kroll 1986.
52. Cavallo 1990; Cavallo and Blumenschine 1989.
53. Potts 1984, 1988.
54. Zihlman 1981.
55. Lewin 1987b; McHenry 1986.
56. Brod 1987; Goleman 1986.

57. Gilligan 1982a.
58. Johanson and Shreeve 1989. New data suggest that the genus *Homo* could have emerged as early as 2.8 to 2.5 million years ago, as evidenced by a new fossil find known as the Ledi jaw (a partial left jaw and five teeth) in Ethiopia (DiMaggio et al. 2015). This individual may have been one of the ancestors of *Homo habilis*.
59. Tobias 1991.
60. Who made the tools and butchered the meat at Olduvai? Although recent data suggests that robust australopithecines could have made and used tools and that these creatures had a bulge in Broca's area in the brain, several lines of evidence suggest that *Homo habilis* individuals made and stored these tools, as well as devised the system of cache sites to butcher meat at Olduvai two million years ago. *(a)* The reduced cheek teeth of *Homo habilis* suggest that these creatures relied on meat (McHenry and O'Brien 1986). *(b)* The increased cranial capacity of this species may even have required the consumption of energy-rich foods such as meat (Ambrose 1986). *(c)* The bones of *Homo habilis* lie in special patterns consistent with those of the stone tools found at Olduvai, and these patterns at Olduvai Gorge fit well with patterns of fossils and tools left at Koobi Fora. *(d)* Several anatomical details of these fossil bones suggest that *Homo habilis* is in the direct line toward humankind.

## CHAPTER 11: WOMEN, MEN, AND POWER

1. Van Allen 1976.
2. Ibid.
3. Van Allen 1976; Okonjo 1976.
4. Discussions of universal male dominance: Anthropologists have proposed several reasons why men universally dominate women. Some have pointed to biology: men are naturally stronger and more aggressive; hence men have always dominated women (Sacks 1979). Some have proposed a psychological explanation: men dominate women to reject the powerful women in their lives (Whiting 1965). Universal male dominance, others say, stems from female reproductive functions. Because women bear children, they are tied to the natural rather than the cultural world (Ortner and Whitehead 1981) or to the private rather than the public sector (Rosaldo 1974). For anthropological discussions of universal male dominance and theories of why gender relations vary cross-culturally, see Dahlberg 1981; Reiter 1975; Etienne and Leacock 1980; Leacock 1981; Friedl 1975; Harris 1977; Sanday 1981; Sacks 1979; Ortner and Whitehead 1981; Rosaldo and Lamphiere 1974; Collier 1988; Konner 2015.
5. Elkin 1939; Hart and Pilling 1960; Rohrlich-Leavitt et al. 1975; Berndt 1981.
6. Montagu 1937, 23.
7. Kaberry 1939; Goodale 1971; Berndt 1981; Bell 1980.
8. Reiter 1975; Slocum 1975.
9. Whyte 1978.
10. Traditional societies with powerful women: Pygmy women of the Congo, Navajo women of the American Southwest, Iroquois women of New York, Tlingit women of southern Alaska, Algonkian women of the American Northeast, Balinese women, Semang women of the tropical forests of the Malay Peninsula, women in Polynesia, women in parts of the Andes, Africa, Southeast Asia, and the Caribbean, Trobriand Islanders of the Pacific, and women in many other societies traditionally wielded substantial economic and social power. See Sanday 1981; Etienne and Leacock 1980; Dahlberg 1981; Reiter 1975; Sacks 1979; Weiner 1976.
11. Leacock 1980, 28.
12. Sanday 1981, 135.
13. Types of power: Power in traditional societies comes in several forms. Sociolo-

gist Robert Alford divides power into three distinct varieties: *(a)* the ability to influence or persuade; *(b)* authority or formal institutionalized command; *(c)* what sociologists sometimes call hegemony, which is almost identical to one meaning of *culture* because it refers to the unquestioned, accepted mores of a culture that bestow power on one gender or individual rather than on another (Alford and Friedland 1985).

14. Friedl 1975; Sacks 1971; Sanday 1974; Whyte 1978.
15. Friedl 1975.
16. Shostak 1981, 243.
17. Rogers 1975.
18. The Human Relations Area File: Many anthropologists regard this file as highly uneven and flawed because the data on each culture are taken by a different ethnographer. Each ethnographer has asked different questions in different ways, recorded his or her perceptions under different circumstances, and had his or her own subjective perspectives. The data in this file were then distilled by Whyte and his colleagues—further reducing the likelihood of accuracy. I use Whyte's analysis here because I do not wish to overlook an available source and because my experience with the ethnographic literature suggests that Whyte's conclusions on this topic represent some general cross-cultural truths.
19. Whyte 1978.
20. Sanday 1981.
21. De Waal 1982, 1989.
22. Fisher 1999.
23. Mazur 1997.
24. Baron-Cohen 2003.
25. De Waal 1996.
26. De Waal 1982, 187.
27. Hrdy 1981; Fedigan 1982.

## CHAPTER 12: ALMOST HUMAN

1. Wrangham 2009, 10.
2. Wrangham 2009.
3. Ibid.
4. Ibid., 109; Aiello and Wheeler 1995.
5. John M. Harris, Rutgers University, personal communication.
6. Wrangham 2009, 42.
7. Brain and Sillen 1988.
8. Klein 1999.
9. Pruetz and LaDuke 2010.
10. Brink 1957.
11. Pruetz and LaDuke 2009.
12. Behrensmeyer 1984.
13. Bramble and Lieberman 2004.
14. Gibbons 1990b.
15. Montagu 1961; Gould 1977; Fisher 1975, 1982; Trevathan 1987.
16. Montagu 1961, 156.
17. Human secondary altriciality: Human newborns are not uniformly altricial; instead, they display a mosaic of features, some of which exhibit more altriciality than others (Gibson 1981). Scientists at present debate whether the "secondary altriciality" of some neonatal traits evolved in response to cephalo-pelvic disproportion (Lindburg 1982). I use the standard explanation that secondary altriciality

*is* a response to cephalo-pelvic disproportion. See Montagu 1961; Gould 1977; Bromage 1987; Trevathan 1987.
18. Klein 1999.
19. Fisher 1975, 1982.
20. Trevathan 1987.
21. Hawkes et al. 1998.
22. De Castro et al. 1999; De Castro et al. 2010; see Dediu and Levinson 2013.
23. Lancaster and Lancaster 1983.
24. Copeland et al. 2011.
25. Wood and Marlowe 2011.
26. Kramer and Greaves 2011.
27. Wrangham 2009, 98.
28. Wrangham 2009.
29. Jia and Weiwen 1990.
30. Klein 1999.

CHAPTER 13: THE FIRST AFFLUENT SOCIETY

1. Conkey 1984.
2. Service 1978; Pfeiffer 1982.
3. Gargett 1989; Chase and Dibble 1987; see Dediu and Levinson 2013.
4. Holloway 1985.
5. Dediu and Levinson 2013.
6. Arensburg et al. 1989.
7. Martínez et al. 2008.
8. Ibid.
9. Steele and Uomini 2009.
10. See Dediu and Levinson 2013; Johansson 2013.
11. See Dediu and Levinson 2013; Johansson 2013.
12. Lupyan and Dale 2010; Dediu and Levinson 2013.
13. Klein 2009.
14. Leroi-Gourhan 1975; Solecki 1971, 1989.
15. Miller 2001.
16. Gargett 1989; Chase and Dibble 1987; Trinkaus and Shipman 1993; d'Errico et al. 2003; d'Errico et al. 2009; Zilhão 2010; see Johansson 2013; Dedie and Levinson 2013.
17. Gibbons 2010; Green et al. 2010.
18. Green et al. 2010.
19. Among the genes that differ between the Neanderthals and modern men and women are some that direct metabolism, skin pigmentation, wound healing, skeletal development, and some associated with cognition. But scientists do not yet know what the genetic variations between these peoples and modern humans actually mean or even if they affect human thinking or behavior (Gibbons 2010). Interestingly, modern humans acquired some genes in the immune system (known as human leukocyte antigen, or HLA genes) from the Neanderthals and their relatives the Denisovans. These alleles help the body recognize foreign microbial invaders; and scientists now believe that the transfer of these genes to modern humans "significantly shaped modern human immune systems" (Abi-Rached 2011, 89) and may have helped our fully modern ancestors survive in European and Asian regions containing unfamiliar pathogens that could have killed them. The Neanderthal and Denisovan versions of these HLA genes have been found in current populations in Europe and Asia. In fact, Peter Parham from the Stanford

University School of Medicine proposes that "Europeans owe 50% of variants of one class of HLA gene to interbreeding, Asians 70–80%, and Papua New Guineans up to 95%"(Callaway 2011, 137).

20. Gibbons 2010, 680.

21. Mellars 1989.

22. It is estimated that the Denisovans split off from the Neanderthals some 400,000 years ago. Genetic evidence of these people comes from two molar teeth and a child's finger bone, all found in Denisova cave in Altai Kria, Russia (Reich et al. 2010). An elegant stone bracelet and several stone tools were found in the same location (Gibbons 2011). Denisovans must have had sex with *Homo sapiens sapiens*, for Denisovan DNA is found today among Papua New Guineans, Australian aborigines, and groups of people in Southeast Asia. Denisova cave was a comfortable three-room cavern with a natural vent for a chimney, so it attracted other visitors as well. Among them were Neanderthals coming from Europe and the Middle East and *Homo sapiens*. All hunted bear, lynx, and wild boar in this part of Siberia some 30,000 to 50,000 years ago. These three types of humanity were not the first to move in, however. This mountainous region was also popular with earlier *Homo erectus* men and women who camped in the Altai Mountains some 800,000 years ago. They abandoned the area when a cold spell became intolerable, but returned some 300,000 years ago. The cave has been used ever since.

23. Gladkih et al. 1984.

24. White 1986; Mellars 1989.

25. White 1989a, 1989b.

26. Early ceramics—a ritual purpose? Archaeological remains from eastern Europe suggest that these figurines were used in ceremonies. On the lower slopes of the Pavlov Hills, in what is today modern Moravia, our ancestors built their homes overlooking the confluence of two meandering rivers some 26,000 years ago. Eighty meters above their village on the rocky slope, they made a circular depression domed on two sides—one of several kilns found in this area. In it were thousands of shattered fragments of hard, durable ceramic figurines made of mammoth fat mixed with bone ash, local loess, and a bit of clay. Only one sculpture from these sites in Moravia remains intact, a wolverine the size of your fist. Either our ancestors were dreadful potters, or they intentionally blew up their art in order to divine or for some other ritual purpose (Vandiver et al. 1989).

27. Fox 1972, 1980; Bischof 1975b; Frayser 1985.

28. Cohen 1964; Fox 1980; Malinowski 1965.

29. Tylor 1889.

30. Inbreeding: It often takes many generations of extremely close inbreeding before harmful genes become selected and dreaded diseases emerge in a family line. In fact, a certain amount of inbreeding is necessary to accentuate positive traits; this is why people breed dogs for temperament or endurance, for example. For good genetic health, a species needs enough inbreeding to fix positive traits and enough outbreeding to mask deleterious recessive genes. So although the incest taboo (mating with nuclear-family members) is universal, marriages between first cousins are obligatory or preferred in many societies (Bischof 1975; Daly and Wilson 1983).

31. Westermarck 1934.

32. Spiro 1958.

33. Shepher 1971, 1983.

34. Bischof 1975b; de Waal 1989.

35. Sade 1968; Bischof 1975b.

36. Bischof 1975b; de Waal 1989; Daly and Wilson 1983.

37. Frayser 1985, 182.

38. Frazer [1922] 1963, 702.
39. Darwin 1871, 47.
40. Fox 1972, 292.
41. Ibid, 287.
42. Damasio et al. 1994.
43. Damon 1988; Kohlberg 1969.
44. Kohlberg 1969; Gilligan and Wiggins 1988; Damon 1988; Kagan and Lamb 1987.
45. See Haidt 2012.
46. See ibid.
47. De Waal, 1996.
48. Ibid., 12.
49. Ibid., 88.
50. Darwin 1871, 493.
51. Haidt 2012, 209.
52. Trinkaus and Shipman 1993, Lebel et al. 2001.

## CHAPTER 14: FICKLE PASSION

1. Shostak 1981; Gregor 1985.
2. Shostak 1981, 226.
3. The Herero are cattle-tending peoples who settled in the area of the Dobe !Kung in the mid-1920s.
4. Private sex: Around the world people seek privacy for coitus. Chimpanzees, baboons, and other primates occasionally usher a partner behind a bush to copulate, but normally primates have intercourse within view of community members. The human drive to seek private, uninterrupted, concealed sex is probably another trait born on the African veldt as our ancient forebears began to pair millions of years ago.
5. Foreplay: The people of Ponape and the Trobriand Islanders of the insular Pacific spend hours at foreplay, whereas the Lepcha of Sikkim do almost no precopulatory caressing. The amount of foreplay varies from one society to the next. From a survey of worldwide studies of foreplay, Goldstein (1976a) lists types of precoital contact in descending order of worldwide prevalence. General body fondling is most important; we seem instinctively to hug, pat, and stroke before making love. "Simple kissing," mouth-to-mouth contact, was next, although new data suggest that kissing has not been as prevalent as was once thought (Ford and Beach 1951; Jankowiak et al. in press, 2015). Fondling the woman's breasts comes next, then touching the woman's genitals, oral stimulation of her breasts, caressing the man's genitals, fellatio, cunnilingus, anilingus, and, last, painful stimulations of body parts (B. Goldstein 1976). Other species also engage in foreplay. Birds tap their bills together. Dogs lick. Whales stroke each other with their flippers. Most birds and mammals engage in some sort of pre-copulatory fondling.
6. Couvade: Several societies in the world have an institution known as the couvade, from the French *couver*, "to incubate or hatch." This custom dictates that the father imitate some of his wife's behavior during and around pregnancy and birth. In some cultures the man acts out the physical pain of childbirth; in others he may simply observe certain dietary taboos. The Mehinaku demand only some dietary restrictions. Occasionally, if the father is not the woman's husband, he will follow the restrictions of the couvades; more often he forgoes these traditions, lest he reveal his relationship with the newborn's mother.
7. Puberty rituals: Most cultures mark puberty with ceremonies for both boys and girls, so it is likely that in our ancestry both genders underwent puberty rituals

prior to wedding. Because arranged first marriages are also common around the world, it is probable that among our ancestors, parents regularly selected the *first* spouse for an adolescent child. See Frayser 1985.

8. Premarital sex: In most cultures of the insular Pacific and in many parts of sub-Saharan Africa and Eurasia, people traditionally tolerated premarital sex. In many places around the Mediterranean, premarital sex was traditionally strictly forbidden. In 82% of 61 cultures recorded, the same limitations (or lack of restrictions) applied to both sexes equally; in these societies there was no double standard with regard to premarital sex. In those cultures where there was a double standard, the boy sometimes got harsher punishment than his girlfriend; many of these societies were in sub-Saharan Africa (Frayser 1985, 205).

9. Age at menarche: Today the median age at menarche for American white girls is 12.8; for American black girls it is 12.5. Early puberty is also common in contemporary European populations. Age at menarche has slowly declined over the last 150 years in American and European cultures. In 1840 the average age at menarche was 16.5–17.5 in several European peoples. This is not to suggest that menarche has been getting progressively earlier throughout human evolution. Among the classical Greeks and Romans, girls may have reached menarche as early as age 13 or 14 (Eveleth 1986). As you recall, among hunting-gathering peoples girls generally reach menarche between ages 16 and 17, suggesting that menarche occurred during late teenage in pehistoric populations (Lancaster and Lancaster 1983).

10. Clark 1980; Cohen 1989.

## CHAPTER 15: "TILL DEATH US DO PART"

1. Gregg 1988.
2. Ibid.
3. Nissen 1988; Clark 1980; Lewin 1988a; McCorriston and Hole 1991; Blumler and Byrne 1991.
4. Whyte 1978.
5. Bullough 1976, 53.
6. Abortion was not always illegal in Western history. The ancient Greeks, for example, believed in small families and approved of abortion. Abortion laws have varied dramatically in Western history, according to varying social circumstances.
7. Whyte 1978.
8. Lacey 1973; Gies and Gies 1978; Lampe 1987.
9. Colossians 3:18.
10. Hunt 1959, 22.
11. Whyte 1978.
12. Social subordination of women in agrarian cultures: A survey of 93 preindustrial societies shows that women in peasant farming communities had less domestic authority, less ritual solidarity with other women, and less control over property than did women in gardening and hunting-gathering cultures. Women's work was less valued, and less importance was placed on women's lives (Whyte 1978).
13. Leacock 1972; Etiene and Leacock 1980.
14. Evolution of chiefdoms: Johnson and Earle (1987) argue that European political organization characterized by permanent "big men," or chiefs, arose in the Upper Paleolithic between 35,000 and 12,000 B.P. because of large-scale hunting and territorial defense in highly populated areas of Europe, but that chiefs became commonplace in Europe with the introduction of agriculture.
15. Whyte 1978, 169.
16. See Fisher 1999.

17. See ibid.
18. See ibid.
19. Ibid.
20. Goody 1983, 211; Queen and Habenstein 1974.
21. Bullough 1976; Lacey 1973.
22. Hunt 1959, 63; Carcopino 1973, 60; Phillips 1988.
23. Matthew 19:3–9.
24. Phillips 1988.
25. Gies and Gies 1978; Bell 1973; Bullough 1978; Hunt 1959; Phillips 1988.
26. Gies and Gies 1978, 33.
27. Queen and Habenstein 1974, 265.
28. Gies and Gies 1978, 18; Dupâquier et al. 1981.
29. Bell 1973; Power 1973; Abrams 1973.
30. Phillips 1988.
31. Goody 1983, 211; Dupâquier et al. 1981; Phillips 1988; Stone 1990.

## CHAPTER 16: FUTURE SEX

1. Lucretius 1965.
2. Divorce rate: The divorce rate is much more difficult to estimate than is generally thought. The number of individuals who divorce per year per 1,000 married persons has no direct correlation with your chances of divorcing during the course of your life. To compute divorce rate, demographers use the "life table approach." They examine the lifetime divorce experience of adults in several successive age cohorts and establish all the factors that contributed to the frequency of divorce over time among the individuals in these cohorts. Then they evaluate the present impact of all these factors, anticipate new factors that could contribute to divorce, and compile all these data to estimate how many people will divorce this year and in coming decades (Cherlin 1981, 25).
3. Cherlin 1981, 53; Levitan et al. 1988, 32, 99; Glick 1975, 8; Espenshade 1985; Cherlin 2009.
4. Klinenberg 2012.
5. See Cherlin 2009; Coontz 2005.
6. Cherlin 2009.
7. Harris 1981; Levitan et al. 1988; Coontz 2005.
8. Evans 1987; Harris 1981; Cherlin 1981; Levitan et al. 1988; Cherlin 2009.
9. Cherlin 2009.
10. Cherlin 1981, 35.
11. Harris 1981.
12. Glick 1975; Levitan et al. 1988.
13. Birth control and divorce: Some scientists argue that the introduction of the birth control pill, the intrauterine device, and surgical sterilization all played significant roles in the declining birthrate in the 1960s and subsequent decades. But the birthrate was low during the Great Depression, when couples in economic crisis wanted to postpone family life and these modern means of birth control were not available (Cherlin 1981, 57). Birthrates also fell in the early 1960s, before these contraceptive methods became widely available (Harris 1981). So sociologist Andrew Cherlin (1981) concluded that these forms of contraception were not major forces in the 1960s trend toward later marriage, fewer children, and more divorce. In fact, birthrates have been declining over the last hundred years, long before technological changes in contraception occurred (Goldin 1990). These new forms of birth control may have affected demo-

graphic trends in other ways, however. By using these devices, more unmarried women can avoid pregnancy; thus fewer women may marry very young—probably increasing the average age at first marriage and enabling more women to enter the job market sooner.

14. Harris 1981, 93.
15. Evans 1987.
16. Cherlin 1981; Klinenberg 2012.
17. Cherlin 1981; Klinenberg 2012; Levitan et al. 1988.
18. Cherlin 2009. Although the divorce rate in the U.S. peaked in the late 1970s and early 1980s, it has been declining since then among college-educated couples; today two-thirds of these marriages are likely to remain stable long-term due to several forces. Among them, these men and women tend to marry later; moreover, both spouses share household duties and both work outside the home to create a stable economic unit. Because many of these people live together before marrying, their unhappy relationships tend to dissolve before wedding. And because most of these people practice birth control, "shotgun" marriages are less common. Yet divorce among less educated people is likely to remain high. And divorce rates are likely to continue to be much higher in all socioeconomic classes than during our agrarian past.
19. Cherlin 2009.
20. Kreider 2006.
21. Ibid.
22. Levitan et al. 1988; London and Foley Wilson 1988; Glick 1975; Cherlin 1981; Furstenberg and Spanier 1984.
23. Coontz 2005.
24. "Singles in America:" 2010, 2011, 2012, 2013, 2014.
25. Cherlin 2009, 139.
26. Ibid., 16; Pew Research Center, Feb. 2013.
27. "Singles in America" 2013.
28. Ibid. 2014.
29. Buss 1994.
30. Apostolou 2007.
31. Cherlin 2009, 26.
32. Sassler and Kusi-Appouh 2011.
33. Cherlin 2009.
34. Garcia et al. 2012; Garcia and Fisher 2015.
35. Monto and Carey 2013.
36. Garcia and Reiber 2008.
37. Meston and Buss 2007.
38. Carmichael et al. 1987; Zak 2008, 2012; Young et al. 1998.
39. Hughes et al. 2007.
40. Mead 1966; Kirkendall and Gravatt 1984.
41. Pew Research Center, 2008.
42. Cherlin 2009.
43. O'Leary et al. 2011.
44. Ipsos 2014.
45. Zentner 2005.
46. See Rudder 2013.
47. "Singles in America" 2014.
48. Ibid. 2013.
49. Alexander and Fisher 2003.
50. Whyte 1978.
51. See Fisher 1999; Baumeister 2000; Diamond 2008.

52. Meston and Buss 2007; Baumeister et al. 2001.
53. Gray and Garcia 2013.
54. "Singles in America" 2013.
55. Gray and Garcia 2013, 203.
56. Mah and Binik 2002.
57. "Singles in America" 2014.
58. Ibid. 2014, 2012.
59. Ibid. 2011.
60. Rudder 2014, 180.
61. "Singles in America" 2011, 2012, 2013, 2014.
62. Klinenberg 2012, 100.
63. Pew Research Center 2013.
64. Hatfield and Rapson 1996.
65. "Singles in America" 2014.
66. Ibid. 2011.
67. Ibid. 2012.
68. Ibid. 2011.
69. Klinenberg 2012, 162.
70. Klinenberg 2012.
71. Zeki and Romaya 2010.
72. "Singles in America" 2011.
73. Ibid. 2010, 2011, 2012, 2013, 2014.
74. Klinenberg 2012; Cherlin 2009.
75. Klinenberg 2012.
76. Ibid.
77. Ibid.
78. Ibid.
79. Meston and Frohlic 2000.
80. Fisher and Thomson 2007.
81. These antidepressants may also affect one's feelings of deep *attachment* to a partner, due to their negative effect on the sex drive. Even the newer serotonin boosters, such as Effexor and Cymbalta (which elevate the norepinephrine system as well as serotonin), can interfere with sexual desire, sexual arousal, sexual performance and orgasm. Reports suggest that as many as 73% of patients taking serotonin-enhancing antidepressants suffer one or more of these sexual side effects (Montejo et al. 2001). These sexual side effects can have serious ramifications. With orgasm, men and women experience a flood of oxytocin and vasopressin—chemicals that produce feelings of trust and attachment. No sex; no orgasm; no flood of these cuddle chemicals. Moreover, a woman does not reach orgasm with every coupling and I am among those who believe this fickle female response is an adaptive mechanism by which a woman distinguishes a patient, empathic Mr. Right from a self-centered Mr. Wrong. These pills may jeopardize a woman's ability to select a suitable mate. Last, with orgasm, a man deposits seminal fluid in the vaginal canal—fluid that contains dopamine, norepinephrine, oxytocin, vasopressin, and other chemicals that can potentially push a woman over the threshold into falling in love or feeling deep attachment for her partner. No male orgasm; no hidden persuaders; no new girlfriend. As these drugs alter an individual's courtship and mating tactics, they can potentially affect their genetic future too.
82. Morais 2004, 120.
83. Earp et al. forthcoming.
84. Young 2009, 148.
85. Bohannan 1985.

# BIBLIOGRAPHY

Abi-Rached, L., M. J. Jobin, S. Kulkaini, et al. 2011. The Shaping of Modern Human Immune Systems by Multiregional Admixture with Archaic Humans. *Science* 334: 89.

Abrams, A. 1973. Medieval women and trade. In *Women: From the Greeks to the French Revolution*, ed. S. G. Bell. Stanford: Stanford Univ. Press.

Abu-Lughod, L. 1986. *Veiled sentiments: Honor and poetry in a Bedouin society.* Berkeley: Univ. of California Press.

———. 1987. Bedouin blues. *Natural History*, July, 24–34.

Acevedo, B., and A. Aron. 2009. Does a long-term relationship kill romantic love? *Review of General Psychology* 13(1): 59–65.

Acevedo, B., A. Aron, H. Fisher, L. Brown. 2011. Neural correlates of long-term intense romantic love. *Social Cognitive and Affective Neuroscience* doi: 10.1093/scan/nsq092.

——— 2012a. Neural correlates of marital satisfaction and well-being: Reward, empathy, and affect. *Clinical Neuropsychiatry*, 9 (1): 20–31.

——— 2012b. Neural correlates of long-term intense romantic love. *Social Cognitive and Affective Neuroscience* 7:145–59.

Ackerman, C. 1963. Affiliations: Structural determinants of differential divorce rates. *American Journal of Sociology* 69:13–20.

Ackerman, D. 1990. *The natural history of the senses.* New York: Random House.

Ackerman, S. 1989. European history gets even older. *Science* 246:28–29.

Adams, D. B., A. R. Gold, and A. D. Burt. 1978. Rise in female-initiated sexual activity at ovulation and its suppression by oral contraceptives. *New England Journal of Medicine* 299:1145–50.

Adams, V. 1980. Getting at the heart of jealous love. *Psychology Today*, May, 38–48.

Aharon, I., N. Etcoff, D. Ariely, et al. 2001. Beautiful Faces have Variable Reward Value: fMRI and Behavioral Evidence. *Neuron* 32:537–551.

Aiello, L. C., and P. Wheeler. 1995. The expensive tissue hypothesis: the brain and digestive system in human and primate evolution. *Current Anthropology* 36:199–221.

Ainsworth, M. D. S., M. C. Blehar, E. Waters, and S. Wall. 1978. *Patterns of Attachment: A psychological study of the strange situation.* Hillsdale, NJ: Erlbaum.

Alcock, J. 1987. Ardent adaptationism. *Natural History*, April, 4.

Alemseged, Z., F. Spoor, W. H. Kimbel, et al. 2006. A juvenile early hominin skeleton from Dikika, Ethiopia. *Nature* 443:296–310.

Alexander, M. G., and T. D. Fisher. 2003. Truth and consequences: using the bogus pipeline to examine sex difference in self-reported sexuality. *Journal of Sex Research* 40(1):27–35.

Alexander, R. D. 1974. The evolution of social behavior. *Annual Review of Ecology and Systematics* 5:325–83.

———. 1987. *The biology of moral systems.* New York: Aldine de Gruyter.

———. 1990. *How did humans evolve?* Museum of Zoology, University of Michigan, Special Publication no. 1.

Alexander, R. D., and K. M. Noonan. 1979. Concealment of ovulation, parental care and human social evolution. In *Evolutionary Biology and Human Social Behavior,* ed. N. A. Chagnon and W. Irons. North Scituate, MA: Duxbury Press.

Alford, R. R., and R. Friedland. 1985. *Powers of theory: Capitalism, the state, and democracy.* New York: Cambridge Univ. Press.

Allen, E. S., and D. H. Baucom. 2001. *Patterns of infidelity.* Poster presented at the annual meeting of the Association for Advancement of Behavior Therapy, Philadelphia, PA, November.

Allen, E. S., G. K. Rhoades, S. M. Stanley, et al. 2008. Premarital precursors of marital infidelity. *Family Process* 47: 243–59.

Allen, L. L., P. S. Bridges, D. L. Evon, et al. 1982. Demography and human origins. *American Anthropologist* 84:888–96.

Allen, M. 1981. Individual copulatory preference and the "Strange female effect" in a captive group-living male chimpanzee *(Pan troglodytes). Primates* 22:221–36.

Altschuler, M. 1971. Cayapa personality and sexual motivation. In *Human Sexual Behavior,* ed. D. S. Marshall and R. C. Suggs. Englewood Cliffs, NJ: Prentice-Hall.

Amato, P. R., and C. Dorius. 2010. Fathers, children, and divorce. In *The role of the father in child development.* 5th edition ed. M. E. Lamb, 177–200. New York: John Wiley & Sons.

Ambrose, S. H. 1986. Comment on: H. T. Bunn and E. M. Kroll, Systematic butchery by Plio/Pleistocene hominids at Olduvai Gorge, Tanzania. *Current Anthropology* 27:431–53.

Andersson, M. 1994. *Sexual selection.* Princeton, NJ: Princeton Univ. Press.

Andrews, P. 1981. Species diversity and diet in monkeys and apes during the Miocene. In *Aspects of human evolution,* ed. C. B. Stringer. London: Taylor and Francis.

Andrews, P., and J. E. Cronin. 1982. The relationships of *Sivapithecus* and *Ramapithecus* and the evolution of the orang-utan. *Nature* 297:541–46.

Andrews, P., and J. A. H. Van Couvering. 1975. Palaeoenvironments in the East African Miocene. In *Approaches to primate paleobiology,* ed. F. S. Szalay. Basel: S. Karger.

Andrews, P. W., J. A. Thomson Jr., A. Amstadter, and M. C. Neale. 2012. Primum non nocere: an evolutionary analysis of whether antidepressants do more harm than good. *Frontiers in Evolutionary Psychology* 3:117.

Angier, N. 1990. Mating for life? It's not for the birds or the bees. *New York Times,* August 21.

Apicella, C. L., D. R. Feinberg, and F. W. Marlow. 2007. Voice pitch predicts reproductive success in male hunter-gatherers. *Biology Letters* 3:682–84.

Apostolou, M. 2007. Sexual selection under parental choice: The role of parents in the evolution of human mating. *Evolution and Human Behavior* 28(6): 403–9.

Arensburg, B., A. M. Tillier, B. Vandermeersch, et al. 1989. A middle paleolithic human hyoid bone. *Nature* 338:758–60.

Aron, A., E. Aron, and C. C. Norman. 2001. Self-expansion model of motivation and cognition in close relationships and beyond. In *Blackwell handbook of social psychology: Interpersonal processes*, ed. G. J. O. Fletcher and M. Clark, 478–501. Malden, MA: Blackwell.

Aron, A., H. E. Fisher, D. J. Mashek, et al. 2005. Reward, Motivation and Emotion Systems Associated with Early-Stage Intense Romantic Love: An fMRI study. *Journal of Neurophysiology* 94:327–37.

Aron, E. and A. Aron. 1996. Love and expansion of the self: The state of the model. *Personal Relationships* 3:45–58.

Atwater, L. 1987. College students extramarital involvement. *Sexuality Today*, Nov. 30, 2.

Avery, C. S. 1989. How do you build intimacy in an age of divorce? *Psychology Today*, May, 27–31.

Axelrod, D. I., and P. H. Raven. 1977. Late Cretaceous and tertiary vegetation history in Africa. In *Biogeography and ecology of southern Africa*, ed. M. J. A. Werger. The Hague: Junk.

Badrian, A., and N. Badrian. 1984. Social organization of *Pan paniscus* in the Lomako Forest, Zaire. In *The pygmy chimpanzee*, ed. R. L. Susman. New York: Plenum Press.

Badrian, N., and R. K. Malenky. 1984. Feeding ecology of *Pan paniscus* in the Lomako Forest, Zaire. In *The pygmy chimpanzee*, ed. R. L. Susman. New York: Plenum Press.

Bailey, J. M., and R. C. Pillard. 1991. A genetic study of male sexual orientation. *Archives of General Psychiatry* 48(12): 1089–96.

Bailey, N. W., and M. Zuk. 2009. Same sex sexual behavior and evolution. *Trends in Ecology and Evolution* 24(8): 439–46.

Baker, R. 1996. Sperm wars: the science of sex. New York: Basic Books.

Baker, R. R. and M. A. Bellis. 1995. *Human sperm competition*. London: Chapman and Hall.

Balsdon, J. P. V. D. 1973. Roman women: Their history and habits. In *Women: From the Greeks to the French Revolution*, ed. S. G. Bell. Stanford, CA: Stanford Univ. Press.

Barash, D. P. 1977. *Sociology and behavior*. New York: Elsevier.

Bardis, P. 1963. Main features of the ancient Roman family. *Social Science* 38 (Oct.): 225–40.

Barnes, J. 1967. The frequency of divorce. In *The craft of social anthropology*, ed. A. L. Epstein. London: Tavistock.

Baron-Cohen S. 2003a. *The essential difference: Men, women and the extreme male brain*. London: Allen Lane.

———. 2003b. The extreme male brain theory of autism. *Trends in Cognitive Sciences* 6: 248–54.

Baron-Cohen, S., R. C. Knickmeyer, and M. K. Belmonte. 2005. Sex differences in the brain: Implications of explaining autism. *Science* 310: 819–23.

Barraza, J., and P. J. Zak. 2009. Empathy toward strangers triggers oxytocin release and subsequent generosity. *Annuals of the New York Academy of Sciences* 1167:182–89.

Barrett, N. 1987. Women and the economy. In *The American woman, 1987–88*, ed. Sara E. Rix. New York: W. W. Norton.

Barringer, F. 1989a. U.S. birth level nears 4 million mark. *New York Times*, Oct. 31.

———. 1989b. Divorce data stir doubt on trial marriage. *New York Times*, June 9.

———. 1991. Changes in U.S. households: Single parents amid solitude. *New York Times*, June 7.

Bartels, A., and S. Zeki. 2000. The neural basis of romantic love. *NeuroReport* 11:3829–34.

———. 2004. The neural correlates of maternal and romantic love. *NeuroImage* 21: 1155–66.

Bateman, A. J. 1948. Intra-sexual selection in drosophila. *Heredity* 2:349–68.

Baumeister, R. F. 2000. Gender differences in erotic plasticity: The female sex drive as socially flexible and responsive. *Psychological Bulletin* 126:347–74.

Baumeister, R. F., K. R. Catanese, and K. D. Vohs. 2001. Is there a gender difference in strength of sex drive? Theoretical views, conceptual distinctions, and a review of relevant evidence. *Personality and Social Psychology Reviews* 5:242–73.

Baumeister, R. F., S. R. Wotman, and A. M. Stillwell. 1993. Unrequited love: On heartbreak, anger, guilt, scriptlessness and humiliation. *Journal of Personality and Social Psychology* 64:377–94.

Beals, R. L. 1946. *Cherán: A Sierra Tarascan village*. Smithsonian Institution, Institute of Social Anthropology, Publication no. 2. Washington, DC: Government Printing Office.

Beardsley, R. K., J. W. Hall, and R. E. Ward. 1959. *Village Japan*. Chicago: Univ. of Chicago Press.

Behrensmeyer, K. 1984. Taphonomy and the fossil record. *American Scientist* 72:558–66.

Behrensmeyer, K., and A. P. Hill. 1980. *Fossils in the making*. Chicago: Univ. of Chicago Press.

Belkin, L. 1989. Bars to equality of sexes seen as eroding, slowly. *New York Times*, Aug. 20.

Bell, A. P., and S. Weinberg. 1978. *Homosexualities: A study of diversity among men and women*. New York: Simon and Schuster.

Bell, D. 1980. Desert politics: Choices in the "marriage market." In *Women and Colonization*, ed. Mona Etienne and Eleanor Leacock. New York: Praeger.

Bell, J. 1995. Notions of love and romance among the Taita of Kenya. In *Romantic Passion: A universal experience?* ed. W. Jankowiak. New York: Columbia Univ. Press.

Bell, S. G., ed. 1973. *Women: From the Greeks to the French Revolution*. Stanford, CA: Stanford Univ. Press.

Benbow, C. P., and J. C. Stanley. 1980. Sex differences in mathematical ability: Fact or artifact. *Science* 210:1234–36.

———. 1983. Sex differences in mathematical reasoning ability: More facts. *Science* 222:1029–31.

Benderly, B. L. 1987. *The myth of two minds: What gender means and doesn't mean*. New York: Doubleday.

———. 1989. Don't believe everything you read: A case study of how the politics of sex differences research turned a small finding into a major media flap. *Psychology Today*, Nov., 63–66.

Benshoof, L., and R. Thornhill. 1979. The evolution of monogamy and concealed ovulation in humans. *Journal of Social and Biological Structures* 2:95–106.

Berger, J. 1986. *Wild horses of the Great Basin: Social competition and population size.* Chicago: Univ. of Chicago Press.

Berggren, W. A., and C. D. Hollister. 1977. Plate tectonics and paleocirculation—Commotion in the ocean. *Tectonophysics* 38:11–48.

Bernard, J. 1964. The adjustment of married mates. In *Handbook of marriage and the family,* ed. H. I. Christensen. Chicago: Rand McNally.

Berndt, C. H. 1981. Interpretations and "facts" in aboriginal Australia. In *Woman the gatherer,* ed. F. Dahlberg. New Haven: Yale Univ. Press.

Bernor, R. L. 1985. Neogene palaeoclimatic events and continental mammalian response: Is there global synchroneity? *South African Journal of Science* 81:261.

Berremann, G. 1962. Pahari polyandry: A comparison. *American Anthropologist* 64:60–75.

Bertram, B. C. R. 1975. Social factors influencing reproduction in wild lions. *Journal of Zoology* 177:463–82.

Bester-Meredith, J. K., L. J. Young, and C. A. Marler. 1999. Species differences in paternal behavior and aggression in *Peromyscus* and their associations with vasopressin immunoreactivity and receptors. *Hormones and Behavior* 36: 25–38, 212–21.

Betzig, L. L. 1982. Despotism and differential reproduction: A cross-cultural correlation of conflict asymmetry, hierarchy and degree of polygyny. *Ethology and Sociobiology* 3:209–21.

———. 1986. *Despotism and differential reproduction: A Darwinian view of history.* Hawthorne, NY: Aldine.

———. 1989. Causes of conjugal dissolution: A cross-cultural study. *Current Anthropology* 30:654–76.

Betzig, L., A. Harrigan, and P. Turke. 1989. Childcare on Ifaluk. *Zeitschrift für Ethnologie* 114:161–77.

Bieber, I., H. J. Dain, P. R. Dince, et al. 1962. *Homosexuality: A psychoanalytic study of male homosexuals.* New York: Basic Books.

Binford, L. R. 1981. *Bones: Ancient men and modern myths.* New York: Academic Press.

———. 1985. Human ancestors: Changing views of their behavior. *Journal of Anthropological Archaeology* 4:292–327.

———. 1987. The hunting hypothesis: Archaeological methods and the past. *Yearbook of Physical Anthropology* 30:1–9.

Birdsell, J. B. 1968. Some predictions for the Pleistocene based on equilibrium systems among recent hunter-gatherers. In *Man the Hunter,* ed. R. B. Lee and I. DeVore. New York: Aldine.

———. 1979. Ecological influences on Australian aboriginal social organization. In *Primate ecology and human origins,* ed. I. S. Bernstein and E. O. Smith. New York: Garland STPM Press.

Birkhead, T., and A. P. Moller. 1998. Sperm competition and sexual selection. New York: Academic Press.

Bischof, N. 1975a. A systems approach toward the functional connections of attachment and fear. *Child Development* 46:801–17.

———. 1975b. Comparative ethology of incest avoidance. In *Biosocial anthropology*, ed. R. Fox. London: Malaby Press.

Blake, J. 1989a. *Family size and achievement.* Berkeley: Univ. of California Press.

———. 1989b. Number of siblings and educational attainment. *Science* 245:32–36.

Blumenschine, R. J. 1986. *Early hominid scavenging opportunities: Implications for carcass availability in the Serengeti and Ngorongoro ecosystems.* British Archaeological Reports International Series, no. 283. Oxford: BAR.

———. 1987. Characteristics of an early hominid scavenging niche. *Current Anthropology* 28:383–407.

———. 1989. A landscape taphonomic model of the scale of prehistoric scavenging opportunities. *Journal of Human Evolution* 18:345–71.

Blumler, M. A., and R. Byrne. 1991. The ecological genetics of domestication and the origins of agriculture. *Current Anthropology* 32:23–54.

Blumstein, P., and P. Schwartz. 1983. *American couples: Money, work, sex.* New York: William Morrow.

Blurton-Jones, N. G. 1984. A selfish origin for human sharing: Tolerated theft. *Ethology and Sociobiology* 5:1–3.

Boesch, C., and A. Boesch. 1984. Mental map in wild chimpanzees: An analysis of hammer transports for nut cracking. *Primates* 25:160–70.

Bohannan, P. 1985. *All the happy families: Exploring the varieties of family life.* New York: McGraw-Hill.

Bonnefille, R. 1985. Evolution of the continental vegetation: The palaeobotanical record from East Africa. *South African Journal of Science* 81:267–70.

Borgerhoff Mulder, M. 1990. Kipsigis women's preferences for wealthy men: Evidence for female choice in mammals? *Behavioral Ecology and Sociobiology* 27:255–64.

Botwin, C. 1988. *Men who can't be faithful.* New York: Warner Books.

Bower, B. 1984. Fossil find may be earliest known hominid. *Science News* 125:230.

———. 1985. A mosaic ape takes shape. *Science News* 127:26–27.

———. 1986. The math gap: Puzzling sex differences. *Science News* 130:357.

———. 1988a. Ancient human ancestors got all fired up. *Science News* 134:372.

———. 1988b. Retooled ancestors. *Science News* 133:344–45.

———. 1989. Conflict enters early European farm life. *Science News* 136:165.

———. 1990. Average attractions: Psychologists break down the essence of physical beauty. *Science News* 137:298–99.

———. 1991. Darwin's minds. *Science News* 140:232–34.

Bowlby, J. 1969. *Attachment and loss.* Vol. 1, *Attachment.* New York: Basic Books.

———. 1973. *Attachment and loss.* Vol. 2, *Separation.* New York: Basic Books.

Brain, C. K. 1981. *The hunters or the hunted? An introduction to African cave taphonomy.* Chicago: Univ. of Chicago Press.

Brain, C. K., and A. Sillen. 1988. Evidence from the Swartkrans cave for the earliest use of fire. *Nature*, 336:464–66.

Bramble, D. M., and D. E. Lieberman. 2004. Endurance running and the evolution of *Homo. Nature* 432:345–52.

Brand, R. J., C. M. Markey, A. Mills, and S. D. Hodges. 2007. Sex differences in self-reported infidelity and its correlates. *Sex Roles,* 57:101–9.

Brandwein, N., J. MacNeice, and P. Spiers. 1982. *The group house handbook: How to live with others (and love it).* Reston, VA: Acropolis.

Bray, O. E., J. J. Kennelly, and J. L. Guarino. 1975. Fertility of eggs produced on territories of vasectomized red-winged blackbirds. *Wilson Bulletin* 87:187–95.

Briggs, J. L. 1970. *Never in anger: Portrait of an Eskimo family.* Cambridge, MA: Harvard Univ. Press.

Brink, A. S. 1957. The spontaneous fire-controlling reactions of two chimpanzee smoking addicts. *South African Journal of Science* 53:241–47.

Brod, H. 1987. Who benefits from male involvement in wife's pregnancy? *Marriage and Divorce Today* 12 (46): 3.

Bromage, T. G. 1987. The biological and chronological maturation of early hominids. *Journal of Human Evolution* 16:257–72.

Brown, E. 1987. The hidden meaning: An analysis of different types of affairs. *Marriage and Divorce Today* 12 (44): 1.

Brown, F., J. Harris, R. Leakey et al. 1985. Early *Homo erectus* skeleton from West Lake Turkana, Kenya. *Nature* 316:788–92.

Brown, L. L., B. P. Acevedo, and H. E. Fisher. 2013. Neural correlates of four broad temperament dimensions: Testing predictions for a novel construct of personality. *PLoS One* 8(11): e78734.

Brown, P. 1988. *The Body and Society: Men, women and sexual renunciation in early Christianity.* New York: Columbia Univ. Press.

Bullough, V. L. 1976. *Sexual variance in society and history.* Chicago: Univ. of Chicago Press.

Bullough, V. L., and B. Bullough. 1987. *Women and prostitution: A social history.* Buffalo, NY: Prometheus.

Bunn, H. T., and E. M. Kroll. 1986. Systematic butchery by Plio/Pleistocene hominids at Olduvai Gorge, Tanzania. *Current Anthropology* 27:431–53.

Burch, E. S., Jr., and T. C. Correll. 1972. Alliance and conflict: Interregional relations in north Alaska. In *Alliance in Eskimo society*, ed. L. Guemple. Seattle: Univ. of Washington Press.

Burgess, E. W., and L. S. Cottrell. 1939. *Predicting success and failure in marriage.* New York: Prentice-Hall.

Burleson, M. H., and W. R. Trevathan. 1990. Non-ovulatory sexual activity: Possible physiological effects on women's lifetime reproductive success. Paper presented at the annual meeting of the Human Behavior and Evolution Society, Los Angeles.

Burley, N. 1979. The evolution of concealed ovulation. *American Naturalist* 114:835–58.

Burns, G. 1990. The 21st Century Family. *Newsweek Special Edition*, Winter/Spring, 10.

Burton, F. D. 1971. Sexual climax in female *Macaca mulatta*. In *Proceedings of the Third International Congress of Primatology, Zurich 1970*, 3:180–91. Basel: Karger.

Buss, D. M. 1989. Sex differences in human mate preferences: Evolutionary hypotheses tested in 37 cultures. *Behavioral and Brain Sciences* 12:1–49.

———.1994. *The Evolution of Desire: Strategies of human mating.* New York: Basic Books.

———. 2000. *The dangerous passion: Why jealousy is as necessary as love and sex.* New York: Free Press.

Bygott, J. D. 1974. Agonistic behavior and dominance in wild chimpanzees. PhD thesis, Univ. of Cambridge.

———. 1979. Agonistic behavior, dominance and social structure in wild chimpanzees of the Gombe National Park. In *The Great Apes*, ed. D. A. Hamburg and E. R. McCown. Menlo Park, CA: Benjamin/Cummings.

Byrne, G. 1989. Overhaul urged for math teaching. *Science* 243:597.

Cacioppe, S, F. Bianchi-Demicheli, C. Frum, J. G. Pfaus, and J. W. Lewis. 2012. The common neural bases between sexual desire and love: a multilevel kernel density fMRI analysis. *J. S. Med.* 9(4): 1048–54.

Callaway, E. 2011. Ancient DNA reveals secrets of human history: Modern humans may have picked up key genes from extinct relatives. *Nature* 476:136–37.

Campbell, B., ed. 1972. *Sexual selection and the Descent of man, 1871–1971*. Chicago: Aldine.

Camperio-Ciani, A., and E. Pellizzari. 2012. Fecundity of paternal and maternal non-parental female relatives of homosexual and heterosexual men. *PLoS One* 7(12): e51088. doi:10.1371/journal.pone.0051088.

Camperio-Ciani, A., F. Corna, and C. Capiluppi. 2004. Evidence for maternally inherited factors favouring male homosexuality and promoting female fecundity. Royal Society: *Biological Sciences* 271, no. 1554 (Nov. 7, 2004): 2217–21.

Cant, J. G. H. 1981. Hypothesis for the evolution of human breasts and buttocks. *American Naturalist* 117:199–204.

Capellanus, A. 1959. *The art of courtly love*. Trans. J. Parry. New York: Ungar.

Carcopino, J. 1973. The emancipation of the Roman matron. In *Women: From the Greeks to the French Revolution*, ed. S. G. Bell. Stanford: Stanford Univ. Press.

Carmichael, M. S., R. Humbert, J. Dixen, et al. 1987. Plasma oxytocin increases in the human sexual response. *Journal of Clinical Endocrinology and Metabolism* 64(1): 27–31.

Carneiro, R. L. 1958. Extra-marital sex freedom among the Kuikuru Indians of Mato Grosso. *Revista do Museu Paulista* (São Paulo) 10:135–42.

———. 1981. The chiefdom: Precursor of the state. In *The Transition to Statehood in the New World*, ed. G. D. Jones and R. R. Kautz. New York: Cambridge Univ. Press.

———. 1987. Cross-currents in the theory of state formation. *American Ethnologist* 14:756–70.

———. 1991. The nature of the chiefdom as revealed by evidence from the Cauca Valley of Colombia. In *Profiles in cultural evolution*, ed. A. T. Rambo and K. Gillogly. Anthropology Papers, Museum of Anthropology, University of Michigan, no. 85: 167–90.

Carretero, M., J. M. Bermúdez de Castro, and E. Carbonell. 2004. Auditory capacities in Middle Pleistocene humans from the Sierra de Atapuerca in Spain. *Proceedings of the National Academy of Sciences* 101 (27): 9976–81.

———. 1998. Neuroendocrine perspectives on social attachment and love. *Psychoneuroendocrinology* 23: 779–818.

Carter, C. S. 1992. Oxytocin and sexual behavior. *Neuroscience and Biobehavioral Reviews* 1(16): 131–44.

Cavallo, J. A. 1990. Cat in the human cradle. *Natural History*, Feb., 53–60.

Cavallo, J. A., and R. Blumenschine. 1989. Tree stored leopard kills: Expanding the hominid scavenging niche. *Journal of Human Evolution* 18:393–99.

Cetron, M., and O. Davies. 1989. *American renaissance: Our life at the turn of the 21st century.* New York: St. Martin's Press.

Chagnon, N. 1982. Sociodemographic attributes of nepotism in tribal populations: Man the rule breaker. In *Current Problems in Sociobiology,* ed. B. Bertram. Cambridge, UK: Cambridge Univ. Press.

Chance, M. R. A. 1962. Social behavior and primate evolution. In *Culture and the evolution of man,* ed. M. F. A. Montagu. New York: Oxford Univ. Press.

Chance, N. A. 1966. *The Eskimo of North Alaska.* New York: Holt, Rinehart and Winston.

Chase, P. G., and H. L. Dibble. 1987. Middle Paleolithic symbolism: A review of current evidence and interpretations. *Journal of Anthropological Archaeology* 6:263–96.

Cherlin, A. J. 1978. Women's changing roles at home and on the job. *Proceedings of a conference on the national longitudinal surveys of mature women in cooperation with the employment and training administration.* Department of Labor Special Report, no. 26.

———. 1981. *Marriage, divorce, remarriage.* Cambridge, MA: Harvard Univ. Press.

———. 1987. Women and the family. In *The American woman, 1987–88,* ed. S. E. Rix. New York: Norton.

———. 2009. The marriage go-round: The state of marriage and the family in America today. New York: Knopf.

Chesters, K. I. M. 1957. The Miocene flora of Rusinga Island, Lake Victoria, Kenya. *Palaeontographica* 101B:30–67.

Chin, P. 1978. *The family.* Trans. S. Shapiro. Peking: Foreign Languages Press.

Chivers, D. J. 1978. Sexual behavior of the wild siamang. In *Recent advances in primatology.* Vol. 1, *Behavior,* ed. D. J. Chivers and J. Herbert. New York: Academic Press.

Chute, M. 1949. *Shakespeare of London.* New York: E. P. Dutton.

Ciochon, R. L., and J. G. Fleagle. 1987. Part V: *Ramapithecus* and human origins. In *Primate evolution and human origins,* ed. R. L. Ciochon and J. G. Fleagle. New York: Aldine de Gruyter.

Clark, G. 1980. *Mesolithic prelude.* Edinburgh: Edinburgh Univ. Press.

Cohen, M. N. 1977. *The Food crisis in prehistory: Overpopulation and the origins of agriculture.* New Haven: Yale Univ. Press.

———. 1980. Speculations on the evolution of density measurement and population regulation in *Homo sapiens.* In *Biosocial mechanisms of population regulation,* ed. M. N. Cohen, R. S. Malpass, and H. G. Klein. New Haven: Yale Univ. Press.

———. 1989. *Health and the rise of civilization.* New Haven: Yale Univ. Press.

Cohen, R. 1971. *Dominance and defiance: A study of marital instability in an Islamic African society.* Washington, DC: American Anthropological Association.

Cohen, Y. A. 1964. *The transition from childhood to adolescence: Cross-cultural studies of initiation ceremonies, legal systems, and incest taboos.* Chicago: Aldine.

Collier, J. F. 1988. *Marriage and inequality in classless societies.* Stanford, CA: Stanford Univ. Press.

Conkey, M. W. 1983. On the origins of Paleolithic art: A review and some critical thoughts. In *The Mousterian legacy,* ed. E. Trinkaus. Oxford: British Archaeological Reports.

————. 1984. To find ourselves: Art and social geography of prehistoric hunter gatherers. In *Past and present in hunter gatherer societies*, ed. C. Schrire. New York: Academic Press.

Conoway, C. H., and C. B. Koford. 1964. Estrous cycles and mating behavior in a free-ranging band of rhesus monkeys. *Journal of Mammalogy* 45:577–88.

Conroy, G. E., M. W. Vannier, and P. V. Tobias. 1990. Endocranial features of *Australopithecus africanus* revealed by 2 and 3-D computed tomography. *Science* 247:838–41.

Constantine, L. L., and J. N. Constantine. 1973. *Group marriage: A study of contemporary multilateral marriage*. New York: Macmillan.

Coolidge, H. J. 1933. *Pan paniscus*, pygmy chimpanzee from south of the Congo River. *American Journal of Physical Anthropology* 18:1–59.

Coontz, S. 2005. *Marriage: A history*. New York: Viking.

Cooper, J. C., S. Dunne, T. Furey, and J. P. O'Doherty. 2012. Dorsomedial prefrontal cortex mediates rapid evaluations predicting the outcome of romantic interactions. *Journal of Neuroscience* 32(45):15647–56.

Copeland S. R., M. Sponheimer, D. J. de Ruiter, et al. 2011. Strontium isotope evidence for landscape use by early hominins. *Nature* 474:76–78.

Corruccini, R. S., R. L. Ciochon, and H. M. McHenry. 1976. The postcranium of Miocene hominoids: Were Dryopithecines merely "dental apes"? *Primates* 17:205–23.

Corruccini, R. S., and H. M. McHenry. 1979. Morphological affinities of *Pan paniscus*. *Science* 204:1341–42.

Cowan, A. L. 1989. Women's gains on the job: Not without a heavy toll. *New York Times*, Aug. 2.

Cronin, J. E. 1983. Apes, humans and molecular clocks: A reappraisal. In *New Interpretations of Ape and Human Ancestry*, ed. R. L. Ciochon and R. S. Corruccini. New York: Plenum Press.

Crook, J. H., and S. J. Crook. 1988. Tibetan polyandry: Problems of adaptation and fitness. In *Human Reproductive Behaviour*, ed. L. Betzig, M. B. Mulder, and P. Turke. Cambridge, UK: Cambridge Univ. Press.

Cutler, W. B., G. Preti, A. Krieger, et al. 1986. Human axillary secretions influence women's menstrual cycles: The role of donor extract from men. *Hormones and Behavior* 20: 463–73.

Dahlberg, F., ed. 1981. *Woman the gatherer*. New Haven: Yale Univ. Press.

Daly, M. 1978. The cost of mating. *American Naturalist* 112:771–74.

Daly, M., and M. Wilson, 1978. *Sex, evolution, and behavior: Adaptations for reproduction.* North Scituate, MA: Duxbury Press.

————. 1983. *Sex, evolution, and behavior*. Boston: Willard Grant Press.

————. 1988. *Homicide*. New York: Aldine de Gruyter.

Damasio, H., T. Grabowski, R. Frank, et al. 1994. The Return of Phineas Gage: Clues about the brain from the skull of a famous patient. *Science*, New Series, 264 (5162): 1102–5.

Damon, W. 1988. *The moral child: Nurturing children's natural moral growth*. New York: Free Press.

Daniels, D. 1983. The evolution of concealed ovulation and self-deception. *Ethology and Sociobiology* 4:69–87.

Darwin, C. 1859. *The Origin of Species*. New York: Modern Library.

———. 1871. *The descent of man and selection in relation to sex*. New York: Modern Library.

———. [1872] 1965. *The expression of the emotions in man and animals*. Chicago: Univ. of Chicago Press.

———. 1911. Letter to Asa Gray, 3 April 1860. In *The life and letters of Charles Darwin*, ed. F. Darwin, Vol. 2, 90–91. New York and London: D. Appleton.

Davidson, R. J. 1994. Complexities in the search for emotion-specific physiology. In *The nature of emotion: Fundamental questions*, ed. P. Ekman and R. J. Davidson. New York: Oxford Univ. Press.

Davis, D. E. 1964. The physiological analysis of aggressive behavior. In *Social behavior and organization among vertebrates*, ed. W. Etkin. Chicago: Univ. of Chicago Press.

Davis, E. 1971. *The first sex*. Harmondsworth, UK: Penguin.

Dawkins, R. 1976. *The Selfish Gene*. Oxford: Oxford Univ. Press.

De Castro, J. M. B., M. Martinón-Torres, L. Prado, et al. 2010. New immature hominin fossil from European Lower Pleistocene shows the earliest evidence of a modern human dental development pattern. *Proceedings of the National Academy of Sciences* 107: 11739–44.

De Castro, J. M. B., A. Rosas, E. Carbonell, et al. 1999. A modern human pattern of dental development in lower pleistocene hominids from Atapuerca-TD6 (Spain). *Proceedings of the National Academy of Sciences* 96: 4210–13.

Dediu, D., and S. C. Levinson. 2013. On the antiquity of language: the reinterpretation of Neanderthal linguistic capacities and its consequences. *Frontiers in Psychology* 4 (397): 1–16.

Degler, C. N. 1991. *In search of human nature: The decline and revival of Darwinism in American social thought*. New York: Oxford Univ. Press.

de Lacoste-Utamsing, C., and R. L. Holloway. 1982. Sexual dimorphism in the human corpus callosum. *Science* 216:1431–32.

Delgado, M. R., L. E. Nystrom, C. Fissel, et al. 2000. Tracking the hemodynamic responses to reward and punishment in the striatum. *Journal of Neurophysiology* 84: 3072–77.

Delson, E., ed. 1985. *Ancestors: The hard evidence*. New York: Alan R. Liss.

De Rougemont, D. 1983. *Love in the Western world*. New York: Schocken.

d'Errico, F., C. Henshilwood, G. Lawson, et al. 2003. Archaeological evidence for the emergence of language, symbolism, and music—an alternative multidisciplinary perspective. *Journal of World Prehistory* 17: 1–70.

d'Errico, F., M. Vanhaeren, C. Henshilwood, et al. 2009. From the origin of language to the diversification of languages: What can archaeology and palaeoanthropology say? In *Becoming eloquent: Advances in the emergence of language, human cognition, and modern cultures*, ed. F. d'Errico & J.-M. Hombert, 13–68. Amsterdam: John Benjamins.

De Vos, G. J. 1983. Social behavior of black grouse: An observational and experimental field study. *Ardea* 71:1–103.

De Waal, F. 1982. *Chimpanzee politics: Power and sex among apes.* New York: Harper and Row.

———. 1987. Tension regulation and nonreproductive functions of sex in captive bonobos *(Pan paniscus). National Geographic Research* 3:318–35.

———. 1989. *Peacemaking among primates.* Cambridge, MA: Harvard Univ. Press.

———. 1996. *Good natured: The origins of right and wrong in humans and other animals.* Cambridge, MA: Harvard Univ. Press.

Diamond, L. M. 2008. *Sexual fluidity.* Cambridge, MA: Harvard Univ. Press.

Diamond, M. 1980. The biosocial evolution of human sexuality. Reply to precis of *The evolution of human sexuality,* by Donald Symons. *Behavioral and Brain Sciences* 3:171–214.

Diana, L. n.d. Extra-marital sex in Italy: A family responsibility. Social Science Program, Virginia Commonwealth Univ.

Diana, M. 2013. The addicted brain. *Frontiers in Psychiatry* 4:40.

Dickemann, M. 1979. The ecology of mating systems in hypergynous dowry societies. *Social Science Information* 18:63–95.

Dionne, E. J. 1989. Struggle for work and family fueling women's movement. *New York Times,* Aug. 22.

Dissanayake, E. 1988. *What is art for?* Seattle: Univ. of Washington Press.

Dixson, A. F. 1999. *Primate sexuality.* New York: Oxford Univ. Press.

———. 2009. *Sexual selection and the origins of human mating systems.* New York: Oxford Univ. Press.

Dobs, A. S., A. M. Matsumoto, C. Wang, and M. S. Kipnes. 2004. Short-term pharmacokinetic comparison of a novel testosterone buccal system and a testosterone gel in testosterone deficient men. *Current Medical Research and Opinion* 5:729–38.

Domes, G., M. Heinrichs, A. Michel, et al. 2007. Oxytocin improves "mind-reading" in humans. *Biological Psychiatry* 61: 731–33.

Donaldson, F. 1971. Emotion as an accessory vital system. *Perspectives in Biology and Medicine* 15:46–71.

Dougherty, E. G. 1955. Comparative evolution and the origin of sexuality. *Systematic Zoology* 4:145–69.

Douglas, C. 1987. The beat goes on. *Psychology Today,* Nov., 37–42.

Dozier, R. W. 2002. *Why we hate: Understanding, curbing, and eliminating hate in ourselves and our world.* New York: Contemporary Books.

Draper, P. 1985. Two views of sex differences in socialization. In *Male-female differences: A bio-cultural perspective,* ed. R. L. Hall, et al. New York: Praeger.

Dupâquier, J., E. Hélin, P. Laslett, et al. 1981. *Marriage and remarriage in populations of the past.* New York: Academic Press.

Durden-Smith, J., and D. Desimone. 1983. *Sex and the brain.* New York: Arbor House.

Dychtwald, K., and J. Flower. 1989. *Age wave: The challenges and opportunities of an aging america.* Los Angeles: Jeremy P. Tarcher.

Earp, B. D., A. Snadberg and J. Savulescu. Forthcoming. The medicalization of love. *Cambridge Quarterly of Health Care Ethics.*

East, R. 1939. *Akiga's story: The Tiv tribe as seen by one of its members.* London: Oxford Univ. Press.

Easterlin, R. A. 1980. *Birth and fortune: The impact of numbers on personal welfare.* New York: Basic Books.

Eberhard, W. G. 1985. *Sexual selection and animal genitalia.* Cambridge, MA: Harvard Univ. Press.

———. 1987. Runaway sexual selection. *Natural History*, Dec., 4–8.

———. 1990. Animal genitalia and female choice. *American Scientist* 87:134–41.

Eibl-Eibesfeldt, I. 1970. *Ethology: The biology of behavior.* New York: Holt, Rinehart and Winston.

———. 1989. *Human ethology.* New York: Aldine de Gruyter.

Eisenberger, N. I., M. D. Lieberman, and K. D. Williams. 2003. Does rejection hurt? An FMRI study of social exclusion. *Science* 302:290–92.

Ekman, P. 1980. *The face of man.* New York: Garland STPM Press.

———. 1985. *Telling lies: Clues to deceit in the marketplace, politics, and marriage.* New York: W. W. Norton.

Ekman, P. E., R. Sorenson, and W. V. Friesen. 1969. Pan-cultural elements in facial displays of emotion. *Science* 164:86–88.

Elkin, A. P. 1939. Introduction to *Aboriginal woman: Sacred and profane*, by P. M. Kaberry. London: Routledge and Kegan Paul.

Elliott, R., J. L. Newman, O. A. Longe, and J. F. W. Deakin. 2003. Differential response patterns in the striatum and orbitofrontal cortex to financial reward in humans: A parametric functional magnetic resonance imaging study. *Journal of Neuroscience* 23(1): 303–7.

Ellis, B., and D. Symons. 1990. Sex differences in sexual fantasy: An evolutionary psychological approach. Paper presented at the annual meeting of the Human Behavior and Evolution Society, Los Angeles.

Ellison, P. 2001. *On fertile ground.* Cambridge, MA: Harvard Univ. Press.

Ember, M., and C. R. Ember. 1979. Male–female bonding: A cross-species study of mammals and birds. *Behavior Science Research* 14:37–56.

Emlen, S. T., and L. W. Oring. 1977. Ecology, sexual selection and the evolution of mating systems. *Science* 197:215–23.

Engels, F. [1884] 1954. *Origin of the family, private property, and the state.* Trans. Ernest Untermann. Moscow: Foreign Languages Publishing House.

Epstein, C. 1988. *Deceptive Distinctions: Sex, gender and the social order.* New York: Russell Sage.

Espenshade, T. J. 1985. Marriage trends in America: Estimates, implications, and underlying causes. *Population and Development Review* 11 (2): 193–245.

Etienne, M., and E. Leacock, eds. 1980. *Women and colonization: Anthropological perspectives.* New York: Praeger.

Evans, M. S. 1987. Women in twentieth-century America: An overview. In *The American Woman: 1987–88*, ed. S. E. Rix. New York: W. W. Norton.

Eveleth, P. B. 1986. Timing of menarche: Secular trend and population differences. In *School-age pregnancy and parenthood: Biosocial dimensions*, ed. J. B. Lancaster and B. A. Hamburg. New York: Aldine de Gruyter.

Fabre-Nys, C. 1997. Male faces and odors evoke differential patterns of neurochemical release in the mediobasal hypothalamus of the ewe during estrus: an insight into sexual motivation. *European Journal of Neuroscience* 9:1666–77.

———. 1998. Steroid control of monoamines in relation to sexual behavior. *Reviews of Reproduction* 3(1): 31–41.

Farah, M. 1984. *Marriage and sexuality in Islam: A translation of al-Ghazālī's Book on the Etiquette of Marriage from the Ihyā*. Salt Lake City: Univ. of Utah Press.

Fedigan, L. M. 1982. *Primate paradigms: Sex roles and social bonds*. Montreal: Eden Press.

Fehrenbacker, G. 1988. Moose courts cows, and disaster. *Standard-Times* (New Bedford, MA), Jan. 23.

Feinman, S., and G. W. Gill. 1978. Sex differences in physical attractiveness preferences. *Journal of Social Psychology* 105:43–52.

Feld, A., ed. 1990. How to stay married in the 90s. *Bride's*, Dec., 126.

Fennema, E. 1990. Justice, equity and mathematics education. In *Mathematics and gender*, ed. E. Fennema and G. C. Leder. New York: Teachers College Press.

Fennema, E. and G. C. Leder, eds. 1990. *Mathematics and gender*. New York: Teachers College Press.

Field, T. M., R. Woodson, R. Greenberg, et al. 1982. Discrimination and imitation of facial expressions by neonates. *Science* 218:179–81.

Finkel, E. J., P. W. Eastwick, B. R. Karney, et al. 2012. Online Dating: A critical analysis from the perspective of psychological science. *Psychological Science in the Public Interest*. 13: 3–66.

Finn, M. V., and B. S. Low. 1986. Resource distribution, social competition and mating patterns in human societies. In *Ecological Aspects of Social Evolution*, ed. D. I. Rubenstein and R. W. Wrangham. Princeton: Princeton Univ. Press.

Fisher, H. E. 1975. The loss of estrous periodicity in hominid evolution. PhD diss., Univ. of Colorado, Boulder.

———. 1982. *The sex contract: The evolution of human behavior*. New York: William Morrow.

———. 1987. The four-year itch. *Natural History*, Oct., 22–33.

———. 1989. Evolution of human serial pairbonding. *American Journal of Physical Anthropology* 78:331–54.

———. 1991. Monogamy, adultery and divorce in cross-species perspective. In *Man and Beast Revisited*, ed. M. H. Robinson and L. Tiger. Washington, DC: Smithsonian Institution Press.

———. 1992. *Anatomy of love: The natural history of monogamy, adultery, and divorce*. New York: Norton.

———. 1998. Lust, attraction, and attachment in mammalian reproduction. *Human Nature*, 9(1): 23–52.

———. 1999. *The first sex: The natural talents of women and how they are changing the world*. New York: Random House.

———. 2004. *Why we love: The nature and chemistry of romantic love*. New York: Henry Holt.

———. 2006. The drive to love: The neural mechanism for mate choice. In *The Psy-

*chology of Love*, 2nd edition, ed. J. R. Sternberg and M. L. Barnes. New Haven: Yale Univ. Press.

———. 2009. *Why him? Why her?* New York: Henry Holt.

———. 2012. We have chemistry! The role of four primary temperament dimensions in mate choice and partner compatibility. *The Psychotherapist* 52 (Autumn 2012): 8–9.

———. 2014. The Tyranny of love: Love addiction—an anthropologist's view. In *Behavioral addictions: Criteria, evidence and treatment.* K. P. Rosenberg and L. C. Feder, eds. 237–60. New York: Elsevier.

———. 2015. Slow love: How casual sex may be improving America's marriages. *Nautilus*, March 5.

———. In preparation. Human divorce patterns: An update.

Fisher, H. E., A. Aron, and L. L. Brown. 2005. Romantic love: An fMRI study of a neural mechanism for mate choice. *Journal of Comparative Neurology* 493:58–62.

———. 2006. Romantic love: A mammalian brain system for mate choice. In "The Neurobiology of Social Recognition, Attraction and Bonding, ed. Keith Kendrick, *Philosophical Transactions of the Royal Society: Biological Sciences* 361:2173–86.

Fisher, H. E., A. Aron, D. Mashek, H. Li, G. Strong, and L. L. Brown. 2002. The neural mechanisms of mate choice: A hypothesis. *Neuroendocrinology Letters* Suppl 4, 23:92–97.

Fisher, H. E., A. Aron, D. Mashek, et al. 2003. Early stage intense romantic love activates cortical-basal-ganglia reward/motivation, emotion and attention systems: an fMRI study of a dynamic network that varies with relationship length, passion intensity and gender. Poster presented at the Annual Meeting of the *Society For Neuroscience*, New Orleans, November 11.

Fisher, H. E., and J. A. Thomson, Jr. 2007. Lust, romance, attachment: Do the side-effects of serotonin-enhancing antidepressants jeopardize romantic love, marriage and fertility? In *Evolutionary Cognitive Neuroscience*, ed. S. M. Platek, J. P. Keenan, and T. K. Shakelford, 245–83. Cambridge, MA: MIT Press.

Fisher, H. E., L. L. Brown, A. Aron, et al. 2010. Reward, addiction, and emotion regulation systems associated with rejection in love. *J. Neurophysiology* 104:51–60.

Fisher, H. E., H. D. Island, J. Rich, D. Marchalik, and L. L. Brown. 2015. Four broad temperament dimensions: Description, convergent validation correlations, and comparison with the Big Five. *Frontiers in Psychology: Personality and Social Psychology* 6:1098.

Fisher, H. E., J. Rich, H. D. Island, and D. Marchalik. 2010. The second to fourth digit ratio: A measure of two hormonally-based temperament dimensions. *Journal of Personality and individual differences* 49 (7):773–77.

Fishman, S. M., and D. V. Sheehan. 1985. Anxiety and panic: Their cause and treatment. *Psychology Today*, April, 26–32.

Flinn, M. V., and B. S. Low. 1986. Resource distribution, social competition and mating patterns in human societies. In *Ecological aspects of social evolution*, ed. D. I. Rubenstein and R. W. Wrangham. Princeton: Princeton Univ. Press.

Foley, R. A., and P. C. Lee. 1989. Finite social space, evolutionary pathways, and reconstructing hominid behavior. *Science* 243:901–6.

Ford, C. S., and F. A. Beach. 1951. *Patterns of sexual behavior.* New York: Harper and Brothers.

Forsyth, A. 1985. Good scents and bad. *Natural History*, Nov., 25–32.

Fortune, R. 1963. *Sorcerers of Dobu*. New York: Dutton.

Fossey, D. 1979. Development of the mountain gorilla *(Gorilla gorilla beringei):* The first thirty-six months. In *The great apes*, ed. D. A. Hamburg and E. R. McCown. Menlo Park, CA: Benjamin/Cummings.

———. 1983. *Gorillas in the mist*. Boston: Houghton Mifflin.

Foucault, M. 1985. *The History of sexuality*. Vol. 2, *The use of pleasure*. Trans. R. Hurley. New York: Pantheon.

Fouts, D. 1983. Louis tries his hand at surgery. *Friends of Washoe* 3(4).

Fox, R. 1972. Alliance and constraint: Sexual selection in the evolution of human kinship systems. In *Sexual selection and the descent of man*, ed. B. Campbell. Chicago: Aldine.

———. 1980. *The Red lamp of incest*. New York: E. P. Dutton.

Fraley, R. C., and P. R. Shaver. 2000. Adult romantic attachment: Theoretical developments, emerging controversies, and unanswered questions. *Review of General Psychology* 4:132–54.

Frank, R. 1985. *Choosing the right pond: Human behavior and the quest for status*. New York: Oxford Univ. Press.

Frascella, J., M. N. Potenza, L. L. Brown, and A. R. Childress. 2010. Shared brain vulnerabilities open the way for nonsubstance addictions: Carving addiction at a new joint? *Annals of the New York Academy of Sciences*, 1187:294–315.

Frayer, D. W., and M. H. Wolpoff. 1985. Sexual Dimorphism. *Annual Review of Anthropology* 14:429–73.

Frayser, S. 1985. *Varieties of sexual experience: An anthropological perspective on human sexuality*. New Haven: HRAF Press.

Frazer, J. G. [1922] 1963. *The golden bough*. New York: Macmillan.

Freud, S. 1918. *Totem and taboo*. Trans. A. A. Brill. New York: Moffat, Yard.

Friedl, E. 1975. *Women and men: An anthropologist's view*. New York: Holt, Rinehart and Winston.

Frisch, R. E. 1978. Population, food intake and fertility. *Science* 199:22–30.

———. 1984. Body fat, puberty, and fertility. *Biological Reviews* 59:161–88.

Frisch, R. E., and R. Revelle. 1970. Height and weight at menarche and a hypothesis of critical weights and adolescent events. *Science* 169:397–99.

Fuller, C. J. 1976. *The Nayars today*. Cambridge, UK: Cambridge Univ. Press.

Furstenberg, F. F., Jr. 1981. Remarriage and intergenerational relations. In *Aging: Stability and changes in the family*. ed. R. W. Fogel et al. New York: Academic Press.

Furstenberg, F. F., Jr., and G. B. Spanier. 1984. *Recycling the family: Remarriage after divorce*. Beverly Hills, CA: Sage Publications.

Gage, R. L. 1979. *Fox family*. New York: Weatherhill/Heibonsha.

Galdikas, B. M. F. 1979. Orangutan adaptation at Tanjung Putting Reserve: Mating and ecology. In *The Great Apes*, ed. D. A. Hamburg and E. R. McCown. Menlo Park, CA: Benjamin/Cummings.

———. 1989. Body weight and reproduction. *Science* 246:432.

———. 1995. *Reflections of Eden: My years with Orangutans of Borneo*. Boston: Little Brown. 144–45.

Galdikas, B. M. F., and J. W. Wood. 1990. Birth spacing patterns in humans and apes. *American Journal of Physical Anthropology* 83:185–91.

Gallup, G. G. 1982. Permanent breast enlargement in human females: A socio-biological analysis. *Journal of Human Evolution* 11:597–601.

Gangestad, S. W., and R. Thornhill. 1997. The evolutionary psychology of extra-pair sex: the role of fluctuating asymmetry. *Evolution and Human Behavior* 18(2): 69–88.

Gangestad, S. W., R. Thornhill, and R. A. Yeo. 1994. Facial attractiveness, developmental stability, and fluctuating asymmetry. *Ethology and Sociobiology* 15:73–85.

Garcia, J. R., and H. E. Fisher. 2015. Why we hook up: Searching for sex or looking for love. In *Gender, sex, and politics: In the streets and between the sheets in the 21st century*, ed. S. Tarrant. New York: Routledge.

Garcia, J. R., J. MacKillop, E. L. Aller, et al. 2010. Associations between the dopamine D4 receptor gene variation with both infidelity and sexual promiscuity. PLoS ONE 5:e14162.

Garcia, J. R., and C. Reiber. 2008. Hook-up behavior: A biopsychosocial perspective. *Journal of Social, Evolutionary and Cultural Psychology* 2(4): 192–208.

Garcia, J. R., C. Reiber, S. G. Massey, and A. M. Merriwether. 2012. Sexual hook-up culture: A review. *Review of General Psychology* 16:161–76.

Gargett, R. H. 1989. Grave shortcomings: The evidence for Neanderthal burial. *Current Anthropology* 30:157–90.

Garver-Apgar, C. E., S. W. Gangestad, R. Thornhill, et al. 2006. "Major histocompatibility complex alleles, sexual responsivity, and unfaithfulness in romantic couples." *Psychological Science* 17 (10): 830–35.

Gaulin, S. J., and J. Boster. 1985. Cross-cultural differences in sexual dimorphism: Is there any variance to be explained? *Ethology and Sociobiology* 6:219–25.

Gaulin, S. J., and R. W. FitzGerald. 1989. Sexual selection for spatial-learning ability. *Animal Behavior* 37:322–31.

Gaulin, S. J., and M. J. Konner. 1977. On the natural diet of primates, including humans. In *Nutrition and the brain*. Vol. 1, ed. R. and J. Wurtman. New York: Raven Press.

Gehlback, F. R. 1986. Odd couples of suburbia. *Natural History*, July, 56–66.

Geschwind, N. 1974. The anatomical basis of hemispheric differentiation. In *Hemispheric function of the human brain*, ed. S. J. Dimond and J. G. Beaumont. New York: John Wiley.

Geschwind, N. G., and A. M. Galaburda. 1985. Cerebral lateralization. Biological mechanisms, associations and pathology: A hypothesis and a program for research. *Archives of Neurology* 42: 428–59.

Gibbons, A. 1990a. Our chimp cousins get that much closer. *Science* 250:376.

———. 1990b. Paleontology by bulldozer. *Science* 247:1407–9.

———. 1991. First hominid finds from Ethiopia in a decade. *Science* 251:1428.

———. 2010. Close encounters of a prehistoric kind. *Science* 328:680–84.

———. 2011. Who were the Denisovans? *Science* 333:1084–87.

Gibbs, H. L., P. J. Weatherhead, P. T. Boag, et al. 1990. Realized reproductive success of polygynous redwinged blackbirds revealed by DNA markers. *Science* 250:1394–97.

Gibson, K. R. 1981. Comparative neuroontogeny, its implications for the development of human intelligence. In *Infancy and epistemology*, ed. G. Butterworth. Brighton, UK: Harvester Press.

Gies, F., and J. Gies. 1978. *Women in the Middle Ages*. New York: Barnes and Noble.

Giese, J. 1990. A communal type of life, and dinner's for everyone. *New York Times*, Sept. 27.

Gilligan, C. 1982a. *In a different voice*. Cambridge, MA: Harvard Univ. Press.

———. 1982b. Why should a woman be more like a man? *Psychology Today*, June, 70–71.

Gilligan, C., and G. Wiggins. 1988. The origins of morality in early childhood relationships. In *Mapping the moral domain*, ed. C. Gilligan, et al. Cambridge, MA: Harvard Univ. Press.

Gingrich, B., Y. Liu, C. Cascio, et al. 2000. D2 receptors in the nucleus accumbens are important for social attachment in female prairie voles (Microtus ochrogaster). *Behavioral Neuroscience* 114(1): 173–83.

Givens, D. B. 1983. *Love signals: How to attract a mate*. New York: Crown.

———. 1986. The big and the small: Toward a paleontology of gesture. *Sign Language Studies* 51:145–70.

Gladkih, M. I., N. L. Kornieta, and O. Soffer. 1984. Mammoth-bone dwellings on the Russian plain. *Scientific American* 251 (5): 164–75.

Glass, S., and T. Wright. 1985. Sex differences in type of extramarital involvement and marital dissatisfaction. *Sex Roles* 12:1101–20.

———. 1992. Justifications for extramarital relationships: The association between attitudes, behaviors, and gender. *Journal of Sex Research* 29:361–87.

Glenn, N., and M. Supancic. 1984. The social and demographic correlates of divorce and separation in the United States: An update and reconsideration. *Journal of Marriage and the Family* 46:563–75.

Glick, P. C. 1975. Some recent changes in American families. *Current Population Reports*, Social Studies Series P-23, no. 52. Washington, DC: U.S. Bureau of the Census.

Goldberg, S. 1973. *The inevitability of patriarchy*. New York: William Morrow.

Goldin, C. 1990. *Understanding the gender gap: An economic history of American women*. New York: Oxford Univ. Press.

———. 1991. A conversation with Claudia Goldin. *Harvard Gazette*, Feb. 1, 5–6.

Goldizen, A. W. 1987. Tamarins and marmosets: Communal care of offspring. In *Primate Societies*, ed. B. B. Smuts et al. Chicago: Univ. of Chicago Press.

Goldstein, B. 1976. *Human sexuality*. New York: McGraw-Hill.

Goldstein, M. C. 1976. Fraternal polyandry and fertility in a high Himalayan village in N. W. Nepal. *Human Ecology* 4 (3): 223–33.

———. 1987. When brothers share a wife. *Natural History*, March, 39–49.

Goleman, D. 1981. The 7,000 faces of Dr. Ekman. *Psychology Today*, Feb., 43–49.

———. 1986. Two views of marriage explored: His and hers. *New York Times*, April 1.

———. 1989. Subtle but intriguing differences found in the brain anatomy of men and women. *New York Times*, April 11.

Golombok, S., and F. Tasker. 1996. Do parents influence the sexual orientation of their children. *Developmental Psychology* 32 (1): 3–11.

Goodale, J. C. 1971. *Tiwi wives: A study of the women of Melville Island, North Australia.* Seattle: Univ. of Washington Press.

Goodall, J. 1968. The behavior of free-ranging chimpanzees in the Gombe Stream Reserve. *Animal Behavior Monographs* 1:161–311.

———. 1970. Tool-using in primates and other vertebrates. *Advanced Studies of Behavior* 3:195–249.

———. 1977. Watching, watching, watching. *New York Times,* Sept. 15.

———. 1986. *The chimpanzees of Gombe: Patterns of behavior.* Cambridge, MA: Belknap Press/Harvard Univ. Press.

———. 1988. *In the shadow of man.* Rev. ed. Boston: Houghton Mifflin.

Goodall, J., A. Bandora, E. Bergmann, et al. 1979. Intercommunity interactions in the chimpanzee population of the Gombe National Park. In *The great apes,* ed. D. A. Hamburg and E. R. McCown. Menlo Park, CA: Benjamin/Cummings.

Goodenough, W. H. 1970. *Description and comparison in cultural anthropology.* Chicago: Aldine.

Goody, J. 1969. Inheritance, property, and marriage in Africa and Eurasia. *Sociology* 3:55–76.

———. 1983. *The Development of the family and marriage in Europe.* Cambridge, UK: Cambridge Univ. Press.

Gordon, A. D. 2006. Scaling of size and dimorphism in primates II: Macroevolution. *International Journal of Primatology* 27: 63–105.

Gorer, G. 1938. *Himalayan village: An account of the Lepchas of Sikkim.* London: Michael Joseph.

Gough, E. K. 1968. The Nayars and the definition of marriage. In *Marriage, family, and residence,* ed. P. Bohannan and J. Middleton. Garden City, NY: Natural History Press.

Gould, J. L. 1982. *Ethology: The mechanisms and evolution of behavior.* New York: W. W. Norton.

Gould, J. L., and C. G. Gould. 1989. *The ecology of attraction: Sexual selection.* New York: W. H. Freeman.

Gould, S. J. 1977. *Ontogeny and phylogeny.* Cambridge, MA: Harvard Univ. Press.

———. 1981. *The mismeasure of man.* New York: W. W. Norton.

———. 1987a. Freudian slip. *Natural History,* Feb., 14–19.

———. 1987b. Steven Jay Gould replies to John Alcock's "Ardent Adaptationism." *Natural History,* April, 4.

Gove, C. M. 1989. Wife lending: Sexual pathways to transcendence in Eskimo culture. In *Enlightened Sexuality,* ed. G. Feuerstein. Freedom, CA: Crossing Press.

Graham, C. A., and W. C. McGrew. 1980. Menstrual synchrony in female undergraduates living on a coeducational campus. *Psychoneuroendocrinology* 5:245–52.

Gray, J. P., and L. D. Wolfe. 1983. Human female sexual cycles and the concealment of ovulation problem. *Journal of Social and Biological Structures* 6:345–52.

Gray, P. B., and J. R. Garcia. 2013. *Evolution and human sexual behavior.* Cambridge, MA: Harvard Univ. Press.

Greeley, A. 1994. Marital infidelity. *Society* 31: 9–13.

Green, R. E., J. Krause, A. Briggs, et al. 2010. A draft sequence of the Neanderthal genome. *Science* 328: 710–26.

Greenfield, L. O. 1980. A late-divergence hypothesis. *American Journal of Physical Anthropology* 52:351–66.

———. 1983. Toward the resolution of discrepancies between phenetic and paleontological data bearing on the question of human origins. In *New Interpretations of Ape and Human Ancestry,* ed. R. L. Ciochon and R. S. Corruccini. New York: Plenum Press.

Gregersen, E. 1982. *Sexual practices: The story of human sexuality.* London: Mitchell Beazley.

Gregg, S. A. 1988. *Foragers and farmers: Population interaction and agricultural expansion in prehistoric Europe.* Chicago: Univ. of Chicago Press.

Gregor, T. 1985. *Anxious pleasures: The sexual lives of an Amazonian people.* Chicago: Univ. of Chicago Press.

Griffin, D. R. 1984. *Animal thinking.* Cambridge, MA: Harvard Univ. Press.

Griffin-Shelley, E. 1991. Sex and love: Addiction, treatment and recovery. Westport, CT: Praeger.

Grine, F. E. 1989. *Evolutionary history of the robust Australopithecines.* New York: Aldine de Gruyter.

Gubernick, D. J. Forthcoming. Biparental care and male-female relations in mammals. In *Infanticide and Parental Care,* ed. S. Parmigiana and F. S. vom Saal. London: Harwood Academic.

Guttentag, M., and P. F. Secord. 1983. *Too many women? The sex ratio question.* Beverly Hills, CA: Sage Publications.

Hagen, E. H. 2011. Evolutionary theories of depression: A critical review. *Canadian Journal of Psychiatry* 56:716–26.

Haidt, J. 2012. The righteous mind: Why good people are divided by politics and religion. New York: Pantheon.

Hall, E. T. 1959. *The silent language.* New York: Doubleday.

———. 1966. *The hidden dimension.* New York: Anchor.

———. 1976. *Beyond Culture.* New York: Doubleday/Anchor.

Hall, J. A. 1984. *Nonverbal sex differences.* Baltimore: Johns Hopkins Univ. Press.

———. 1978. Decoding wordless messages. *Human Nature,* May, 68–75.

Hall, J. A., R. Rosenthal, D. Archer, et al. 1977. The profile of nonverbal sensitivity. In *Advances in Psychological Assessment.* Vol. 4, ed. P. McReynolds. San Francisco: Jossey-Bass.

Hall, R. L. 1982. *Sexual dimorphism in Homo Sapiens: A question of size.* New York: Praeger.

Hall, T. 1987. Infidelity and women: Shifting patterns. *New York Times,* June 1.

Halpern, H. M. 1982. How to break your addiction to a person. New York: McGraw-Hill.

Hamer, D. H., S. Hu, V. L. Magnuson, et al. 1993. A Linkage between DNA markers on the X chromosome and male sexual orientation. *Science* 261: 321–27.

Hames, R. B. 1988. The allocation of parental care among the Ye'kwana. In *Human reproductive behavior: A Darwinian perspective,* ed. L. Betzig, M. Borgerhoff Mulder, and P. Turke. New York: Cambridge Univ. Press.

Hamilton, W. D. 1964. The genetical evolution of social behaviour: I. and II. *Journal of Theoretical Biology* 7:1–52.

———. 1980. Sex versus non-sex versus parasite. *Oikos* 35:282–90.

Hamilton, W. D., P. A. Henderson, and N. A. Moran. 1981. Fluctuation of environment and coevolved antagonist polymorphism as factors in the maintenance of sex. In *Natural Selection and Social Behavior*, ed. R. D. Alexander and D. W. Tinkle. New York: Chiron Press.

Hamilton, W. D., and M. Zuk. 1982. Heritable true fitness and bright birds: A role for parasites? *Science* 218:384–87.

Hammock, E. A., and L. J. Young. 2002. Variation in the vasopressin V1a receptor promoter and expression: Implications for inter- and intraspecfiic variation in social behaviour. *European Journal of Neuroscience* 16:399–402.

Harcourt, A. H. 1979a. Social relationships between adult male and female mountain gorillas in the wild. *Animal Behavior* 27:325–42.

———. 1979b. The social relations and group structure of wild mountain gorillas. In *The Great Apes*, ed. D. A. Hamburg and E. R. McCown. Menlo Park, CA: Benjamin/Cummings.

Harris, H. 1995. Rethinking Heterosexual Relationships in Polynesia: A Case Study of Mangaia, Cook Island. In *Romantic Passion: A Universal Experience?* ed. W. Jankowiak. New York: Columbia Univ. Press.

Harris, John M. Rutgers University. Personal communication.

Harris, M. 1977. Why men dominate women. *New York Times Magazine*, Nov. 13, 46, 115–23.

———. 1981. *America now: The anthropology of a changing culture*. New York: Simon and Schuster.

Harrison, R. J. 1969. Reproduction and reproductive organs. In *The biology of marine mammals*, ed. H. T. Andersen. New York: Academic Press.

Harrison, T. 2010. Apes among the tangled branches of human origins. *Science* 327:532–533.

Hart, C. W. M., and A. R. Pilling. 1960. *The Tiwi of North Australia*. New York: Holt, Rinehart and Winston.

Harwood, D. M. 1985. Late Neogene climate fluctuations in the southern high-latitudes: Implications of a warm Pliocene and deglaciated Antarctic continent. *South African Journal of Science* 81:239–41.

Hassan, F. 1980. The growth and regulation of human population in prehistoric times. In *Biosocial Mechanism of Population Regulation*, ed. M. N. Cohen et al. New Haven: Yale Univ. Press.

Hatfield, E. 1988. Passionate and companionate love. In *The Psychology of Love*, ed. R. J. Sternberg and M. L. Barnes, 191. New Haven: Yale Univ. Press.

Hatfield, E., and R. Rapson. 1987. Passionate love/sexual desire: Can the same paradigm explain both? *Archives of Sexual Behavior* 16:259–78.

———. 1996. *Love and sex: Cross-cultural perspectives*. Needham Heights, MA: Allyn and Bacon.

Hatfield, E. and S. Sprecher. 1986. Measuring passionate love in intimate relationships. *Journal of Adolescence* 9:383–410.

Hausfater, G., and S. B. Hrdy. 1984. *Infanticide: Comparative and evolutionary perspectives.* New York: Aldine.

Hawkes, K., K. Hill, and J. F. O'Connell. 1982. Why hunters gather: Optimal foraging and the Ache of eastern Paraguay. *American Ethnologist* 9:379–98.

Hawkes, K., J. F. O'Connell, N. G. Blurton Jones, et al. 1998. Grandmothering, menopause, and the evolution of human life histories. *Proceedings of the National Academy of Sciences* 95 (3): 1336–39.

Hay, R. L., and M. D. Leakey. 1982. The fossil footprints of Laetoli. *Scientific American,* Feb., 50–57.

Hazan, C., and L. M. Diamond. 2000. "The place of attachment in human mating." *Review of General Psychology* 4:186–204.

Hazan, C., and P. R. Shaver. 1987. Romantic love conceptualized as an attachment process. *Journal of Personality and Social Psychology* 52:511–24.

Heider, K. G. 1976. Dani sexuality: A low energy system. *Man* 11:188–201.

Henley, N. 1977. *Body politics: Power, sex and nonverbal communication.* Englewood Cliffs, NJ: Prentice-Hall.

Henrich, J., R. Boyd, and P. J. Richerson. 2012. The puzzle of monogamous marriage. *Philosophical Transactions of the Royal Society, B: Biological Sciences,* 367ff.

Henry, D. J. 1985. The little foxes. *Natural History,* Jan., 46–56.

Henry, J. 1941. *Jungle people.* New York: J. J. Augustine.

Hess, E. H. 1975. *The tell-tale eye.* New York: Van Nostrand Reinhold.

Hewlett, B. S. 1991. Demography and childcare in preindustrial societies. *Journal of Anthropological Research* 47:1–37.

———. ed. 1992. *Father child relations.* New York: Aldine de Gruyter.

Hiatt, L. R. 1989. On cuckoldry. *Journal of Social and Biological Structures* 12:53–72.

Hill, K. R., R. S. Walter, M. Bozicevic, et al. 2011. Co-residence patterns in hunter-gatherer societies show unique human social structure. *Science* 331:1286–89.

Hite, S. 1981. *The Hite report on male sexuality.* New York: Ballantine.

Hochschild, A., with A. Machung. 1989. *The second shift.* New York: Viking.

Holloway, R. L. 1985. The poor brain of *Homo sapiens neanderthalensis:* See what you please. . . . In *Ancestors: The hard evidence,* ed. E. Delson. New York: Alan R. Liss.

Hopson, J. L. 1979. *Scent signals: The silent language of sex.* New York: William Morrow.

———. 1980. Scent: Our hot-blooded sense. *Science Digest Special,* Summer, 52–53, 110.

Howell, J. M. 1987. Early farming in northwestern Europe. *Scientific American* 257:118–24, 126.

Howell, N. 1979. *Demography of the Dobe !Kung.* New York: Academic Press.

Hrdy, S. B. 1981. *The woman that never evolved.* Cambridge, MA: Harvard Univ. Press.

———. 1983. Heat loss. *Science* 83, Aug., 73–78.

———. 1986. Empathy, polyandry, and the myth of the coy female. In *Feminist approaches to science,* ed. R. Bleier. New York: Pergamon Press.

Hughes, S. M., F. Dispenza, and G. G. Gallup. 2004. Ratings of voice attractiveness predict sexual behavior and body configuration. *Evolution and Human Behavior* 25:295–304.

Hughes, S. M., M. A. Harrison, and G. G. Gallup. 2007. Sex differences in romantic kissing among college students: An evolutionary perspective. *Evolutionary Psychology* 5 (3): 617–31.

Human Genome Project. 2014.

Hunt, M. M. 1959. *The natural history of love.* New York: Alfred A. Knopf.

———. 1974. *Sexual behavior in the 1970s.* Chicago: Playboy Press.

Hunter, M. S., C. Nitschke, and L. Hogan. 1981. A scale to measure love addiction. *Psychological Reports* 48:582.

Ingalhalikar, M., A. Smith, D. Parker, et al. 2014. Sex differences in the structural connectome of the human brain. *Proceedings of the National Academy of Sciences* 111(2):823–28.

Ingmanson, Ellen, anthropologist, personal communication.

Ipsos Poll. 2014.

Isaac, B. L., and W. E. Feinberg. 1982. Marital form and infant survival among the Mende of rural upper Bambara chiefdom, Sierra Leone. *Human Biology* 54:627–34.

James, S. R. 1989. Hominid use of fire in the Lower and Middle Pleistocene: A review of the evidence. *Current Anthropology* 30:1–26.

Jankowiak, W. R. 1992. *Sex, death and hierarchy in a Chinese city: An anthropological account.* New York: Columbia Univ. Press.

Jankowiak, W. R., and E. F. Fischer. 1992. A cross-cultural perspective on romantic love. *Ethnology* 31 (2): 149–55.

Jankowiak, W. R., and M. D. Hardgrave. 2007. Individual and societal responses to sexual betrayal: A view from around the world. *Electronic Journal of Human Sexuality* 10.

Jankowiak, W. R., S. L. Volsche and J. R. Garcia. 2015. In press. Is the romantic/sexual kiss a near human universal? *American Anthropologist* 117 (3): 535–39.

Jarman, M. V. 1979. Impala social behavior: Territory, hierarchy, mating and use of space. *Fortschritte Verhaltensforschung* 21:1–92.

Jenni, D. A. 1974. Evolution of polyandry in birds. *American Zoology* 14:129–44.

Jespersen, O. [1922] 1950. *Language: Its nature, development and origin.* London: George Allen and Unwin.

Jia, L., and H. Weiwen. 1990. *The story of Peking Man: From archaeology to mystery.* New York: Oxford Univ. Press.

Johanson, D. C., ed. 1982. Pliocene hominid fossils from Hadar, Ethiopia. *American Journal of Physical Anthropology* 57:373–402.

Johanson, D. C., and M. Edey. 1981. *Lucy: The beginnings of humankind.* New York: Simon and Schuster.

Johanson, D. C., and J. Shreeve. 1989. *Lucy's child: The discovery of a human ancestor.* New York: William Morrow.

Johanson, D. C., and T. D. White. 1979. A systematic assessment of early African hominids. *Science* 203:321–30.

Johansson, S. 2013. The talking Neanderthals: What do fossils, genetics, and archeology say? *Biolinguistics* 7:35–74.

Johnson, A. W., and T. Earle. 1987. *The evolution of human societies: From foraging group to agrarian state.* Stanford, CA: Stanford Univ. Press.

Johnson, L. L. 1989. The Neanderthals and population as prime mover. *Current Anthropology* 30:534–35.

Johnson, R. A. 1983. *We: Understanding the psychology of romantic love.* San Francisco: Harper and Row.

Johnson, S. C. 1981. Bonobos: Generalized hominid prototypes or specialized insular dwarfs? *Current Anthropology* 22:363–75.

Jones, E., and K. Hill. 1993. Criteria of facial attractiveness in five populations. *Human Nature* 4:271–96.

Jorgensen, W. 1980. *Western Indians.* San Francisco: W. H. Freeman.

Jost, A. 1972. A new look at the mechanisms controlling sex differentiation in mammals. *Johns Hopkins Medical Journal* 130:38–53.

Jungers, W. 1988. Relative joint size and hominoid locomotor adaptations. *Journal of Human Evolution* 17:247.

Kaberry, P. M. 1939. *Aboriginal woman: Sacred and profane.* London: Routledge and Kegan Paul.

Kagan, J., and S. Lamb, eds. 1987. *The emergence of morality in young children.* Chicago: Univ. of Chicago Press.

Kagan, J., J. S. Reznick, and N. Snidman. 1988. Biological Bases of Childhood Shyness. *Science* 240:167–71.

Kano, T. 1979. A pilot study on the ecology of pygmy chimpanzees, *Pan paniscus.* In *The great apes,* ed. D. A. Hamburg and E. R. McCown. Menlo Park, CA: Benjamin/Cummings.

———. 1980. Social behavior of wild pygmy chimpanzees *(Pan paniscus)* of Wamba: A preliminary report. *Journal of Human Evolution* 9:243–60.

Kano, T., and M. Mulavwa. 1984. Feeding ecology of the pygmy chimpanzees *(Pan paniscus)* of Wamba. In *The pygmy chimpanzee,* ed. R. L. Susman. New York: Plenum Press.

Kantrowitz, B., and P. Wingert. 1990. Step by step. *Newsweek Special Edition,* Winter/Spring, 24–34.

Kapit, W., R. I. Macey, and E. Meisami. 2000. *The physiology coloring book.* New York: Addison Wesley Longman.

Kay, R. F. 1981. The nut-crackers: A new theory of the adaptations of the Ramapithecinae. *American Journal of Physical Anthropology* 55:141–51.

Kelly, R. 1995. *The foraging spectrum.* Washington, DC: Smithsonian Press.

Kimura, D. 1983. Sex differences in cerebral organization for speech and praxic functions. *Canadian Journal of Psychology* 37:19–35.

———. 1989. How sex hormones boost or cut intellectual ability. *Psychology Today,* Nov., 63–66.

Kinsey, A. C., W. B. Pomeroy, and C. E. Martin. 1948. *Sexual behavior in the human male.* Philadelphia: W. B. Saunders.

Kinsey, A. C., W. B. Pomeroy, C. E. Martin, and P. H. Gebhard. 1953. *Sexual behavior in the human female.* Philadelphia: W. B. Saunders.

Kinzey, W. G. 1987. Monogamous primates: A primate model for human mating systems. In *The Evolution of Human Behavior,* ed. W. G. Kinzey. Albany: State Univ. of New York Press.

Kirkendall, L. A., and A. E. Gravatt. 1984. Marriage and family: Styles and forms. In *Marriage and the family in the year 2000,* ed. L. A. Kirkendall and A. E. Gravatt. Buffalo, NY: Prometheus.

Kleiman, D. G. 1977. Monogamy in mammals. *Quarterly Review of Biology* 52:39–69.

Kleiman, D. G., and J. F. Eisenberg. 1973. Comparisons of child and felid social systems from an evolutionary perspective. *Animal Behavior* 21:637–59.

Kleiman, D. G., and J. R. Malcolm. 1981. The evolution of male parental investment in mammals. In *Parental care in mammals,* ed. D. J. Gubernick and P. H. Klopfer. New York: Plenum Press.

Klein, L. 1980. Contending with colonization: Tlingit men and women in change. In *Woman and colonization,* ed. M. Etienne and E. Leacock. New York: Praeger.

Klein, Laura. Pacific University. Personal communication.

Klein, R. G. 1999. *The human career: Human biological and cultural origins,* 2nd edition. Chicago: Univ. of Chicago Press.

Klinenberg, E. 2012. *Going solo: The extraordinary rise and surprising appeal of living alone.* New York: Penguin.

Knickmeyer, R., S. Baron-Cohen, P. Raggatt, et al. 2006. Fetal testosterone and empathy. *Hormones and Behavior* 49: 282–92.

Kohlberg, L. 1969. Stage and sequence: The cognitive-developmental approach to socialization. In *Handbook of socialization theory and research,* ed. D. A. Goslin. Chicago: Rand McNally.

Kohler, W. 1925. *The mentality of apes.* London: Routledge and Kegan Paul. Reprint, New York: Liveright, 1976.

Konner, M. J. 1982. *The tangled wing: Biological constraints on the human spirit.* New York: Harper and Row.

———. 1988. Is orgasm essential? *Sciences,* March–April, 4–7.

Konner, M. J. 2015. *Women after all: Sex, evolution and the end of male supremacy.* New York: W. W. Norton.

Konner, M. J., and C. Worthman. 1980. Nursing frequency, gonadal function, and birth spacing among !Kung hunter-gatherers. *Science* 207:788–91.

Koob, G. F., and N. D. Volkow. 2010. Neurocircuitry of addiction. *Neuropsychopharmacology* 35:217–38.

Kramer, K. L., and R. D. Greaves. 2011. Postmarital residence and bilateral kin associations among hunter-gatherers: Pumé foragers living in the best of both worlds. *Hum Nat* 22:41–63.

Kreider, R. 2006. *Remarriage in the United States.* Poster presented at the annual meeting of the American Sociological Association, Montreal, August 10–14.

Krier, B. A. 1988. Why so many singles? *Los Angeles Times,* June 26.

Kristof, N. D. 1991. Love, the starry-eyed kind, casts spell on China. *New York Times,* March 6.

Kruuk, H. 1972. *The spotted hyena: A study of predation and social behavior.* Chicago: Univ. of Chicago Press.

Kummer, H. 1968. *Social organization of Hamadryas baboons.* Chicago: Univ. of Chicago Press.

Kuroda, S. 1984. Interaction over food among pygmy chimpanzees. In *The pygmy chimpanzee*, ed. R. L. Susman. New York: Plenum Press.

Lacey, W. K. 1973. Women in democratic Athens. In *Women: From the Greeks to the French Revolution*. ed. S. G. Bell. Stanford, CA: Stanford Univ. Press. '

Lack, D. 1968. *Ecological adaptations for breeding in birds*. London: Methuen.

Laitman, J. T. 1984. The anatomy of human speech. *Natural History*, Aug., 20–27.

Laitman, J. T., R. C. Heimbuch, and E. S. Crelin. 1979. The basicranium of fossils hominids as an indicator of their upper respiratory system. *American Journal of Physical Anthropology* 51:15–34.

Lampe, P. E., ed. 1987. *Adultery in the United States: Close encounters of the sixth (or seventh) kind*. Buffalo: Prometheus.

Lancaster, J. B. 1979. Sex and gender in evolutionary perspective. In *Human sexuality*, ed. M. Katchadourian. Berkeley: Univ. of California Press.

———. 1986. Human adolescence and reproduction: An evolutionary perspective. In *School-age pregnancy and parenthood*, ed. J. B. Lancaster and B. A. Hamburg. New York: Aldine de Gruyter.

———. 1992. Parental investment and the evolution of the juvenile phase of the human life course. In *The Origins of Humanness*, ed. A. Brooks. Washington, DC: Smithsonian Institution Press.

Lancaster, J. B., and C. S. Lancaster. 1983. Parental investment: The hominid adaptation. In *How humans adapt: A biocultural odyssey*, ed. D. J. Ortner. Washington, DC: Smithsonian Institution Press.

Langlois, J. H., L. A. Roggman, R. J. Casey, et al. 1987. Infant preferences for attractive faces: Rudiments of a stereotype. *Developmental Psychology* 23:363–69.

Latimer, B. M., T. D. White, W. H. Kimbel, et al. 1981. The pygmy chimpanzee is not a living missing link in human evolution. *Journal of Human Evolution* 10:475–88.

Laumann, E. O., J. H. Gagnon, R. T. Michael, and S. Michaels. 1994. *The social organization of sexuality: Sexual practices in the United States*. Chicago: Univ. of Chicago Press.

Lawrence, R. J. 1989. *The poisoning of eros: Sexual values in conflict*. New York: Augustine Moore Press.

Lawson, A. 1988. *Adultery: An analysis of love and betrayal*. New York: Basic Books.

Leacock, E. B. 1980. Montagnais women and the Jesuit program for colonization. In *Women and colonization*, ed. M. Etienne and E. Leacock. New York: Praeger.

———. 1981. *Myths of male dominance*. New York: Monthly Review Press.

———. ed. 1972. *The origins of the family, private property and the state, by Frederick Engels with an introduction by Eleanor Burke Leacock*. New York: International Publishers.

Leakey, M. D. 1971. *Olduvai Gorge*. Vol. 3. London: Cambridge Univ. Press.

Leakey, M. D., and R. L. Hay. 1979. Pliocene footprints in the Laetolil beds at Laetoli, northern Tanzania. *Nature* 278:317–23.

Leakey, M. D., R. L. Hay, G. H. Curtis, et al. 1976. Fossil hominids from the Laetolil Beds. *Nature* 262:460–66.

Lebel, S., E. Trinkaus, M. Faure, et al. 2001. Comparative morphology and paleobiology of Middle Pleistocene human remains from the Bau del l'Aubesier, Vaucluse, France. *Proceedings of the National Academy of Sciences* 98, 11097–102.

LeBoeuf, B. J. 1974. Male–male competition and reproductive success in elephant seals. *American Zoologist* 14:163–76.

Le Clercq, C. 1910. *New relation of Gaspesia*, ed. W. F. Ganong. Toronto: Champlain Society.

Leder, G. C. 1990. Gender differences in mathematics: An overview. In *Mathematics and gender*, ed. E. Fennema and G. C. Leder. New York: Teachers College Press.

Lee, R. B. 1968. What hunters do for a living, or, How to make out on scarce resources. In *Man the hunter*, ed. R. B. Lee and I. DeVore. New York: Aldine.

———. 1980. Lactation, ovulation, infanticide, and women's work: A study of hunter-gatherer population regulation. In *Biosocial mechanisms of population regulation*, ed. M. N. Cohen et al. New Haven: Yale Univ. Press.

Lehrman, N. S. 1962. Some origins of contemporary sexual standards. *Journal of Religion and Health* 1:362–86.

———. 1963. Moses, monotheism and marital fidelity. *Journal of Religion and Health* 3:70–89.

Leroi-Gourhan, A. 1975. The flowers found with Shanidar IV: A Neanderthal burial in Iraq. *Science* 190:562–64.

LeVay, S. 1991. A difference in hypothalamic structure between heterosexual and homosexual men. *Science* 253:1034–37.

Levinger, G. 1968. Marital cohesiveness and dissolution: An integrative review. In *Selected studies in marriage and the family*, ed. R. R. Winch and L. L. Goodman. 3rd ed. New York: Holt, Rinehart and Winston.

Lévi-Strauss, C. 1985. *The view from afar*. New York: Basic Books.

Levitan, S. A., R. S. Belous, and F. Gallo. 1988. *What's happening to the American family?* Baltimore: Johns Hopkins Univ. Press.

Lewin, R. 1982. How did humans evolve big brains? *Science* 216:840–41.

———. 1983a. Fossil Lucy grows younger, again. *Science* 219:43–44.

———. 1983b. Is the orangutan a living fossil? *Science* 222:1222–23.

———. 1985. Surprise findings in the Taung child's face. *Science* 228:42–44.

———. 1987a. Africa: Cradle of modern humans. *Science* 237:1292–95.

———. 1987b. Four legs bad, two legs good. *Science* 235:969–71.

———. 1988a. A revolution of ideas in agricultural origins. *Science* 240:984–86.

———. 1988b. Conflict over DNA clock results. *Science* 241:1598–1600.

———. 1988c. DNA clock conflict continues. *Science* 241:1756–59.

———. 1988d. Subtleties of mating competition. *Science* 242:668.

———. 1989. Species questions in modern human origins. *Science* 243:1666–67.

Lewis, H. T. 1989. Reply to Hominid use of fire in the Lower and Middle Pleistocene: A review of the evidence, by S. R. James. *Current Anthropology* 30:1–26.

Lewis, R. A., and G. B. Spanier. 1979. Theorizing about the quality and stability of marriage. In *Contemporary theories about the family*, ed. W. Burr, R. Hill, F. Nye, and I. Reiss. New York: Free Press.

Lewis, T., F. Amini, and R. Lannon. 2000. *A general theory of love*. New York: Random House.

Lieberman, P. 1984. *The biology and evolution of language.* Cambridge, MA: Harvard Univ. Press.

Liebowitz, M. R. 1983. *The chemistry of love.* Boston: Little, Brown.

Lim, M. M., A. Z. Murphy, and L. J. Young. 2004. Ventral striatopallidal oxytocin and vasopressin V1a receptors in the monogamous prairie vole *(Microtus ochrogaster). Journal of Comparative Neurology* 468: 555–70.

Lim, M. M., and L. J. Young. 2004. "Vasopressin-dependent neural circuits underlying pair bond formation in the monogamous prairie vole." *Neuroscience,* 125: 35–45.

Lindburg, D. G. 1982. Primate obstetrics: The biology of birth. *American Journal of Primatology,* Supplement 1:193–99.

Lloyd, E. A. 2005. *The case of the female orgasm.* Cambridge, MA: Harvard Univ. Press.

Lloyd, H. G. 1980. *The red fox.* London: Batsford.

Lloyd, P. 1968. Divorce among the Yoruba. *American Anthropologist* 70:67–81.

London, K. A., and B. Foley Wilson. 1988. D-i-v-o-r-c-e. *American Demographics,* Oct., 22–26.

Lovejoy, C. O. 1981. The origin of man. *Science* 211:341–50.

———. 2009. Re-examining human origins in light of *Ardipithecus ramidus* and the paleobiology of early hominins. *Science* 326:74–8, 85–93.

———. 2010. An enlarged postcranial sample confirms *Australopithecus afarensis* dimorphism was similar to modern humans. *Philosophical Transactions of the Royal Society B,* 365: 3355–63.

Low, B. S. 1979. Sexual selection and human ornamentation. In *Evolutionary biology and human social behavior,* ed. N. A. Chagnon and W. Irons. North Scituate, MA: Duxbury Press.

Low, B. S., R. D. Alexander, and K. M. Noonan. 1987. Human hips, breasts and buttocks: Is fat deceptive? *Ethology and Sociobiology* 8 (4): 249–58.

Lucretius. 1965. *On the nature of the universe.* New York: Frederick Ungar.

Lupyan, G., and R. Dale. 2010. Language structure is partly determined by social structure. *PLoS ONE* 5 (1): e8559. doi:10.1371/journal.pone.0008559.

Maccoby, E. E., and C. N. Jacklin. 1974. *The psychology of sex differences.* Stanford, CA: Stanford Univ. Press.

MacDonald, G., and M. R. Leary. 2005. Why does social exclusion hurt? The relationship between social and physical pain. *Psychological Bulletin* 131(2): 202–23.

Mace, D., and V. Mace. 1959. *Marriage: East and West.* Garden City, NY: Doubleday/ Dolphin.

MacKinnon, J. 1979. Reproductive behavior in wild orangutan populations. In *The great apes,* ed. D. A. Hamburg and E. R. McCown. Menlo Park, CA: Benjamin/ Cummings.

MacLean, P. D. 1973. *A triune concept of the brain and behaviour.* Toronto: Toronto Univ. Press.

Maglio, V. J. 1978. Patterns of faunal evolution. In *Evolution of African mammals,* ed. V. J. Maglio and H. B. S. Cooke. Cambridge, MA: Harvard Univ. Press.

Mah, K., and Y. M. Binik. 2002. Do all orgasms feel alike? Evaluating a two-dimensional model of the orgasm experience across gender and sexual context. *Journal of Sex Research* 39: 104–13.

Malinowski, B. 1965. *Sex and repression in savage society*. New York: World.

Manning, J. T. 2002. *Digit ratio: A pointer to fertility, behavior, and health*. New Brunswick, NJ: Rutgers Univ. Press.

Manning, J. T., S. Baron-Cohen, S. Wheelwright, and G. Sanders. 2001. The 2nd to 4th digit ratio and autism. *Developmental Medicine and Child Neurology* 43: 160–64.

Manning, J. T. and D. Scutt. 1996. Symmetry and ovulation in women. *Human Reproduction* 11:2477–80.

Manning J. T., D. Scutt, G. H. Whitehouse, et al. 1996. Asymmetry and menstrual cycle in women. *Ethology and Sociobiology* 17:129–43.

Mansperger, M. C. 1990. The precultural human mating system. *Journal of Human Evolution* 5:245–59.

Marazziti, D., H. S. Akiskal, A. Rossi and G. B. Cassano. 1999. Alteration of the platelet serotonin transporter in romantic love. *Psychological Medicine* 29:741–45.

Marks, J. 1989. The hominin clad. *Science* 246:1645.

Marlowe, F. 1998. The nobility hypothesis: The human breast as an honest signal of residual reproductive value. *Human Nature* 9:263–71.

———. 2000. Paternal investment and the human mating system. *Behavioural Processes* 51: 45–61.

———. 2004. Marital residence among foragers. *Current Anthropology* 45:277–84.

———. 2005. Hunter-gatherers and human evolution. *Evolutionary Anthropology* 14:54–67.

———. 2010. The Hadza: Hunter-gatherers of Tanzania. Berkeley: Univ. of California Press.

*Marriage and Divorce Today*. 1987. The hidden meaning: An analysis of different types of affairs. June 1, 1–2.

———. 1986. May 12, 1.

Martin, M. K., and B. Voorhies. 1975. *Female of the species*. New York: Columbia Univ. Press.

Martin, R. D. 1982. Human brain evolution in an ecological context. 52nd James Arthur Lecture on the Evolution of the Human Brain, American Museum of Natural History, New York.

Martínez, I., J. L. Arsuaga, R. Quam, et al. 2008. Human hyoid bones from the Middle Pleistocene site of the Sima de los Huesos (Sierra de Atapuerca, Spain). *Journal of Human Evolution* 54: 118–24.

Mascia-Lees, F. E., J. H. Relethford, and T. Sorger. 1986. Evolutionary perspectives on permanent breast enlargement in human females. *American Anthropologist* 88:423–29.

Maxwell, M. 1984. *Human evolution: A philosophical anthropology*. New York: Columbia Univ. Press.

Maynard Smith, J. 1978. *The evolution of sex*. Cambridge, UK: Cambridge Univ. Press.

Mazur, A., Susman, E. J., and S. Edelbrock. 1997. Sex differences in testosterone response to a video game contest. *Evolution and Human Behavior* 18(5): 317–26.

McClintock, M. K. 1971. Menstrual synchrony and suppression. *Nature* 229:244–45.

McCorriston, J., and F. Hole. 1991. The ecology of seasonal stress and the origins of agriculture in the Near East. *American Anthropologist* 93:46–69.

McCullough, D. 2001. *John Adams.* New York: Simon and Schuster.

McGinnis, P. R. 1979. Sexual behavior in free-living chimpanzees: Consort relationships. In *The great apes,* ed. D. A. Hamburg and E. R. McCown. Menlo Park, CA: Benjamin/Cummings.

McGrew, W. C. 1974. Tool use by wild chimpanzees in feeding upon driver ants. *Journal of Human Evolution* 3:501–8.

———. 1979. Evolutionary implications of sex differences in chimpanzee predation and tool use. In *The great apes,* ed. D. A. Hamburg and E. R. McCown. Menlo Park, CA: Benjamin/Cummings.

———. 1981. The female chimpanzee as a human evolutionary prototype. In *Woman the gatherer,* ed. F. Dahlberg. New Haven: Yale Univ. Press.

McGuinness, D. 1976. Perceptual and cognitive differences between the sexes. In *Explorations in Sex Differences,* ed. B. Lloyd and J. Archer. New York: Academic Press.

———. 1979. How schools discriminate against boys. *Human Nature,* Feb., 82–88.

———. 1985. Sensory biases in cognitive development. In *Male-female differences: A bio-cultural perspective.* ed. R. L. Hall, et al. New York: Praeger.

McGuinness, D., and K. H. Pribram. 1979. The origin of sensory bias in the development of gender differences in perception and cognition. In *Cognitive growth and development,* ed. M. Bortner. New York: Brunner/Mazel.

McGuire, M., M. Raleigh, and G. Brammer. 1982. Sociopharmacology. *Annual Review of Pharmacology and Toxicology* 22:643–61.

McHenry, H. M. 1986. The first bipeds. *Journal of Human Evolution* 15:177.

McHenry, H. M., and C. J. O'Brien. 1986. Comment on H. T. Bunn and E. M. Kroll, Systematic butchery by Plio/Pleistocene hominids at Olduvai Gorge, Tanzania. *Current Anthropology* 27:431–53.

McMillan, V. 1984. Dragonfly monopoly. *Natural History,* July, 33–38.

McWhirter, N., and R. McWhirter. 1975. *Guinness book of world records.* New York: Sterling.

Mead, M. 1935. *Sex and temperament in three primitive societies.* New York: William Morrow.

———. 1949. *Male and female.* New York: William Morrow.

———. 1966. Marriage in two steps. *Redbook,* July, 47–49, 84, 86.

Mealey, L. 1985. The relationship between social status and biological success: A case study of the Mormon religious hierarchy. *Ethology and Sociobiology* 6:249–57.

Mearns, J. 1991. Coping with a breakup: Negative mood regulation expectancies and depression following the end of a romantic relationship. *Journal of Personality and Social Psychology* 60:327–34.

Meggitt, M. J. 1962. *Desert people: A study of the Walbiri aborigines of central Australia.* Chicago: Univ. of Chicago Press.

Melis, M., S. Spiga, and M. Diana. 2005. The dopamine hypothesis of drug addiction: hypodopaminergic state. *International Review of Neurobiology.* 63:101–54.

Mellars, P. 1989. Major issues in the emergence of modern humans. *Current Anthropology* 30:349–85.

Mellen, S. L. W. 1981. *The evolution of love.* San Francisco: W. H. Freeman.

Mellody, P., A. W. Miller, and J. K. Miller. 1992. *Facing love addiction*. New York: HarperCollins.

Meloy, J. R., ed. 1998. The psychology of stalking: Clinical and forensic perspectives. San Diego, CA: Academic Press.

Meloy, J. R., B. Davis, and J. Lovette. 2001. Risk factors for violence among stalkers. *Journal of Threat Assessment* 1:1–16.

Meloy, J. R., and H. E. Fisher. 2005. Some thoughts on the neurobiology of stalking. *Journal of Forensic Sciences* 50(6):1472–80.

Meston, C. M., and D. M. Buss. 2007. *Why women have sex: Understanding sexual motivations from adventure to revenge (and everything in between)*. New York: Henry Holt.

Meston, C. M., and P. F. Frohlic. 2000. "The Neurobiology of Sexual Function." *Archives of General Psychiatry* 57:1012–30.

Michod, R. E. 1989. What's love got to do with it? *The Sciences,* May–June, 22–28.

Michod, R. E., and B. R. Levin, eds. 1987. *The evolution of sex: An examination of current ideas*. Sunderland, MA: Sinauer.

Miller, A. J., S. Sassler, and D. Kusi-Appouh. 2011. The specter of divorce: Views from working- and middle-class cohabitors. *Family Relations* 60:602–16.

Miller, G. F. 2000. *The mating mind: How sexual choice shaped the evolution of human nature*. New York: Doubleday.

Miller, J. A. 1983. Masculine/feminine behavior: New views. *Science News* 124:326.

Mitterauer, M., and R. Sieder. 1982. *The European family: Patriarchy to partnership from the Middle Ages to the present*. Chicago: Univ. of Chicago Press.

Miyamoto, M. M., J. L. Slightom, and M. Goodman. 1987. Phylogenetic relations of humans and African apes from DNA sequences in the ψη-globin region. *Science* 238:369–72.

Mock, D. W., and M. Fujioka. 1990. Monogamy and long-term pair bonding in vertebrates. *Trends in Ecology and Evolution* 5 (2): 39–43.

Moir, A., and D. Jessel. 1989. *Brain sex: The real differences between men and women*. London: Michael Joseph.

Moller, A. P. 1988. Ejaculate quality, testes size and sperm competition in primates. *Journal of Human Evolution* 17:479.

Money, J. 1980. *Love and love sickness: The science of sex, gender difference, and pair-bonding*. Baltimore: Johns Hopkins Univ. Press.

———. 1986. *Lovemaps: Clinical concepts of sexual/erotic health and pathology, paraphilia, and gender transposition in childhood, adolescence and maturity*. New York: Irvington.

Money, J., and A. A. Ehrhardt. 1972. *Man and woman, boy and girl: The differentiation and dimorphism of gender identity from conception to maturity*. Baltimore: Johns Hopkins Univ. Press.

Montagu, A. 1937. *Coming into being among the Australian aborigines*. London: Routledge.

———. 1961. Neonatal and infant immaturity in man. *Journal of the American Medical Association* 178:56–57.

———. 1971. *Touching: The human significance of the skin*. New York: Columbia Univ. Press.

————. 1981. *Growing young.* New York: McGraw-Hill.

Montejo, A. L., G. Llorca, J. A. Izquierdo, and F. Rico-Vallademoros. 2001. Incidence of sexual dysfunction associated with antidepressant agents: A prospective multicenter study of 1022 outpatients. *Journal of Clinical Psychiatry* 62 (3): 1020.

Monto, M., and A. Carey. 2013. A New Standard of Sexual Behavior? Are Claims Associated with the "Hookup Culture" supported by Nationally Representative Data? Paper presented at the American Sociological Association 108th Annual Meeting, Aug. 13.

Morais, R. C. 2004. Prozac Nation: Is the party over? *Forbes*, Sept. 6, 119–24.

Morgan, L. H. 1877. *Ancient society.* New York: World.

Morris, D. 1967. *The naked ape.* New York: McGraw-Hill.

————. 1971. *Intimate behavior.* New York: Bantam.

Morrison, P. 1987. Review of *Dark caves, bright visions: Life in Ice Age Europe* by Randall White. *Scientific American* 256 (3): 26–27.

Morton, Eugene. Dept. of Ornithology, Smithsonian Institution. Personal communication.

Moss, C. 1988. *Elephant memories: Thirteen years in the life of an elephant family.* New York: William Morrow.

Murdock, G. P. 1949. *Social structure.* New York: Free Press.

————. 1965. Family stability in non-European culture. In *Culture and society*, ed. G. P. Murdock. Pittsburgh: Univ. of Pittsburgh Press.

————. 1967. *Ethnographic Atlas.* Pittsburgh: Univ. of Pittsburgh Press.

Murdock, G. P., and D. R. White. 1969. Standard cross-cultural sample. *Ethnology* 8:329–69.

Nadel, S. F. 1942. *A black Byzantium: The kingdom of Nupe in Nigeria.* London: Oxford Univ. Press.

Nadler, R. D. 1975. Sexual cyclicity in captive lowland gorillas. *Science* 189:813–14.

————. 1988. Sexual aggression in the great apes. In *Human sexual aggression*, ed. R. A. Prentky and V. L. Quinsey. *Annals of the New York Academy of Sciences* 528:154–61.

Najib, A., J. P. Lorberbaum, S. Kose, et al. 2004. Regional brain activity in women grieving a romantic relationship breakup. *American Journal of Psychiatry* 161(12): 2245–56.

Nemeroff, C. B. 1998. The neurobiology of depression. *Scientific American* 278:42–49.

Nimuendaju, C. 1946. *The eastern Timbira.* Trans. R. H. Lowie. Univ. of California Publications in American Archaeology and Ethnology, vol. 41. Berkeley: Univ. of California Press.

Nishida, T. 1979. The social structure of chimpanzees of the Mahali Mountains. In *The great apes*, ed. D. A. Hamburg and E. R. McCown. Menlo Park, CA: Benjamin/ Cummings.

Nissen, H. J. 1988. *The early history of the ancient Near East, 9000–2000* B.C. Chicago: Univ. of Chicago Press.

Nolen-Hoeksema, S., J. Larson, and C. Grayson. 1999. Explaining the gender difference in depressive symptoms. *Journal of Personality and Social Psychology* 77:1061–72.

Oakley, K. P. 1956. Fire as a Paleolithic tool and weapon. *Proceedings of the Prehistoric Society* 21:36–48.

O'Brien, E. M. 1984. What was the acheulean hand ax? *Natural History*, July, 20–4.

Okonjo, K. 1976. The dual-sex political system in operation: Igbo women and community politics in Midwestern Nigeria. In *Women in Africa: Studies in social and economic change*, ed. N. J. Hafkin and E. G. Bay. Stanford, CA: Stanford Univ. Press.

O'Leary, K. D., B. P. Acevedo, A. Aron, et al. 2011. Is long-term love more than a rare phenomenon?: If so,what are its correlates? *Social Psychological and Personality Science*, 3(2):241–49.

Ophir, A.'G., J. O. Wolff, and S. M. Phelps. 2008. Variation in the neural V1aR predicts sexual fidelity and space use among male prairie voles in semi-natural settings. *Proceedings of the National Academy of Sciences* 105:1249–54.

Orians, G. H. 1969. On the evolution of mating systems in birds and mammals. *American Naturalist* 103:589–603.

Ortigue, S., F. Bianchi-Demichelli, S. T. Grafton, et al. 2007. The neural basis of love as a subliminal prime: An event-related functional magnetic resonance imaging study. *Journal of Cognitive Neuroscience* 19:1218–30.

Ortner, S. B., and H. Whitehead. 1981. Introduction: Accounting for sexual meanings. In *Sexual meanings*, ed. S. B. Ortner and H. Whitehead. Cambridge, UK: Cambridge Univ. Press.

Orzeck, T., and E. Lung. 2005. Big-five personality differences of cheaters and non-cheaters. *Current Psychology* 24: 274–86.

Otten, C. M. 1985. Genetic effects on male and female development and on the sex ratio. In *Male–female differences: A bio-cultural perspective*, ed. R. H. Hall et al. New York: Praeger.

Pagels, E. 1988. *Adam, Eve and the Serpent*. New York: Vintage.

Palombit, R. A., R. M. Seyfarth, and D. L. Cheney. 1997. The adaptive value of "friendships" to female baboons: Experimental and observational evidence. *Animal Behavior* 54:599–614.

Panksepp, J. 1998. *Affective neuroscience: The foundations of human and animal emotions*. New York: Oxford Univ. Press.

———. 2003. Neuroscience: Feeling the pain of social loss. *Science* 302:237–9.

Parker, G. A., R. R. Baker, and V. G. F. Smith. 1972. The origin and evolution of gamete dimorphism and the male–female phenomenon. *Journal of Theoretical Biology* 36:529–53.

Pavelka, M. S., and L. M. Fedigan. 1991. Menopause: A comparative life history perspective. *Yearbook of Physical Anthropology* 34:13–38.

Peck, J. R., and M. W. Feldman. 1988. Kin selection and the evolution of monogamy. *Science* 240:1672–74.

Pedersen, C. A., J. D. Caldwell, G. F. Jirikowsk, and T. R. Insel, eds. 1992. *Oxytocin in maternal, sexual and social behaviors*. New York: New York Academy of Sciences.

Peele, S. 1975. Love and addiction. New York: Taplinger.

*People*. 1986. Unfaithfully yours: Adultery in America. Aug. 18, 85–95.

Perper, T. 1985. *Sex signals: The biology of love*. Philadelphia: ISI Press.

Pew Research Center: Social and Demographic Trends. 2010. The decline of marriage and rise of new families. Nov. 18 http://pewsocialtrends.org/2010/11/18.

———. 2013. Love and Marriage. Feb. 13. http://pewsocialtrends.org/2013/2/13.

Pfaff, D. W., and H. E. Fisher. 2012. Generalized brain arousal mechanisms and other biological, environmental and psychological mechanisms that contribute to libido. In *From the couch to the lab: Trends in Neuropsychoanalysis*, ed. A. Fotopoulou et al. 65–84. Cambridge, UK: Cambridge Univ. Press.

Pfeiffer, J. E. 1982. *The creative explosion: An inquiry into the origins of art and religion.* New York: Harper and Row.

Phillips, R. 1988. *Putting asunder: A history of divorce in Western society.* Cambridge, UK: Cambridge Univ. Press.

Pilbeam, D. 1985. Patterns of hominoid evolution. In *Ancestors: The hard evidence*, ed. E. Delson. New York: Alan R. Liss.

Pinker, S. 2014. The village effect. New York: Spiegel and Grau.

Pitkow, L. J., C. A. Sharer, X. Ren, et al. 2001. Facilitation of affiliation and pair-bond formation by vasopressin receptor gene transfer into the ventral forebrain of a monogamous vole. *Journal of Neuroscience* 21:7392–96.

Pittman, F. 1989. *Private lies: Infidelity and the betrayal of intimacy.* New York: W. W. Norton.

Plavcan, J. M. 2012. Sexual size dimorphism, canine dimorphism and male–male competition in primates. Where do humans fit in? *Human Nature* 23:45–67.

Plooij, F. X. 1978. Tool-use during chimpanzee's bushpig hunt. *Carnivore* 1:103–6.

Posner, R. A. 1992. *Sex and reason.* Cambridge, MA: Harvard Univ. Press.

Potts, R. 1984. Home bases and early hominids. *American Scientist* 72:338–47.

———. 1988. *Early hominid activities at Olduvai.* New York: Aldine de Gruyter.

———. 1991. Untying the knot: Evolution of early human behavior. In *Man and beast revisited*, ed. M. H. Robinson and L. Tiger. Washington, DC: Smithsonian Institution Press.

Power, E. 1973. The position of women. In *Women: From the Greeks to the French Revolution.* ed. S. G. Bell. Stanford, CA: Stanford Univ. Press.

Preti, G., W. B. Cutler, C. R. Garcia, et al. 1986. Human axillary secretions influence women's menstrual cycles: The role of donor extract of females. *Hormones and Behavior* 20:474–82.

Price, D., and J. A. Brown, eds. 1985. *Prehistoric hunter-gatherers: The emergence of cultural complexity.* New York: Academic Press.

Pruetz, J. D. and T. C. LaDuke. 2010. Brief communication: reaction to fire by savanna chimpanzees (*Pan troglodytes verus*) at Fongoli, Senegal: conceptualization of "Fire Behavior" and the case for a chimpanzee model. *American Journal of Physical Anthropology* 141:646–50.

Pusey, A. E. 1979. Intercommunity transfer of chimpanzees in Gombe National Park. In *The great apes*, ed. D. A. Hamburg and E. R. McCown. Menlo Park, CA: Benjamin/ Cummings.

———. 1980. Inbreeding avoidance in chimpanzees. *Animal Behavior* 28:543–52.

Quadagno, D. M., H. E. Shubeita, J. Deck, and D. Francoeur. 1981. Influence of male social contacts, exercise and all-female living conditions on the menstrual cycle. *Psychoneuroendocrinology* 6:239–44.

Queen, S. A., and R. W. Habenstein. 1974. *The family in various cultures.* Philadelphia: J. B. Lippincott.

Quinlan, R., and M. Quinlan. 2008. Human lactation, pair-bonds and alloparents: A cross-cultural analysis. *Human Nature* 19:87–102.

Radcliffe-Brown, A. R. 1922. *The Andaman Islanders.* Cambridge, UK: Cambridge Univ. Press.

Raleigh, M., M. T. McGuire, G. L. Brammer, et al. Forthcoming. Serotonergic mechanisms promote dominance acquisition in adult male vervet monkeys. *Brain Research.*

Rancourt-Laferriere, D. 1983. Four adaptive aspects of the female orgasm. *Journal of Social and Biological Structures* 6:319–33.

Rawson, B., ed. 1986. *The family in ancient Rome: New perspectives.* Ithaca, NY: Cornell Univ. Press.

Rebhun, L. A. 1995. Language of love in northeast Brazil. In *Romantic Passion: A Universal Experience?* ed. W. Jankowiak, 252. New York: Columbia Univ. Press.

Reich, D., R. E. Green, M. Kircher, et al. 2010. Genetic history of an archaic hominin group from Denisova Cave in Siberia. *Nature* 468: 1053–60.

Reichard, G. S. 1950. *Navaho Religion.* New York: Bollingen Foundation.

Reik, T. 1964. *The need to be loved.* New York: Bantam.

Reiter, R. R. 1975. Introduction to *Toward an anthropology of women,* ed. R. R. Reiter. New York: Monthly Review Press.

———, ed. 1975. *Toward an Anthropology of Women.* New York: Monthly Review Press.

Reno, P. L., R. S. Meindl, M. A. McCollum, and C. O. Lovejoy. 2003. Sexual dimorphism in *Australopithecus afarensis* was similar to that of modern humans. *Proceedings of the National Academy of Sciences USA* 100: 9404–09.

Repenning, C. A., and O. Fejfar. 1982. Evidence for early date of Ubeidiya, Israel, hominid site. *Nature* 299:344–47.

Retallack, G. J., D. P. Dugas, and E. A. Bestland. 1990. Fossil soils and grasses of the Middle Miocene East African grassland. *Science* 247:1325.

Reynaud, M., L. Karila, L. Blecha, and A. Benyamina. 2010. Is love passion an addictive disorder? *American Journal of Drug and Alcohol Abuse* 36(5): 261–67.

Roberts, L. 1988. Zeroing in on the sex switch. *Science* 239:21–23.

Rodman, P. S. 1988. Orangutans. *Institute of Human Origins Newsletter* 6 (1): 5.

Rogers, S. C. 1975. Female forms of power and the myth of male dominance: A model of female/male interaction in peasant society. *American Ethnologist* 2:727–56.

Rohrlich-Leavitt, R., B. Sykes, and E. Weatherford. 1975. Aboriginal woman: Male and female, anthropological perspectives. In *Toward an anthropology of women,* ed. R. R. Reiter. New York: Monthly Review Press.

Rosaldo, M. Z. 1974. Woman, culture, and society: A theoretical overview. In *Woman, culture, and society,* ed. M. Z. Rosaldo and L. Lamphere. Stanford: Stanford Univ. Press.

Rosaldo, M. Z., and L. Lamphere, eds. 1974. *Women, Culture, and Society.* Stanford, CA: Stanford Univ. Press.

Rose, M., and R. M. Kreider. 2006. *Remarriage in the United States.* Poster presented at the annual meeting of the American Sociological Association, Montreal, Aug. 10–14, by the U.S. Bureau of the Census.

Rose, M. D. 1983. Miocene hominoid postcranial morphology: monkey-like, ape-like, neither, or both? In *New interpretations of ape and human ancestry,* ed. R. L. Ciochon and R. S. Corruccini. New York: Plenum Press.

Rose, R. M., I. S. Bernstein, T. P. Gordon, and S. F. Catlin. 1974. Androgens and aggression: A review and recent findings in primates. In *Primate aggression, territoriality, and xenophobia*, ed. R. L. Holloway. New York: Academic Press.

Rose, R. M., J. W. Holaday, and I. S. Bernstein. 1971. Plasma testosterone, dominance rank and aggressive behavior in male rhesus monkeys. *Nature* 231:366–68.

Rosenberg, L. P., and S. Park. 2002. Verbal and spatial functions across the menstrual cycle in healthy young women. *Psychoneuroendocrinology* 27: 835–41.

Rosenblum, A. 1976. *The natural birth control book*. Philadelphia: Aquarian Research Foundation.

Rosenthal, N. E. 2002. The emotional revolution: How the new science of feelings can transform your life. New York: Citadel Press.

Rossi, A. 1984. Gender and parenthood. *American Sociological Review* 49:1–19.

Rowell, T. E. 1972. Female reproductive cycles and social behavior in primates. In *Advances in the study of behavior*. Vol. 4, ed. D. S. Lehrman et al. New York: Academic Press.

Rudder, C. 2014. *Dataclysm: Who we are when we think no one's looking*. New York: Crown.

Rue, L. L. 1969. *The world of the red fox*. Philadelphia: J. B. Lippincott.

Ruse, M. 1988. *Homosexuality: A philosophical inquiry*. Oxford: Basil Blackwell.

Russell, M. J. 1976. Human olfactory communication. *Nature* 260:520–22.

Russett, C. E. 1989. *Sexual science: The Victorian construction of womanhood*. Cambridge, MA: Harvard Univ. Press.

Rutberg, A. T. 1983. The evolution of monogamy in primates. *Journal of Theoretical Biology* 104:93–112.

Ryan, A. S., and D. C. Johanson. 1989. Anterior dental microwear in *Australopithecus afarensis:* Comparisons with human and nonhuman primates. *Journal of Human Evolution* 18:235–68.

Ryder, N. B. 1974. The family in developed countries. *Scientific American*, March, 123–32.

Sabelli, H. C. 1991. Rapid treatment of depression with selegiline–phenylalanine combination. Letter to the editor. *Journal of Clinical Psychiatry* 52:3.

Sabelli, H. C., L. Carlson-Sabelli, and J. I. Javaid. 1990. The thermodynamics of bipolarity: A bifurcation model of bipolar illness and bipolar character and its psychotherapeutic applications. *Psychiatry* 53:346–68.

Sacks, K. 1971. Comparative notes on the position of women. Paper delivered at the annual meeting of the American Anthropological Association, Washington, DC.

———. 1979. *Sisters and wives: The past and future of sexual equality*. Urbana: Univ. of Illinois Press.

Sade, D. S. 1968. Inhibition of son–mother mating among free-ranging rhesus monkeys. *Science and Psychoanalysis* 12:18–37.

Sahlins, M. 1972. *Stone Age economics*. New York: Aldine.

Sanday, P. R. 1974. Female status in the public domain. In *Woman, culture, and society*, ed. M. Z. Rosaldo and L. Lamphere. Stanford, CA: Stanford Univ. Press.

———. 1981. *Female power and male dominance: On the origins of sexual inequality*. Cambridge, UK: Cambridge Univ. Press.

Sanders, A. R., E. R. Martin, G. W. Beecham, et al. 2015. Genome-wide scan demonstrates significant linkage for male sexual orientation. *Psychological Medicine* 45 (7): 1379–88.

Sapolsky, R. M. 1983. Endocrine aspects of social instability in the olive baboon. *American Journal of Primatology* 5:365–76.

Sarich, V. M., and J. E. Cronin. 1976. Molecular systematics of the primates. In *Molecular anthropology*, ed. M. Goodman and R. E. Tashian. New York: Plenum Press.

Sarich, V. M., and A. C. Wilson. 1967a. Immunological time scale for hominid evolution. *Science* 158:1200–3.

———. 1967b. Rates of albumin evolution in primates. *Proceedings of the National Academy of Sciences* 58:142–48.

Savage-Rumbaugh, E. S., and B. J. Wilkerson. 1978. Socio-sexual behavior in *Pan paniscus* and *Pan troglodytes*: A comparative study. *Journal of Human Evolution* 7:327–44.

Schaef, A. W. 1989. *Escape from intimacy: The pseudo-relationship addictions*. San Francisco: Harper and Row.

Schaller, G. B. 1972. *The Serengeti lion: A study of predator–prey relations*. Chicago: Univ. of Chicago Press.

Schaller, G. B., and G. R. Lowther. 1969. The relevance of carnivore behavior to the study of early hominids. *Southwestern Journal of Anthropology* 25:307–41.

Schlegel, A. 1972. *Male dominance and female autonomy: Domestic authority in matrilineal societies*. New Haven: HRAF Press.

Schmitt, D. P. 2004a. The big five related to risky sexual behavior across 10 world regions: Differential personality associations of sexual promiscuity and relationship infidelity. *European Journal of Personality* 18:301–19.

———. 2004b. Patterns and universals of mate poaching across 53 nations: The effects of sex, culture and personality on romantically attracting another person's partner. *Journal of Personality and Social Psychology* 86:560–84.

Schmitt, D. P., and D. M. Buss. 2001. Human mate poaching: Tactics and temptations for infiltrating existing mateships." *Journal of Personality and Social Psychology* 80: 894–917.

Schneider, H. K. 1971. Romantic love among the Turu. In *Human sexual behavior*, ed. D. S. Marshall and R. C. Suggs. Englewood Cliffs, NJ: Prentice-Hall.

Schrire, C., ed. 1984. *Past and present in hunter-gatherer societies*. New York: Academic Press.

Schultz, W. 2000. Multiple Reward Signals in the Brain. Nature Reviews. *Neuroscience* 1 (Dec. 2000): 199–207.

Sefcek, J. A., B. H. Brumbach, G. Vasquez, and G. F. Miller. 2006. The evolutionary psychology of human mate choice: How ecology, genes, fertility, and fashion influence mating behavior. In *Handbook of the evolution of human sexuality*, ed. M. Knauth, 125–82. Philadelphia: Haworth Press.

Seligman, J. 1990. Variations on a theme. *Newsweek Special Edition*, Winter/Spring, 38–46.

Service, E. R. 1978. The Arunta of Australia. In *Profiles in ethnology*, ed. E. R. Service. 3rd ed. New York: Harper and Row.

*Sexuality Today*. 1988. Approaching the male of the species. March 7, 5.

Shackelford, T. K., Besser, A., and A.T. Goetz. 2008. Personality, marital satisfaction, and probability of marital infidelity. *Individual Differences Research* 6 (1): 13–25.

Shepher, J. 1971. Mate selection among second generation kibbutz adolescents and adults: Incest avoidance and negative imprinting. *Archives of Sexual Behavior* 1:293–307.

———. 1983. *Incest—A biosocial view.* New York: Academic Press.

Sherfey, M. J. 1972. *The nature and evolution of female sexuality.* New York: Vintage.

Sherman, J. 1978. *Sex-related cognitive differences: An essay on theory and evidence.* Springfield, IL: Charles C. Thomas.

Shipman, P. 1984. Scavenger Hunt. *Natural History,* April, 20–27.

———. 1986. Scavenging or hunting in early hominids: Theoretical framework and test. *American Anthropologist* 88:27–43.

———. 1987. Studies of hominid–faunal interaction at Olduvai Gorge. *Journal of Human Evolution* 15:691–706.

Shorey, H. H. 1976. *Animal communication by pheromones.* New York: Academic Press.

Short, R. V. 1976. The evolution of human reproduction. *Proceedings of the Royal Society* B, 195:3–24.

———. 1977. Sexual selection and descent of man. In *Reproduction and evolution,* ed. J. H. Calaby and C. Tyndale-Biscoe. Canberra: Australian Academy of Science.

———. 1984. Breast-feeding. *Scientific American,* April, 35–41.

Shostak, M. 1981. *Nisa: The life and words of a !Kung woman.* New York: Random House.

Sibley, C., and J. Ahlquist. 1984. The phylogeny of hominoid primates, as indicated by DNA–DNA hybridization. *Journal of Molecular Evolution* 20:2–11.

Silverman, I., and M. Beals. 1990. Sex differences in spatial abilities: Evolutionary theory and data. Paper delivered at the annual meeting of the Human Behavior and Evolution Society, Los Angeles.

Silverstein, C. 1981. *Man to man: Gay couples in America.* New York: William Morrow.

Simons, E. L. 1985. Origins and characteristics of the first hominoids. In *Ancestors: The hard evidence.* ed. E. Delson. New York: Alan R. Liss.

———. 1989. Human origins. *Science* 245:1343–50.

Simpson-Hebert, M., and S. L. Huffman. 1981. The contraceptive effect of breast-feeding. In *Breastfeeding,* ed. E. C. Baer and B. Winikoff. Special Issue of *Studies in Family Planning* 12 (4): 125–33.

Sinclair, A. R. E., M. D. Leakey, and M. Norton-Griffiths. 1986. Migration and hominid bipedalism. *Nature* 324:307.

Singh, D. 1993. Adaptive significance of waist-to-hip ratio and female physical attractiveness. *Journal of Personality and Social Psychology* 65:293–307.

———. 2002. Female mate value at a glance: Relationship of waist-to-hip ratio to health, fecundity and attractiveness. *Neuroendocrinology Letters* Suppl. 4, 23:81–91.

Singles in America. 2010, 2011, 2012, 2013, 2014. Attitudes and Behaviors of Singles in America collected annually between 2010–14, using a representative sample based on the U.S. Census (Total 25,000+ singles). Data courtesy of Match.com and Helen Fisher.

Slocum, S. 1975. Woman the gatherer: Male bias in anthropology. In *Toward an anthropology of women,* ed. R. R. Reiter. New York: Monthly Review Press.

Small, M. F. 1988. Female primate sexual behavior and conception: Are there really sperm to spare? *Current Anthropology* 29:81–100.

Smith, B. H. 1986. Dental development in *Australopithecus* and early *Homo*. *Nature* 323:327.

Smith, R. L. 1984. Human sperm competition. In *Sperm competition and the evolution of mating systems*, ed. R. L. Smith. New York: Academic Press.

Smuts, Barbara B. 1985. *Sex and friendship in baboons*. New York: Aldine de Gruyter.

———. 1987. What are friends for? *Natural History*, Feb., 36–44.

———. 1992. Male–infant relationships in nonhuman primates: Parental investment or mating effort? In *Father–child relations*, ed. B. Hewlett. New York: Aldine de Gruyter.

Solar, C., M. Nuñez, R. Gutierrez, et al. 2003. Facial attractiveness in men provides clues to semen quality. *Evolution and Human Behavior* 24:199–207.

Solecki, R. S. 1971. *Shanidar: The first flower people*. New York: Knopf.

———. 1989. On the evidence for Neanderthal burial. *Current Anthropology* 30:324.

Solway, J. S., and R. B. Lee. 1990. Foragers, genuine or spurious? *Current Anthropology* 31:109–46.

Sostek, A. J., and R. J. Wyatt. 1981. The chemistry of crankiness. *Psychology Today*, Oct., 120.

Spencer, R. F. 1959. *The North Alaskan Eskimo: A study in ecology and society*. Washington, DC: Smithsonian Institution Press.

Spiro, M. E. 1958. *Children of the kibbutz*. Cambridge, MA: Harvard Univ. Press.

Springer, S. P., and G. Deutsch. 1985. *Left brain, right brain*. Rev. ed. San Francisco: W. H. Freeman.

Steele, J., and N. Uomini. 2009. Can the archaeology of manual specialization tell us anything about language evolution? A survey of the state of play. *Cambridge Archaeological Journal* 19: 97–110.

Stendhal. [1822] 1975. *Love*. Trans. G. Sale and S. Sale. Harmondsworth, UK: Penguin.

Stephens, W. N. 1963. *The family in cross-cultural perspective*. New York: Holt, Rinehart and Winston.

Stoehr, T., ed. 1979. *Free love in America: A documentary history*. New York: AMS Press.

Stone, L. 1990. *Road to divorce: England, 1530–1987*. New York: Oxford Univ. Press.

Strassman, B. I. 1981. Sexual selection, parental care, and concealed ovulation in humans. *Ethology and Sociobiology* 2:31–40.

Straus, L. G. 1989. On early hominid use of fire. *Current Anthropology* 30:488–89.

Stringer, C. B., and P. Andrews. 1988. Genetic and fossil evidence for the origin of modern humans. *Science* 239:1263–68.

Strum, S. 1990. *Almost human: A journey into the world of baboons*. New York: W. W. Norton.

Suggs, R. C., and D. S. Marshall. 1971. Anthropological perspectives on human sexual behavior. In *Human sexual behavior*, ed. D. S. Marshall and R. C. Suggs. Englewood Cliffs, NJ: Prentice-Hall.

Susman, R. L. 1984. The locomotor behavior of *Pan paniscus* in the Lomako Forest. In *The pygmy chimpanzee*, ed. R. L. Susman. New York: Plenum Press.

———. 1989. New hominid fossils from the Swartkrans formation excavations (1979–1986): Postcranial specimens. *American Journal of Physical Anthropology* 79:451–74.

————. 1990. Evidence for tool behavior in the earliest hominids. Paper delivered at the Anthropology Section of the New York Academy of Sciences, Nov. 19.

Susman, R. L., J. T. Stern, Jr., and W. L. Jungers. 1985. Locomotor adaptations in the Hadar hominids. In *Ancestors: The hard evidence*, ed. E. Delson. New York: Alan R. Liss.

Swami, V., and A. W. Furnham. 2008. The psychology of human attraction. New York: Routledge.

Symons, D. 1979. *The evolution of human sexuality*. New York: Oxford Univ. Press.

————. 1982. Another woman that never existed. *Quarterly Review of Biology* 57:297–300.

Symons, D., and B. Ellis. 1989. Human male–female differences in sexual desire. In *The sociobiology of sexual and reproductive strategies*, ed. A. E. Rasa, C. Vogel, and E. Voland. New York: Chapman and Hall.

Tafoya, M. A., and B. H. Spitzberg. 2007. The dark side of infidelity: Its nature, prevalence, and communicative functions. In *The dark side of interpersonal communication*. 2nd edition, ed. B. H. Spitzberg and W. R. Cupach, 201–42. Mahwah, NJ: Lawrence Erlbaum Associates.

Tanner, N. M. 1981. *On becoming human*. Cambridge, UK: Cambridge Univ. Press.

Tanner, N. M., and A. L. Zihlman. 1976. Women in evolution. Part I: Innovation and selection in human origins. *Signs: Journal of Women in Culture and Society* 1:585–608.

Tavris, C., and S. Sadd. 1977. *The Redbook report on female sexuality*. New York: Delacorte.

Taylor, S. E., L. C. Klein, B. P. Lewis, T. L. Gruenewald, R. A. R. Gurung, and J. A. Updegraff. 2000. Biobehavioral responses to stress in females: Tend-and-befriend, not fight-or-flight. *Psychological Review* 107:751–53.

Teleki, G. 1973a. *The predatory behavior of wild chimpanzees*. Lewisburg, PA: Bucknell Univ. Press.

————. 1973b. The omnivorous chimpanzee. *Scientific American*, Jan., 3–12.

Tennov, D. 1979. *Love and limerence: The experience of being in love*. New York: Stein and Day.

Textor, R. B. 1967. *A cross-cultural summary*. New Haven: HRAF Press.

Thomas, E. M. 1993. *The hidden life of dogs*. New York: Houghton Mifflin.

Thomas, H. 1985. The Early and Middle Miocene land connection of the Afro-Arabian plate and Asia: A major event for hominoid dispersal? In *Ancestors: The hard evidence*, ed. E. Delson. New York: Alan R. Liss.

Thompson, A. P. 1983. Extramarital sex: A review of the research literature. *Journal of Sex Research* 19:1–22.

Thompson-Handler, N., R. K. Malenky, and N. Badrian. 1984. Sexual behavior of *Pan paniscus* under natural conditions in the Lomako Forest, Equateur, Zaire. In *The pygmy chimpanzee*, ed. R. L. Susman. New York: Plenum Press.

Thornhill, R., and J. Alcock. 1983. *The evolution of insect mating systems*. Cambridge, MA: Harvard Univ. Press.

Thornhill, R., and S. W. Gangestad. 1993. Human facial beauty. *Human Nature* 4 (3): 237–69.

Thornhill, R., S. W. Gangestad, and R. Comer. 1995. Human female orgasm and mate fluctuating asymmetry. *Animal Behavior* 50:1601–15.

Tiger, L. 1992. *The pursuit of pleasure*. Boston: Little, Brown.

Tobias, P. V. 1991. *Olduvai Gorge.* Vol. 4, *The skulls, endocasts and teeth of Homo habilis.* New York: Cambridge Univ. Press.

Tofler, A. 1980. *The third wave.* New York: William Morrow.

Torrence, R., ed. 1989. *Time, energy and stone tools.* New York: Cambridge Univ. Press.

Townsend, J. M. 1998. *What women want, what men want.* New York: Oxford Univ. Press.

Trevathan, W. R. 1987. *Human birth: An evolutionary perspective.* New York: Aldine de Gruyter.

Trinkaus, E., and P. Shipman. 1993. *The Neandertals.* London: Pimlico.

Trivers, R. L. 1972. Parental investment and sexual selection. In *Sexual selection and the descent of man, 1871–1971,* ed. B. Campbell. Chicago: Aldine.

———. 1985. *Social evolution.* Menlo Park, CA: Benjamin/Cummings.

Tsapelas, I., H. E. Fisher, and A. Aron. 2010. Infidelity: who, when, why. In *The dark side of close relationships,* Vol. 2, ed. W. R. Cupach and B. H. Spitzberg, 175–96. New York: Routledge.

Tucker, D. M., P. Luu, and D. Derryberry. 2005. Love hurts: The evolution of empathic concern through the encephalization of nociceptive capacity. *Development and Psychopathology* 17:699–713.

Tunnell, G. G. 1990. Systematic scavenging: Minimal energy expenditure at Olare Orok in the Serengeti ecosystem. In *Problem solving in taphonomy,* ed. S. Solomon, I. Davidson, and D. Watson. Santa Lucia, Australia: Univ. of Queensland Press.

Turke, P. W. 1984. Effects of ovulatory concealment and synchrony on protohominid mating systems and parental roles. *Ethology and Sociobiology* 5:33–44.

Turnbull, C. M. 1981. Mbuti womanhood. In *Woman the gatherer,* ed. F. Dahlberg. New Haven: Yale Univ. Press.

Tutin, C. E. G. 1979. Mating patterns and reproductive strategies in a community of wild chimpanzees *(Pan troglodytes schweinfurthii). Behavioral Ecology and Sociobiology* 6:39–48.

Tutin, C. E. G., and R. McGinnis. 1981. Chimpanzee reproduction in the wild. In *Reproductive biology of the great apes,* ed. C. E. Graham. New York: Academic Press.

Tuttle, R. H. 1990. The pitted pattern of Laetoli feet. *Natural History,* March, 61–64.

Tylor, E. B. 1889. On a method of investigating the development of institutions: Applied to laws of marriage and descent. *Journal of the Royal Anthropological Institute* 18:245–69.

Udry, J. R., and N. M. Morris. 1977. The distribution of events in the human menstrual cycle. *Journal of Reproductive Fertility* 51:419–25.

United Nations Statistical Office, Department of Economic and Social Affairs. 1955. Divorce rates per 1000 married couples, 1935–53. *Demographic Yearbook: 1954.* Chart 35. New York: United Nations.

———. 1958. Technical Notes. *Demographic Yearbook: 1954.* New York: United Nations.

———. 1984. *Demographic Yearbook: 1982.* New York: United Nations.

———. 2012a. *Demographic Yearbook: 2012.* New York: United Nations.

———. 2012b. Fertility and family planning section, Table: The World Marriage Data. New York: United Nations.

U.S. Bureau of the Census. 1986. *Statistical Abstract of the United States.* 1985, Chart 124. Washington DC.

Van Allen, J. 1976. "Aba Riots" or Igbo Women's War? Ideology, stratification, and the invisibility of women. In *Women in Africa*, ed. N. J. Hafkin and E. G. Bay. Stanford, CA: Stanford Univ. Press.

Van Couvering, J. A., and J. A. H. Van Couvering. 1975. African isolation and the Tethys seaway. In *Proceedings of the VI Congress of the Regional Committee on Mediterranean Neogene Stratigraphy*. Bratislava: Slovak Academy of Science.

Van Couvering, J. A. H. 1980. Community evolution and succession in East Africa during the Late Cenozoic. In *Bones in the making*, ed. A. Hill and K. Berensmeyer. Chicago: Univ. of Chicago Press.

van den Berghe, P. L. 1979. *Human family systems: An evolutionary view*. Westport, CT: Greenwood Press.

Vandiver, P., O. Soffer, B. Klima, and J. Svoboda. 1989. The origins of ceramic technology at Dolni Vestonice, Czechoslovakia. *Science* 246:1002–8.

Van Gulik, R. 1974. *Sexual life in Ancient China: A preliminary survey of Chinese sex and society from ca. 1500 BC until 1644 AD*. Leiden: E. J. Brill.

Van Hooff, J. A. R. A. M. 1971. *Aspects of the social behavior and communication in human and higher non-human primates*. Rotterdam: Bronder-Offset.

Van Steenberger, H., S. J. E. Langeslag, G. P. H. Band, and B. Hommel. 2013. Reduced cognitive control in passionate lovers. doi 10.1007/s11031-013-9380-3.

Van Valen, L. 1973. A new evolutionary law. *Evolutionary Theory* 1:1–30.

Veit, P. G. 1982. Gorilla society. *Natural History*, March, 48–58.

Velle, W. 1982. Sex, hormones and behavior in animals and man. *Perspectives in Biology and Medicine* 25:295–315.

Verner, J., and M. F. Willson. 1966. The influence of habitats on mating systems of North American passerine birds. *Ecology* 47:143–47.

Villmoare, B., W. H. Kimbel, C. Seyoum, et al. 2015. Early Homo at 2.8 Ma from Ledi-Geraru, Afar, Ethiopia. *Science* 347 (6228): 1352–55.

*Vital Statistics of the United States, 1960*. 1964. Vol. 3. Table 4–7. Washington, DC: National Center for Health Statistics.

———, *1970*. 1974. Vol. 3. Table 2–4. Rockville, MD: National Center for Health Statistics.

———, *1977*. 1981. Vol. 3. Table 2–17. Hyattsville, MD: National Center for Health Statistics.

———, *1979*. 1984. Vol. 3. Table 2–22. Hyattsville, MD: National Center for Health Statistics.

———, *1981*. 1985. Vol. 3. Table 2–13. Hyattsville, MD: National Center for Health Statistics.

———, *1983*. 1987. Vol. 3. Table 2–10. Hyattsville, MD: National Center for Health Statistics.

———, *1986*. 1990. Vol. 3. Table 2–29. Hyattsville, MD: National Center for Health Statistics.

Vrba, E. S. 1985. African Bovidae: Evolutionary events since the Miocene. *South African Journal of Science* 81:263–66.

Wagner, J., ed. 1982. *Sex roles in contemporary American communes*. Bloomington: Indiana Univ. Press.

Walum, H., L. Westberg, S. Henningsson, et al. 2008. Genetic variation in the vasopressin receptor 1a gene (AVPR1A) associates with pair-bonding behavior in humans. *Proceedings of the National Academy of Sciences* 105 (37): 14153–56.

Wang, Z. X., C. F. Ferris, and G. J. De Vries. 1994. The role of septal vasopressin innervation in paternal behavior in prairie voles (*Microtus ochrogaster*). *Proceedings of the National Academy of Sciences* 91, no. 1: 400–4.

Wang, Z., D. Toloczko, L. J. Young, et al. 1997. Vasopressin in the forebrain of common marmosets (*Calithrix jacchus*): Studies with in situ hybridization, immunocytochemistry and receptor autoradiography. *Brain Research* 768:147–56.

Washburn, S. L., and C. S. Lancaster, 1968. The evolution of hunting. In *Man the hunter*, ed. R. B. Lee and I. DeVore. New York: Aldine.

Washburn, S. L., and R. Moore. 1974. *Ape into man: A study of human evolution*. Boston: Little, Brown.

Watanabe, H. 1985. *Why did man stand up?: An ethnoarchaeological model for hominization*. Tokyo: Univ. of Tokyo Press.

Watson, P. J. and P. W. Andrews. 2002. Toward a revised evolutionary adaptationist analysis of depression: The social navigation hypothesis. *Journal of Affective Disorders* 72:1–14.

Watson, J. C., R. C. Payne, A. T. Chamberlain, et al. 2008. The energetic costs of load-carrying and the evolution of bipedalism. *Journal of Human Evolution* 54:675–83.

Wedekind, C., T. Seebeck, F. Bettens, et al. 1995. MHC-dependent mate preferences in humans. *Proceedings of the Royal Society of London*, 260:245–9.

Weiner, A. B. 1976. *Women of value, men of renown: New perspective in Trobriand exchange*. Austin: Univ. of Texas Press.

Weisman, S. R. 1988. Broken marriage and brawl test a cohesive cast. *New York Times*, Feb. 21.

Weiss, R. 1987. How dare we? Scientists seek the sources of risk-taking behavior. *Science News* 132:57–59.

———. 1988. Women's skills linked to estrogen levels. *Science News* 134:341.

Weiss, R. S. 1975. *Marital separation*. New York: Basic Books.

Werner, D. 1984. Paid sex specialists among the Mekranoti. *Journal of Anthropological Research* 40:394–405.

Westermarck, E. 1922. *The history of human marriage*. 5th ed. New York: Allerton.

———. 1934. Recent theories of exogamy. *Sociological Review* 26:22–44.

Westneat, D. F., P. W. Sherman, and M. L. Morton. 1990. The ecology and evolution of extra-pair copulations in birds. In *Current ornithology*. Vol. 7, ed. D. M. Power. New York: Plenum Press.

White, J. M. 1987. Premarital cohabitation and marital stability in Canada. *Journal of Marriage and the Family* 49:641–47.

White, R. 1986. *Dark caves, bright visions: Life in Ice Age Europe*. New York: American Museum of Natural History.

———. 1989a. Visual thinking in the Ice Age. *Scientific American*, July, 92–99.

———. 1989b. Production complexity and standardization in Early Aurignacian bead and pendant manufacture: Evolutionary implications. In *The human revolution*, ed. P. Mellars and C. B. Stringer. Vol. 1. Edinburgh: Edinburgh Univ. Press.

White, T. D. 1977. New fossil hominids from Laetoli, Tanzania. *American Journal of Physical Anthropology* 46:197–229.

———. 1980. Additional fossil hominids from Laetoli, Tanzania: 1976–1979 specimens. *American Journal of Physical Anthropology* 53:487–504.

———. 1985. The hominids of Hadar and Laetoli: An element-by-element comparison of the dental samples. In *Ancestors: The hard evidence*. ed. E. Delson. New York: Alan R. Liss.

White, T. D., B. Asfaw, Y. Beyene, et al. 2009. *Ardipithecus ramidus* and the paleobiology of early hominids. *Science* 326 (5949): 64, 75–86.

Whiting, B. B. 1965. Sex identity conflict and physical violence: A comparative study. *American Anthropologist* 67:123–40.

Whiting, B. B., and J. W. M. Whiting. 1975. *Children in six cultures*. Cambridge, MA: Harvard Univ. Press.

Whitten, R. G. 1982. Hominid promiscuity and the sexual life of proto-savages: Did *Australopithecus* swing? *Current Anthropology* 23:99–101.

Whyte, M. K. 1978. *The status of women in preindustrial societies*. Princeton: Princeton Univ. Press.

———. 1990. *Dating, mating, and marriage*. New York: Aldine de Gruyter.

Wickler, W. 1976. *The ethological analysis of attachment*. Berlin: Verlag Paul Parey.

Wiederman, M. W. 1997. Extramarital sex: Prevalence and correlates in a national survey. *Journal of Sex Research*, 34: 167–74.

Williams, G. C. 1975. *Sex and evolution*. Princeton: Princeton Univ. Press.

Wilmsen. E. N. 1989. *Land filled with flies: A political economy of the Kalahari*. Chicago: Univ. of Chicago Press.

Wilmsen, E. N., and J. R. Denbow. 1990. Paradigmatic history of San-speaking peoples and current attempts at revision. *Current Anthropology* 31:489–524.

Wilson, E. O. 1975. *Sociobiology: The new synthesis*. Cambridge, MA: Belknap Press/Harvard Univ. Press.

Wilson, H. C. 1988. Male axillary secretions influence women's menstrual cycles: A critique. *Hormones and Behavior* 22:266–71.

Wilson, M., and M. Daly. 1991. The man who mistook his wife for a chattel. In *The adapted mind: Evolutionary psychology and the generation of culture*, ed. J. H. Barkow, L. Cosmides, and J. Tooby. New York: Oxford Univ. Press.

Wittenberger, J. F., and R. L. Tilson. 1980. The evolution of monogamy: Hypotheses and evidence. *Annual Review of Ecology and Systematics* 11:197–232.

Wlodarski, R. 2014. What's in a kiss? The effect of romantic kissing on mate desirability. *Evolutionary Psychology* 12 (1): 178–99.

Wlodarski, R., and R. I. M. Dunbar. 2013. Examining the possible functions of kissing in romantic relationships. *Archives of Sexual Behavior* 42(8): 1415–23.

Wolfe, L. 1981. *Women and sex in the 80s: The Cosmo report*. New York: Arbor House.

Wolpoff, M. H. 1980. *Paleo-anthropology*. New York: Alfred A. Knopf.

———. 1982. *Ramapithecus* and hominid origins. *Current Anthropology* 23:501–22.

———. 1984. Evolution of *Homo erectus:* The question of stasis. *Paleobiology* 10: 389–406.

———. 1989. Multiregional evolution: The fossil alternative to Eden. In *The human revolution*, ed. P. Mellars and C. B. Stringer. Vol. 1. Edinburgh: Edinburgh Univ. Press.

Wolpoff, M. H., J. N. Spuhler, F. H. Smith, et al. 1988. Modern human origins. *Science* 241:772–74.

Wood, B. M., and F. W. Marlowe. 2011. Dynamics of post-marital residence among the Hadza: A kin investment model. *Human Nature* 22:128–38.

Woodburn, J. 1968. An introduction to Hadza ecology. In *Man the hunter*, ed. R. B. Lee and I. DeVore. New York: Aldine.

Wrangham, R. W. 1977. Feeding behavior of chimpanzees in Gombe National Park, Tanzania. In *Primate ecology*, ed. T. H. Clutton-Brock. London: Academic Press.

———. 1979a. On the evolution of ape social systems. *Social Science Information* 18:335–68.

———. 1979b. Sex differences in chimpanzee dispersion. In *The great apes*, ed. D. A. Hamburg and E. R. McCown. Menlo Park, CA: Benjamin/Cummings.

———. 2009. *Catching fire: How cooking made us human*. New York: Basic Books.

WuDunn, S. 1991. Romance, a novel idea, rocks marriages in China. *New York Times*, April 17.

Xu, X., A. Aron, L. L. Brown, et al. 2011. Reward and motivation systems: A brain mapping study of early-stage intense romantic love in Chinese participants. *Human Brain Mapping* 32(2): 249–57.

Yerkes, R. M., and J. H. Elder. 1936. Oestrus, receptivity and mating in the chimpanzee. *Comparative Psychology Monographs* 13:1–39.

Young, L. J. 1999. Oxytocin and vasopressin receptors and species-typical social behaviors. *Journal of Hormones and Behavior* 36:212–21.

———. 2009. Love: Neuroscience reveals all. *Nature* 457:148.

Young, L. J., Z. Wang, and T. R. Insel. 1998. Neuroendocrine bases of monogamy. *Trends in Neuroscience* 21:71–5.

Young, L. J., J. T. Winslow, R. Nilsen, and T. R. Insel. 1997. Species differences in V1a receptor gene expression in monogamous and nonmonogamous voles: Behavioral consequences. *Behavioral Neuroscience* 111:599–605.

Zak, P. J. 2008. The neurobiology of trust. *Scientific American* 298 (6): 88–95.

———. 2012. *The moral molecule: The source of love and prosperity*. New York: Dutton.

Zak, P. J., R. Kurzban and W. T. Matzner. 2005. The neurobiology of trust. *Annals of the New York Academy of Sciences* 1032:224–27.

Zak, P. J., A. A. Stanton, and S. Sahmadi. 2007. Oxytocin increases generosity in humans. *PLoS ONE* 2:54–71.

Zeki, S., and J. P. Romaya. 2010. The brain reaction to viewing faces of opposite- and same-sex romantic partners. *PLoS ONE* 5(12): e15802. doi:10.1371.

Zentner, M. R. 2005. Ideal mate personality concepts and compatibility in close relationships: A longitudinal analysis. *Journal of Personality and Social Psychology* 89 (2): 242–56.

Zietsch, B. P., and P. Santtila. 2013. No direct relationship between human female orgasm rate and number of offspring. *Animal Behavior* 89:253–55.

Zihlman, A. L. 1979. Pygmy chimpanzee morphology and the interpretation of early hominids. *South African Journal of Science* 75:165–68.

———. 1981. Women as shapers of the human adaptation. In *Woman the gatherer*, ed. F. Dahlberg. New Haven: Yale Univ. Press.

Zihlman, A. L., J. E. Cronin, D. L. Cramer, and V. M. Sarich. 1987. Pygmy chimpanzee as a possible prototype for the common ancestor of humans, chimpanzees and gorillas. In *Interpretations of ape and human ancestry,* ed. R. L. Ciochon and R. S. Corruccini. New York: Plenum Press.

Zihlman, A. L., and N. Tanner. 1978. Gathering and hominid adaptation. In *Female hierarchies,* ed. L. Tiger and H. Fowler. Chicago: Beresford Book Service.

Zilhão, J. 2010. Neanderthals are us: Genes and culture. *Radical Anthropology* 2010 (4): 5–15.

Zimen, E., ed. 1980. *The red fox: Symposium on behavior and ecology.* The Hague: Junk.

Zuckerman, M. 1971. Dimensions of sensation seeking. *Journal of Consulting and Clinical Psychology* 36:45–52.

Zuckerman, M., M. S. Buchsbaum, and D. L. Murphy. 1980. Sensation seeking and its biological correlates. *Psychological Bulletin* 88:187–214.

Zuckerman, M., J. A. Hall, S. W. DeFrank, and R. Rosenthal. 1976. Encoding and decoding of spontaneous and posed facial expressions. *Journal of Personality and Social Psychology* 34:966–77.

Zuckerman, Sir S. 1932. *The social life of monkeys and apes.* London: Butler and Turner.

## 436 | INDEX

gender differences (*continued*)
    in thinking, 198–99, 201, 202
    in verbal skills, 193–94, 196–97, 199, 201, 202, 203
genes, genetics, 29, 30, 45
    adultery and, 73, 74–75, 77, 78, 355*n*
    of African apes, 110
    art and, 252
    attachment and, 365*n*
    conscience and, 260
    Denovians and, 374*n*
    divorce and, 97
    FOXP2, 250
    gender differences and, 193
    homosexuality and, 348*n*
    inbreeding and, 256, 374*n*
    incest taboo and, 256
    kin selection and, 46–47
    of Neanderthals, 252, 373*n*–74*n*
    possessiveness and, 154
    recombination and, 44
    sexual selection and, 188
    waist-to-hip ratio and, 177
"genetic repair" theory, 350*n*
genetic variability, 77
genetic variety, 139
genitals, 28, 112, 193, 256
    foreplay and, 375*n*
    !Kung and, 266, 267, 270, 271
    Mehinaku and, 275, 276, 277
    stimulation of, 25, 303
    *see also* penis; vagina
George (*Homo habilis* male), 209, 210, 222, 226
Georgia, 242
Gergen, David, xii
Germany, Germanic people, 177, 282, 285, 292, 293, 315
gestures, *see* body talk
gibbons, 48, 153
gifts, 17, 118, 265, 268, 275, 351*n*, 352*n*
    sexual politics and, 218–19
Gilbert, W. S., 202
Gilligan, Carol, 201
Givens, David, 7–11
Glass, S., 73
Glenmullen, Joseph, 318
global empathy, 261
God, 1, 65–68, 83, 292, 293, 294
going on safari, 115, 119, 144

Gombe Stream Reserve, 113–16, 153, 228, 257–58, 362*n*
Goodall, Jane, 113, 116, 258, 362*n*
Goodenough, Ward, 119, 351*n*
good-mother signal, 174
gorillas, 5, 8, 35, 57, 349*n*
    birth spacing in, 364*n*
    humans compared with, 110, 171, 360*n*
    penis of, 171
    sex life of, 104, 105, 108–10, 133, 171, 359*n*–60*n*
    silverback male, 108, 109
    testicles of, 172
grammar, 10, 193
grandmother hypothesis, 237, 369*n*
graves and burials, 250–51, 252, 255
Great Barrier Reef, 46
Great Britain, 177, 293
    in Nigeria, 213–15
Great Depression, 297, 377*n*
Greece, 24
Greeks, ancient, 66, 67, 113, 148, 285, 286
    divorce and, 291
    menarche in, 376*n*
    Zeus and Hera story in, 311
Gregg, Susan, 282–83
Gregor, Thomas, 266, 272, 276, 277, 278
grooming, 114, 118, 119, 203, 227
grooming talk, 9–10
group hunting, 116–17
group marriage (polygynandry), 47, 55–57
group size, hominin, 144, 364*n*
guilt, 260, 261, 264
*Guinness Book of World Records, The*, 50

Hadar River, 124–25
Hadza, 88, 130, 316
Haidt, Jonathan, 263
hair:
    body, 176
    facial, 175, 176
    pubic, 277
Hall, Edward, 12
Hamilton, Gilbert, 69
happiness, 68, 73, 306–8, 314, 319
    love and, 147–48, 155–56, 160
Hardgrave, 153